Enhancing the Role of Ultrasound with Contrast Agents

Riccardo Lencioni (Ed.)

Enhancing the Role of Ultrasound with Contrast Agents

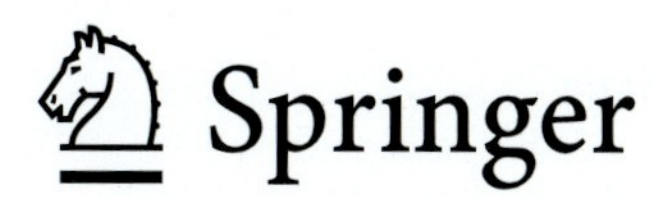

Editor
Prof. Dr. Riccardo Lencioni
Division of Diagnostic and Interventional Radiology
Department of Oncology, Transplants
and Advanced Technologies in Medicine
University of Pisa
Pisa, Italy

CD-ROM edited by
Prof. Dr. Riccardo Lencioni
Dr. Clotilde Della Pina
Division of Diagnostic and Interventional Radiology
Department of Oncology, Transplants
and Advanced Technologies in Medicine
University of Pisa
Pisa, Italy

Library of Congress Control Number: 2006921996

ISBN 10 88-470-0475- 6 Springer Milan Berlin Heidelberg New York
ISBN 13 978-88-470-0475- 7 Springer Milan Berlin Heidelberg New York

Springer is a part of Springer Science+Business Media
springer.com

Printed in Italy

This textbook was funded in part by an educational grant from Bracco. Bracco, however, exercises no editorial comment, review, or any other type of control over the content of this textbook. For any product or type of product, whether a drug or device, referenced in this textbook, physicians should carefully review the product's package insert, instructions for use, or user manual prior to patient administration to ensure proper utilization of the product.

Cover design: Simona Colombo, Milan, Italy
Typesetting: Graphostudio, Milan, Italy
Printing and binding: Arti Grafiche Nidasio, Assago (Milan), Italy

Preface

The introduction of microbubble contrast agents and the development of contrast-specific scanning techniques have opened new prospects in ultrasound. The advent of second-generation agents – that enable real-time contrast-enhanced imaging – has been instrumental in improving the acceptance and the reproducibility of examinations. Contrast ultrasound substantially improves detection and characterization of focal liver lesions with respect to baseline studies, and has already been introduced in international guidelines for the diagnosis of liver tumors. The role of contrast agents in vascular ultrasound is also established, and several new clinical applications are emerging.

This book, written by the leading experts in the field, provides an up-to-date overview on the clinical value of contrast agents in ultrasound. The volume moves from a background section on technique and methodology to the main sections on the clinical application of contrast ultrasound in the liver and in vascular diseases. A final section discusses results and prospects of contrast ultrasound modality in the other fields. A selection of relevant clinical cases is presented in the enclosed CD-ROM.

This volume is the result of the efforts of several world-renowned experts. I am greatly in debt to them for their enthusiastic commitment and support. Also, I would like to thank my mentor, Professor Carlo Bartolozzi, for his precious advice, as well as Drs. Dania Cioni, Laura Crocetti, and Clotilde Della Pina for their contribution to this editorial project. I sincerely hope that the book fulfils the expectations of my colleagues – radiologists, clinicians, and surgeons – who are interested in the very exciting field of contrast ultrasound.

Pisa, March 2006

Riccardo Lencioni

Contents

SECTION IV – New Prospects in Clinical Application of Contrast Ultrasound

Contributors

Luca Aiani
Department of Radiology
Ospedale Valduce
Como, Italy

Thomas Albrecht
Department of Radiology
and Nuclear Medicine
Campus Benjamin Franklin
Charité – Universitätsmedizin Berlin
Berlin, Germany

Eva Bartels
Department of Clinical
Neurophysiology
Georg-August-University
Göttingen, Germany

Carlo Bartolozzi
Division of Diagnostic and
Interventional Radiology
Department of Oncology,
Transplants, and Advanced
Technologies in Medicine
University of Pisa, Italy

Claudia Borghi
Department of Radiology
Ospedale Valduce
Como, Italy

Molly Brewer
Department of Gynecology Oncology
University of Arizona
Arizona Cancer Center
Tucson, USA

Concepcio Bru
Diagnostic Imaging Center
Hospital Clínic
Barcelona, Spain

Dania Cioni
Division of Diagnostic
and Interventional Radiology
Department of Oncology,
Transplants, and Advanced
Technologies in Medicine
University of Pisa
Pisa, Italy

Roberta Chersevani
Department of Diagnostic Imaging
General Hospital
Gorizia, Italy

David Cosgrove
Imaging Sciences Department
Imperial College
Hammersmith Hospital
London, UK

Laura Crocetti
Division of Diagnostic
and Interventional Radiology
Department of Oncology,
Transplants, and Advanced
Technologies in Medicine
University of Pisa
Pisa, Italy

Stefan Delorme
Department of Radiology
German Cancer Research Center
Heidelberg, Germany

Clotilde Della Pina
Division of Diagnostic and
Interventional Radiology
Department of Oncology,
Transplants, and Advanced
Technologies in Medicine
University of Pisa
Pisa, Italy

Christoph F. Dietrich
Department Innere Medizin 2
Caritas Krankenhaus
Bad Mergentheim, Germany

Dirk W. Droste
Department of Neurology
Centre Hospitalier de Luxembourg
Luxembourg
Department of Neurology
University of Münster
Münster, Germany

Robert Eckersley
Imaging Sciences Department
Imperial College
Hammersmith Hospital
London, UK

Thomas Fischer
Department of Radiology
Charité
Universitätsmedizin Berlin
Berlin, Germany

Ferdinand Frauscher
Department of Radiology II
Medical University Innsbruck
Innsbruck, Austria

Paul G. Horgan
Senior Lecturer and Hon Consultant
Surgeon,
University of Glasgow
Glasgow, UK

Andrea S. Klauser
Department of Radiology II
Medical University Innsbruck
Innsbruck, Austria

Martin Krix
Department of Radiology
German Cancer Research Center
Heidelberg, Germany

Tiziana Ierace
Department of Radiology
General Hospital
Busto Arsizio, Italy

Nathalie Lassau
Ultrasonography Unit
and Imaging Laboratory
of Small Animal
Imaging Department
Institut Gustave-Roussy
Villejuif, France

Jérome Leclère
Ultrasonography Unit
Imaging Department
Institut Gustave-Roussy
Villejuif, France

Edward Leen
Consultant Radiologist
Hon Senior Lecturer
University of Glasgow
Glasgow, UK

Riccardo Lencioni
Division of Diagnostic
and Interventional Radiology
Department of Oncology,
Transplants, and Advanced
Technologies in Medicine
University of Pisa
Pisa, Italy

Henri Marret
Department of Gynecology,
Obstetrics, Fetal Medicine
and Human Reproduction
Bretonneau Hospital
CHRU Tours
Tours, France

Alberto Martegani
Department of Radiology
Ospedale Valduce
Como, Italy

Susan Moug
Research Fellow
Department of Surgery
University of Glasgow
Glasgow, UK

Carlos Nicolau
Diagnostic Imaging Center
Hospital Clínic
Barcelona, Spain

Anders Nilsson
Department of Radiology
Ultrasound Unit
Uppsala University Hospital
Uppsala, Sweden

Pierre Péronneau
Imaging Laboratory
of Small Animal
Imaging Department
Institut Gustave-Roussy
Villejuif, France

Giorgio Rizzatto
Department of Diagnostic Imaging
General Hospital
Gorizia, Italy

Stéphane Sauget
Department of Gynecology, Obstetrics,
Fetal Medicine and Human Reproduction
Bretonneau Hospital
CHRU Tours
Tours, France

Luigi Solbiati
Department of Radiology
General Hospital
Busto Arsizio, Italy

Massimo Tonolini
Department of Radiology
General Hospital
Busto Arsizio, Italy

Lars Thorelius
Head of Ultrasound Section
Department of Radiology
Linköping University Hospital
Linköping, Sweden

François Tranquart
Department of Medical Imaging,
Nuclear Medicine and Ultrasound
Bretonneau Hospital
CHRU Tours
Tours, France

SECTION I

Technique and Methodology of Contrast Ultrasound

I.1

Contrast-Enhanced Ultrasound: Basic Physics and Technology Overview

David Cosgrove and Robert Eckersley

Introduction

Microbubbles represent an entirely new class of materials that are mainly used as intravascular contrast agents for US, though they can also be instilled into the urinary bladder to look for ureteric reflux [1] and into the uterus to check tubal patency [2]. Their effect depends on the compressibility of gases, which is markedly different from the near-incompressibility of tissue. Exploiting this difference has led to the development of several multipulse sequences that cancel tissue signals and emphasise those from the microbubbles, thus improving the contrast-to-tissue signal ratio. Overlay or side-by-side displays allow the agent image to be viewed along with the grey-scale image to facilitate locating the region of interest.

Not only can major vessels be displayed, but microbubbles within the microvasculature are also detected (though the capillary bed itself cannot be resolved anatomically), because these methods do not depend on microbubble flow but merely on their presence. In practice, these specific modes have found major clinical application in the liver for the detection and characterisation of focal lesions, although the same principles apply also in the kidneys and spleen. They are also very widely used in echocardiography, for endocardial border detection and to evaluate myocardial perfusion, applications that are beyond the remit of this article.

Conventional Doppler methods also work well and contrast is helpful in peripheral vascular disease (notably for transcranial Doppler, carotid stenosis and in renal artery stenosis) when the unenhanced Doppler signals are too weak to be clinically useful.

Microbubbles are eminently suitable for use as tracers because of the small volumes injected. This has been exploited in the liver to identify conditions characterised by arterio-venous shunting such as cirrhosis and metastases - an early hepatic vein transit time indicates a haemodynamic abnormality.

Microbubble Contrast Agents

Unlike all other imaging technologies, until recently US lacked agents that could be administered to patients to improve or enhance the diagnostic information available. However, this has changed with the recent introduction of microbubble contrast agents [3]. The field is a dynamic one, with many new agents being developed along with new ways to exploit the opportunities they offer [4-8]. Microbubbles are made small enough to cross capillary beds (the pulmonary capillaries have the smallest calibre in the body at 7μm) and are usually given as an intravenous injection (Fig. 1). The discovery of their striking enhancement of US signals dates from a chance observation by a cardiologist, Dr Claude Joyner, who noticed an increase in the signal intensity on an M-mode study of the aortic root each time an injection of an iodinated contrast medium was made for an angiographic cardiac study [9]. Further investigation revealed that the effect was not specific to the X-ray contrast agent, but occurred with any injected liquid and, importantly for the ongoing development of these agents, it was enhanced by first drawing up some of the patient's blood into the syringe. Dr Steve Feinberg found that this improvement resulted from the stabilising effects of serum albumen, and that the enhancement resulted from gas bubbles in the injectate, demonstrated by the fact that the effect was suppressed if the fluid was subjected to high pressure in the syringe. The

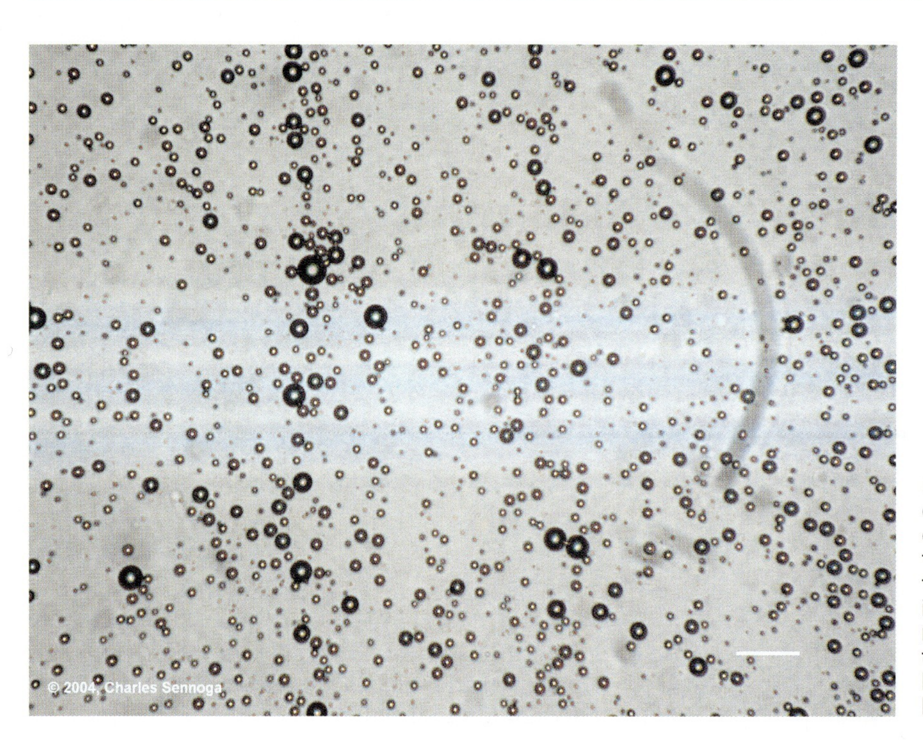

Fig. 1. Light microscope view of a phospholipid-shell microbubble. The size distribution and spherical form of these microbubbles is shown in this micrograph. The scale represents 25μ. (Image courtesy of Dr. Charles Sennoga, Imaging Sciences Department, Imperial College, London)

first clinical applications of the phenomenon used "shaken saline", which was actually injected rapidly from one syringe into another via a three-way tap so that traces of air were incorporated as bubbles, often stabilised by a small amount of the patient's blood. This was used to reveal right-to-left intracardiac shunts, seen as echoes in the left atrium or ventricle following intravenous (iv) injection using M-mode or B-mode scanning. The size of the bubbles thus produced could not be controlled and unfortunately, some serious complications occurred, notably paradoxical cerebral emboli, producing transient or prolonged ischaemic attacks and even an associated death. The development of colour Doppler obviated the need for shaken saline injections for the detection of these shunts. The line of research eventually led to the commercialisation of Albunex, which is produced by high intensity sonication of an albumen solution.

A different line of work cumulated in the development of disaccharide-based microbubbles such as Echovist and Levovist [10, 11]. Development of these agents resulted from the hypothesis that pressure changes in the left ventricle could be estimated by measuring the resonant frequency of microbubbles in the blood because the change in mean diameter would correspond to a change in the acoustic resonance. Many means of making microbubbles were evaluated, including using the ability of rough surfaces to act as nidation sites, much as irregularities on the inside of a glass trigger the formation of bubbles from a carbonated drink. Amongst the materials tried, sugar crystals seemed promising, as they are non-toxic and well characterised. They were ground into a fine powder to produce a matrix of microcrystals. The size of the resultant microbubbles depended on the dimensions of the spaces between the microcrystals. Unfortunately, measuring intracardiac pressure turned out to require an extremely tight microbubble size-range and the original goal was never achieved. However, the microbubbles produced gave strong enhancement. The first agent to enter clinical trials, Echovist, had only a short life in the circulation after iv injection because it was not stable enough to survive cardio-pulmonary transit and thus it could only be used for intracardiac shunt detection. Though safer than shaken saline (because of the controlled microbubble sizes), it too was replaced by colour Doppler for this purpose, though it is still used in US contrast salpingography. The addition of traces of a surfactant (palmitic acid) greatly improved stability so that the bubbles could survive cardio-pulmonary passage to give left-sided heart enhancement, hence its designation as Levovist. It also enhanced the signals from the peripheral vasculature, and was licensed for Doppler enhancement of vessels such as the carotid arteries and the portal system. Unfortunately, it turned out that the enhancement it gave necessitated disruption of the microbubbles (in fact, only the free air bubbles liberated in this process were responsible for the US signals) and therefore, only short duration studies could be performed: the act of imaging these fragile microbubbles destroyed them.

Levovist was found to have one very useful property: it is taken up by the reticulo-endothelial system in the liver and spleen where it persists for several minutes after it has been cleared from the circulating blood pool [12]. This property, which was a chance discovery, proved to be useful for the detection of focal lesions such as metastases that did not contain Kupffer cells, even when they were undetectable on unenhanced scans because of their small size or because of lack of contrast with the surrounding liver (so-called isoechoic metastases). Tissues that were comprised of functioning liver, such as focal fatty change, regenerating nodules and focal nodular hyperplasia, shared this property with the surrounding liver and so disappeared in this late phase rather than becoming prominent as defects against the enhanced liver background, as was the case with metastases. Newer microbubbles share this property to some extent, though it seems likely that they are not specifically taken up by phagocytes, but instead simply float in the high capacity vasculature of the sinusoids in the liver and spleen. The importance of this late sinusoidal phase for the detection of malignancies, first discovered with Levovist, also applies to the newer agents.

As well as reflecting incident US, microbubbles respond to the alternating compression and rarefaction cycles of the US wave by changing diameter, since their gas content is much more compressible than tissue. These oscillations are typically asymmetrical (the gas tends to resist compression but expands more easily) and this "non-linear response" alters the character of the returned signals. Signal processing to select these signals and separate them from tissue echoes has been developed and it permits continuous real-time imaging of the contrast agent as it arrives at a region of interest and then washes out over 2-5 minutes. This allows the arterial and venous phases to be studied. In addition, many agents show an affinity for the liver and spleen, persisting in normal sinusoids for many minutes. This parenchymal 'sinusoidal' or 'late' phase highlights masses that do not contain normal liver tissue and has proven to be particularly valuable for detecting metastases, while the arterial phase helps characterise focal lesions in the liver (and to a lesser extent, in the spleen) by virtue of their vascular supply.

In addition to their value in imaging, microbubbles may be used as tracers to provide information on haemodynamics. An example is the ability to time the delay from their first appearance in the hepatic artery until they arrive in hepatic vein branches. Normally this takes 12 seconds or more, but when there is arterio-venous shunting in the liver this time is greatly shortened. This simple test has been shown to be able to discriminate mild from severe forms of viral hepatitis and to separate both from frank cirrhosis [13, 14]. It seems also to be capable of detecting micrometastases in colorectal cancer [15].

Microbubble Properties

The microbubbles used as contrast agents for US are made to be smaller than 7 µm in diameter so that they can cross capillary beds. When administered intravenously, these agents flood the blood pool and remain within the vascular compartment unless there is active bleeding. Thus, they serve as blood pool agents and their contrast effects are closer to those of the labelled red blood cells used in nuclear medicine studies than to the ionic agents used in X-ray and MR studies; in particular, microbubbles do not cross the endothelium and therefore do not have the interstitial phase that is typical of the conventional contrast agents. Microbubbles do not seem to affect blood flow and generally behave in the same way as red blood cells (with the important exception of when they are phagocytosed by the reticulo-endothelial system, which treats some microbubbles as foreign particles – see below).

They must survive passage through the cardio-pulmonary circulation to produce useful systemic enhancement. Both the gas they contain and their stabilising shell are critical to their effectiveness as contrast agents and to rendering them sufficiently stable, allowing them to persist for several minutes after injection. The first agent for cardiac use, Albunex, has a shell of denatured albumen and contains air. The first widely used agent, Levovist (Schering, Germany), is made of galactose microcrystals whose surfaces provide nidation sites on which air bubbles form when they are suspended in water; they are stabilised by a trace of palmitic acid which acts as a surfactant. An improved version of Albunex, Optison (GE, UK), is filled with perfluoropropane while a family of perfluoro gas-containing agents such as SonoVue (Bracco, Italy) and perflutren (Definity, Bristol Meyers Squibb, USA) that use phospholipids as the membranes are important in clinical practice.

High molecular weight gases are chosen for their slow diffusion through the membrane, prolonging their effective life in the circulation, where they are subject to mechanical trauma by the action of heart valves and by the US beam.

Obviously, the gas should be biologically inert and for this reason, the perfluoro gases have been chosen, in which a carbon chain has its hydrogen atoms completely replaced by elements such as fluorine or sulphur. The perfluorocarbons such as perfluoropropane (a three carbon chain compound used in Definity) have excellent durability and provide strong enhancement. SonoVue contains sulphur hexafluoride, which is characterised by very low solubility in blood and is also a very effective contrast agent.

The membrane is also critical for both longevity and resonance and, naturally, must also be biologically inert. Denatured human serum albumen (HSA) is used in several contrast agents (Albunex and Optison are available for clinical use, but Quantison has been withdrawn from further development). Denatured HSA is sufficiently flexible to allow the bubbles to respond to the acoustic pressure changes when insonated. In general, it is biologically inert, with the denaturation neutralising any immunogenic potential. However, there have been theoretical concerns over the possibility of transmitting viral or prion diseases because of the human origin of the protein. While this is unlikely because of the denaturing process to which the albumen is subjected, there remains a risk, so ethics committees have insisted that the origin of the shell be clearly labelled in patient information sheets, which has resulted in a few patients refusing to have this type of contrast agent.

Many microbubbles use phospholipid-shells. The bubbles are not present in the lyophilised powder that is presented in the vial, but are formed during agitation after the diluent (usually normal saline) has been added. The size of the resulting microbubbles and their shell thickness are critically determined by the exact mixture of the different phospholipids and the associated surfactants. The consistency of the resulting microbubbles is remarkable. Again, the shell properties are important for both the stability and response of the microbubbles.

Microbubble Behaviour

While the classical specific acoustic impedance change between plasma and gas is sufficient to produce strong signals from microbubbles, just as from any other gas, the effect is weak *in vivo* because of the high dilution (for example, a dose of 5mL in around 5 litres of blood, i.e. 1:1000 or more). On intravital microscopic views after injection of clinically equivalent doses, one sees one microbubble pass between several hundred red cells. Using conventional B-mode scanning, the effect can be discerned in large blood spaces such as the cardiac chambers, but not in smaller vessels. Doppler is more sensitive and can be used in clinical practice. The effect is useful for improving the signal-to-noise ratio of studies in situations where the signals are attenuated. This application, known as 'Doppler rescue', is important for transcranial Doppler where the skull attenuates the signals from intracranial arteries. Contrast agents are widely used in neurology centres where monitoring vasospasm after cerebrovascular events is important. It is also useful in otherwise difficult radiological studies, for example, for renal artery stenosis and for Tips shunts in the liver, both of which are situations where attenuation of the Doppler signals frequently impedes unenhanced studies. In 'Doppler rescue', important as these studies may be, essentially no new principles are involved, the microbubbles simply boost the signals from blood.

However, the behaviour of microbubbles in a US field is unique and this can be exploited in entirely new ways to give information of a new order, in particular in detection of the microcirculation. This unique phenomenon results from the high compressibility of the gas of microbubbles: whereas tissue is virtually incompressible (the molecules moving only a few Angstroms as the ultrasonic compression and rarefaction wave passes), microbubbles expand and contract markedly. The extent of the change depends on the acoustic power applied, but at diagnostic levels they may halve and double in size.

Bubbles have a natural oscillation frequency, or resonance, depending on their size. When the driving pressure changes of the US are matched to this resonant frequency, the bubbles become extremely efficient at translating the sound energy from the propagating sound wave into scattered signals. The frequencies used for abdominal US imaging are in the 3-5 MHz range. This corresponds to the resonant frequencies of 3-5 μ microbubbles (5 μ SonoVue microbubbles, for example, resonate at around 5 MHz and those of 2 μ resonate at 7 MHz). This is a coincidence, because different considerations determine the bubble size and the acoustic wavelength needed, but it accounts for the exceptionally strong response of US contrast agents (Fig. 2).

In addition to the resonance effect, the response of the microbubbles to the US wave becomes non-linear at higher acoustic pressures. This behaviour results from the fact that the bubbles are able to expand more easily than they contract because the increasing bubble pressures at smaller volumes resist further compression due to their stiffness, whereas further expansion

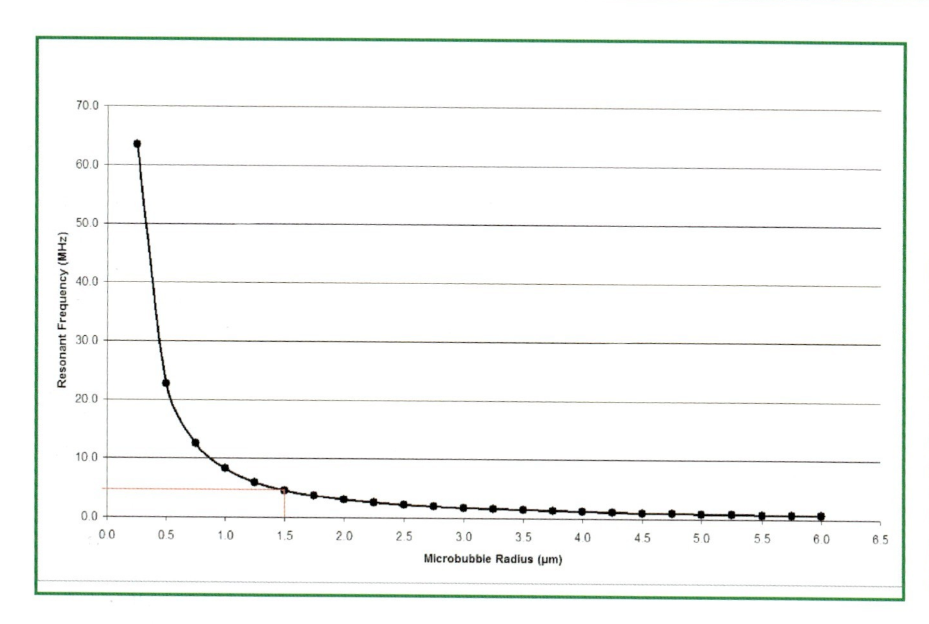

Fig. 2. The calculated resonance frequency plotted against the radius of a microbubble. The chart shows the resonant frequency for the microbubble Sonazoid plotted against the bubble's radius at rest. The red lines indicate that at 5 MHz the resonance corresponds with the median diameter of 5 Ķ. (Figure kindly supplied by Kevin Chetty, Imaging Sciences Department, Imperial College, London)

consumes less energy. This means that their diameter change is asymmetrical about the radius at equilibrium, with larger increases in the rarefaction phase than contractions in the compression phase. Thus, the signals returning from the bubbles are a distorted version of the insonating wave; this is known as a non-linear response. At still higher pressures, the bubble oscillations become more complex, diverging from simple spherical changes and further increasing the non-linear properties of the scattered US.

These non-linearities appear as harmonics (or overtones) of the original transmitted US frequency and can be seen on a frequency spectrum of the returning signals. Usually these are higher frequencies (most prominently the second harmonic at twice the transmitted or fundamental frequency); higher third or fourth order harmonics are typically outside the range of sensitivity of the US transducer and so are undetectable. For higher frequency applications, the second harmonics are very strongly attenuated and often lie outside the band pass of the transducer. An alternative approach to harmonic imaging is to use microbubbles with a second harmonic frequency tuned to the transducer centre frequency and detect the subharmonic signals from the microbubbles, i.e., at half the transmitted frequency. There are also other sources of non-linear behaviour, which occur because of the pressure dependent behaviour and the inertia of the bubble shell. For example, if two similar pulses with differing amplitudes are incident on the microbubbles, the scattered response will not be directly proportional to the difference in the incident pressures. This asymmetrical response is not associated with a change in frequency and these non-linear responses at the fundamental frequency are important because the transducer is at its most sensitive at this point and pulses can be designed to use the full bandwidth of the transducer most efficiently [16]. In practice, a combination of these two sources of non-linearity is employed by modern US scanners to generate contrast-specific images.

A mathematical description of the non-linear response of a microbubble has been devised and is commonly referred to as the modified Rayleigh-Plesset equation. A number of researchers have developed variations on this model, an example described by de Jong is presented in equation (1) [16a]. This model describes the bubble radius as a function of time and accounts for the physical properties of the bubble shell and the effect of the gas within the bubble. The model takes the form of a second order differential equation:

(1)

$$\rho R\ddot{R}+\frac{3}{2}\rho\dot{R}^{2}=p_{go}\left(\frac{R_0}{R}\right)^{3\Gamma}+p_v-p_{lo}-\frac{2\sigma}{R}-2S_p\left(\frac{1}{R_0}-\frac{1}{R}\right)-\delta_{Tot}\omega\rho R\dot{R}-p_{ac}$$

Where R is the instantaneous bubble radius; ρ is the density of the surrounding medium; P_{go} is the initial gas pressure inside the bubble; P_v is the vapour pressure; P_{lo} is the hydrostatic pressure; σ is the surface tension coefficient; δ_{Tot} is the total damping coefficient due to sound radiation, liquid viscosity, heat transport and the viscous resistance of the encapsulating shell; ω is the angular frequency of the incident sound field; P_{ac} is the time varying pressure of the acoustic field; S_p is the shell stiffness parameter and Γ is the polytropic exponent of the gas. '•' denotes differentiation with respect to time. The model is only applicable for low acoustic driving pressures, when the bubble oscillations remain radially symmetrical. At higher pressures, the bubble behaviour becomes more complex and the bubbles will ultimately be disrupted. This disruption can cause fragmentation into smaller bubbles or the release of free gas bubbles; in both cases, the resulting bubbles then dissolve more rapidly.

Methods for Detection of Microbubble Signals

The change in density at the surface of a bubble in plasma represents a major impedance mismatch and the echogenicity this produces is exploited in the uses of microbubbles to improve Doppler studies, so-called 'Doppler rescue'. The increase in the reflectivity of blood thus produced is obvious and useful for Doppler but is not visible on conventional grey-scale imaging because the microbubble concentration is too low.

The harmonics emitted by microbubbles, as described above, can be used to image US contrast agents by tuning the receiver to the harmonic signal (e.g. the second harmonic at double the fundamental frequency), so that the harmonics can be separated from the fundamental signals from tissue.

However, in order to perform a good separation of the harmonic microbubble signals from the linear scattered tissue signals, a longer, narrow band US pulse must be used. This trade-off results in a compromise between sensitivity and specificity to microbubbles versus image resolution. Furthermore, tissues also produce harmonics, especially when higher acoustic powers are used and these contaminate the signals from microbubbles. Tissue harmonics result from distortion of the acoustic wave as it propagates through the tissue and arise because the wave travels slightly faster through the higher density tissue at the high pressure phase of the wave than in the lower density tissue in the rarefaction phase (sound velocity depends on the density of the medium). Thus, the wave of the transmitted pulse is gradually distorted as it propagates through the tissue, i.e. US conduction is non-linear, and this implies that harmonics are added to the signal. The higher the acoustic power, the greater the effect. Tissue harmonics are exploited in conventional B-mode imaging to reduce sidelobe and reverberation artefacts but contaminate the non-linear signals from microbubbles and appear as noise in contrast-only images.

Distinguishing between tissue and microbubble harmonics is challenging; in practice, when using many of the simple contrast modes available, the two signals are inextricably mixed together. The fact that tissue harmonics are stronger when a higher acoustic power is used underlies the use of a low mechanical index (MI) for contrast studies. This has the important added benefit of minimising bubble destruction and so allowing continuous real-time scanning. Inevitably, low MIs are associated with reduced signal-to-noise ratios so the contrast images may become noisy and a compromise may have to be reached.

The goal of separating tissue from microbubble harmonics completely can be achieved in two ways. In the first to be discovered, a high MI beam is used and the microbubbles are deliberately disrupted. Using a multipulse sequence such as standard colour Doppler, the sudden disappearance of a signal from its previous location (loss of correlation between sequential echoes) is seen as a major Doppler shift and is registered as colour signals [12]. This method works well for the more fragile air-based agents such as Levovist, and modified colour Doppler signal processing has been developed to optimise the display, particularly by improving spatial resolution. This approach, often known a Stimulated Acoustic Emission (SAE), is particularly successful in the late phase of contrast agents that show liver/spleen tropism a few minutes after injection. Lesions that do not contain functioning tissue, such as malignancies, are shown as voids in the colour map, because Levovist highlights the normal liver and spleen. This method has the advantage of high sensitivity (it can probably detect a single microbubble being disrupted) and of showing the microbubble signature exclusively in the colour layer of the registered image with the conventional grey-scale image as an underlayer or on a split screen display for navigation purposes. However, because the contrast agent is rapidly destroyed, real-time scanning cannot be used, so a rather clumsy sweep-and-review approach has to be adopted [17].

The alternative approach, and now the mode of choice for contrast studies, relies on the fact that newer microbubbles, particularly those with phospholipid-shells, can be driven to generate non-linear signals at much lower acoustic powers than those necessary to generate tissue harmonics [18, 19]. Thus, if a very low acoustic power can be used without the image disappearing into noise, only the microbubbles produce non-linear signals and these can be separated from the tissue signals. An important step in the progress to this ideal was the development of the pulse inversion mode (PIM), which evolved from the desire to detect microbubble harmonics but to avoid frequency filtering [20] (Fig. 3). In this mode a pair of pulses is sent sequentially along each scan line, the second being inverted in polarity from the first. The returning echoes from the pair are summed so that the linear echoes cancel because they are completely out-of-phase, leaving only non-linear components for image formation. Spatial resolution is not impaired because the transmitted pulses are the same as those used for conventional imaging. PIM gives excellent quality images in both vascular and late phases and, like the high MI modes, detects the presence of microbubbles without relying on their motion. Thus, both these modes can detect contrast within the microcirculation though, of course, vessels smaller than the resolution limit of US – some 200 μm at best – cannot be resolved as discrete structures.

In its initial implementation, PIM deployed relatively high MIs, resulting in contamination of the microbubble signals by tissue harmonics. Special approaches are required to operate at the low powers needed to avoid tissue harmonics without too much image degradation. One method is to send a stream of alternating phase inverted pulses and use colour Doppler circuitry to pick out the harmonics; essentially this method (known as Power Pulse-Inversion, PPI) exploits the high sensitivity of Doppler to overcome the signal-to-noise limitation [20]. By using the Doppler circuitry to depict the microbubble signature, the B-mode tissue image can be displayed as a background image, just as in colour Doppler. In a similar approach to PPI, the direction of flow of the microbubbles (and therefore of blood) in larger vessels is detected with low MI velocity Doppler, while slow moving and stationary microbubbles are shown in green using a pulse inversion sequence. This combined mode, known as Vascular Recognition Imaging (Toshiba), also allows the microbubble signature to be displayed separately from, or combined with, the B-mode and provides additional information on the flow direction in larger vessels.

Another approach also uses a series of pulses, though only three per line, but as well as inverting the phase, the amplitude of the pulses is changed and this preserves more of the non-linear content of the received signals and thus improves sensitivity [21, 22]. Implemented as Contrast Pulse Sequences (CPS, Siemens Acuson), the non-linear microbubble signals are displayed in a colour tint over the B-mode picture or as a split screen so that both can be viewed as required.

All of these modes operate at very low transmit powers (MI <0.2) and, as well as not producing tissue harmonics, this has the important advantage that bubble destruction is minimised so that real-time scanning can be used. This makes contrast studies much easier to perform since no special scanning techniques are required.

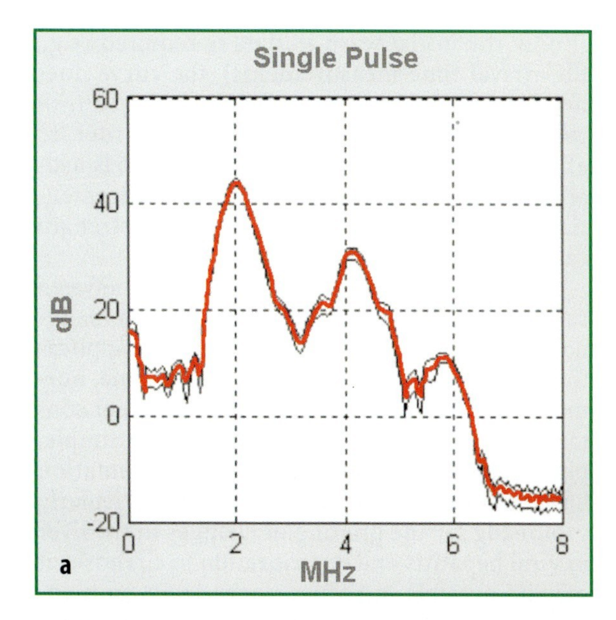

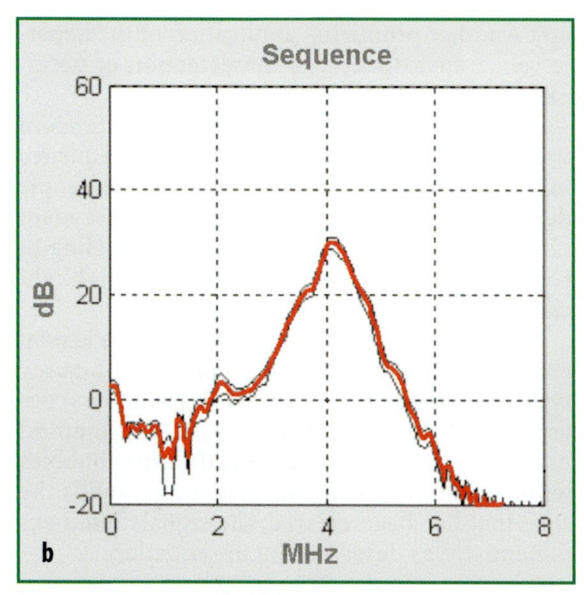

Fig. 3. *Frequency Spectra of Microbubbles.* In these charts the frequencies emitted by the microbubbles in a water tank is plotted on the X-axis with the signal strength on the Y-axis. **a** Shows the spectrum using a single pulse of 2 MHz frequency, as used in conventional B-mode imaging. The fundamental signal at 2 MHz is dominant but there are also second and third harmonics at 4 and 6 MHz. In **b**, a phase inversion sequence was used: the fundamental (and the third harmonics) have been suppressed, leaving only the second harmonic. This approach allows the microbubble signals to be separated from tissue signals. (The *red lines* are the averages of repeated measurements and the *black lines* indicate the standard deviation of the measurements) (Modified from [16])

Functional Studies

The use of microbubbles for functional studies employs analytical techniques originally developed for nuclear medicine, CT and MRI [23]. Essentially, following a bolus injection, the arrival and wash-out of the microbubbles is tracked in a region of interest, for example, a major vessel or a tissue region. The way the contrast signal changes with time is plotted as a time-intensity curve from which a variety of features can be extracted. These divide into two families, those relating to the timing of the changes and those relating to the amount of enhancement: some features such as the full-width-at-half-maximum value, incorporate both temporal and quantitative values. The quantitative features depend on a fixed relationship between the amount of microbubbles in the region of interest and their signal strength [24]. This has been demonstrated to be largely true for Levovist under clinically relevant concentrations using the spectral Doppler signal strength [25] and with colour Doppler for other microbubbles [26], but not for non-linear modes with newer types of microbubble. It seems certain that this predictable relationship will breakdown when the concentration of the microbubbles is high because they self-shadow, an effect that is obvious in clinical studies of the left ventricle of the heart. It is also likely that the relationship varies with the region's depth in the body, because of simple attenuation, so that comparison for regions at different depths may not be valid.

However, these limitations do not apply to the temporal features, which are therefore likely to be more robust. Examples of these are the time from injection to arrival or to peak enhancement (e.g., in a tumour) and the delay between the appearances in related vessels (e.g., the hepatic or renal artery and vein).

Measurement of the signal strength can be made off-line and much pioneer work in this field was carried out with the audio output from spectral Doppler, which can easily be digitised by a computer equipped with a sound card. The two-dimensional data can also be analysed, either using digital cine clips, despite the fact that they are usually too short, or from videotaped sequences. Software to perform the analyses on this data has been developed by several academic laboratories and is frequently found built-in to modern clinical US scanners. This has the advantage of allowing the data used for analysis to be corrected for scanner settings such as gain and TGC. In practice, these applications offer a tool with which a series of regions of interest can be drawn on screen, and offer a selection of other analytical tools. Some also incorporate motion tracking [22], which helps to correct for the effects of respiratory motion. For cardiac use, ECG gating is essential.

The raw time-intensity curves are usually noisy, with cardiac fluctuations superimposed on the slower wash-in and wash-out data (as well as other forms of noise and clutter) and usually require smoothing before they can be analysed. If only the initial wash-in data is required (e.g., for arrival time measurements), the curve does not need further manipulation, but the effects of recirculation must be corrected in order to analyse the decay parts of the curve. This is usually done by applying a γ-variate fit which essentially strips out late surges in the signal strength caused by recirculation [27].

The best features for discriminating between various pathologies, such as benign from malignant, are still being worked out. In some applications, such as the hepatic vein transit time, normal values and the effects of using different contrast agents have been established and simple, practicable methods for clinical implementation have been developed. This method is particularly promising for the grading of changes in the liver in viral hepatitis and deterioration to cirrhosis; it may be possible to reduce dependence on biopsies to assess the best time to offer antiviral therapy. Another promising application of the hepatic vein transit time is in the detection of occult metastases.

Another way to use the dynamic data from tissue regions is to assemble the image sequence into functional (parametric) images, for example depicting the time to arrival of the contrast agent [28]. This approach is particularly promising in tumours, since it could be expected to highlight chaotic flow in malignancies.

A unique way to obtain excellent bolus arrival characteristics exploits the fragility of many types of microbubble in the sound field. First developed for the myocardium [29], this method uses a high MI beam to destroy the microbubbles within a slice of tissue. As the contrast refills the slice that has been cleared, the signals build exponentially, as described by the equation:

$$I = A(1 - e^{-\beta t})$$

where I = signal intensity and t is the pulsing interval. The slope of the exponent (β) is proportional to the speed of flow into the slice while the peak signal strength, A, is proportional to the fractional vascular volume. The product of these two parameters is an indirect measure of tissue perfusion. This provides the opportunity to compare perfusion in adjacent tissue regions.

A practical way to generate reperfusion curves is to switch the scanner to a high MI mode (often this uses colour Doppler beams) for a second or so and then to a low MI contrast mode to observe the tissue refill in real-time. Assumptions involved include the supposition that the low MI beam is non-destructive (probably this is unachievable), that microbubble destruction is complete within the slice, and that the circulating concentration is steady. It also assumes that the tissue does not move across the scanned beam.

Reperfusion Kinetics using this technique have been applied to the heart [29] and the brain [30] and the resulting perfusion overlay images are impressive, though this has not yet become accepted as a clinical tool. A small study in the kidney using the destruction-reperfusion method with Levovist infusion in normal volunteers showed a good correlation between cortical flow increases produced by administration of dopamine and total renal blood flow, measured as the clearance of radio-labelled paramino hippurate (PAH) clearance [31]. The fractional vascular volume did not change. Though this was a small study, it convincingly demonstrated that non-invasive renal blood flow measurements are feasible.

Targeted Microbubbles

Despite the apparent simplicity of their shells, ligands can be attached to microbubbles to target them to specific cell membrane molecules for diagnostic or therapeutic purposes [32, 33]. A common way to effect this is to exploit the biotin-avidin conjugation system. Avidin, found in egg albumen, has high affinity for biotin, a vitamin, and proteins bind to the complex [34, 35]. Antibodies or protein ligands for example, can be attached to activated endothelium in this way. Microbubbles modified in this way selectively bind to e-selectin that is expressed on endothelium that has been activated (for example, by inflammatory processes including atheroma), but not on normal endothelium. They remain acoustically active and emit harmonics when insonated. Thus, they can be used to detect activated endothelium. Other potentially useful ligands include monoclonal antibodies directed against malignant cells and against activated platelets that are found in fresh thrombus [33, 36].

Drug Delivery

The potential for drug and gene delivery using US and microbubbles is a research arena of great interest [37]. The process is twofold: US, even at diagnostic power levels, produces transient gaps in cell membranes that facilitate ingress of molecules present in the interstitial fluid [38]. This process is known as sonoporation. The cell wall defects close spontaneously within hours or minutes of turning off the US field and, provided the acoustic power is low, do not seem to cause permanent damage to the cells. This enhancement of incorporation of ambient molecules is improved if microbubbles are also present, presumably because of the mechanical effects of the microbubble oscillation as they resonate in the sound field. Thus, microbubbles can be used to potentiate incorporation of molecules into cells. Even large molecules such as genetic material can be incorporated in this way, a process known as transduction. Furthermore, genetic material incorporated in this way remains active and can synthesise copies of functioning enzymes [39]. A hope is that further selectivity can be achieved by using targeted microbubbles.

Safety of Microbubbles

The safety of microbubbles needs to be assessed both in terms of their effects on the body, in the same way as any administered substance, as well as for effects associated with their response to US energy [40, 41]. Overall, the fact that several microbubble preparations have gained approval by regulatory bodies following extensive phase three clinical trials underlies their safety in clinical practice. Minor adverse effects of contrast agents are reported in less than 5% of subjects and typically include transient discomfort at the injection site, taste aberrations and vaso vagal attacks. Some serious adverse events have been reported in post-marketing surveillance by manufacturers, including premature ventricular contractions (PVCs) during echocardiography [42]. These occur when US at high MIs is used at end systole (a particularly sensitive phase of the cardiac cycle) and the effect is reproducible in animal studies. It is increased when high doses of contrast are used, leading to the obvious recommendation to use low MIs and low doses for echocardiography.

Rare adverse events emerge for all drugs that are used extensively and, for US contrast agents, these include allergic or hypersensitivity reactions that cannot be predicted from the clinical trials. Three deaths have been reported following contrast echocardiograph studies, all in patients with severe coronary artery disease. Though the temporal relationship and the underlying clinical instability of these patients suggested that the deaths were not related to the contrast agent used, the agent was withdrawn temporarily and caution was advised for patients with angina when it was later reintroduced.

Clinicians using microbubble contrast agents need to be trained to deal with such rare but serious adverse events, as recommended by the European Federation for Ultrasound in Medicine and Biology [43]: *"It is recommended that investigators wishing to undertake UCA examinations should gain experience by observing contrast studies being performed in a department with expertise in this area. They should also ensure that their equipment is optimized for contrast examination by discussion with their equipment manufacturers. It is also important that in their own department there are adequate numbers of examinations being performed and different types of pathological processes being observed to acquire and maintain their skills. Practitioners need to be competent in the administration of contrast agents, familiar with any contra-indications and be able to deal with any possible adverse effect, within the medical and legal framework of their country."*

In vitro studies show that US from clinical scanners produces effects such as sonoporation, detachment from glass substrates, haemolysis and cell death in the presence of microbubbles at diagnostic concentrations. These effects seem to be mechanical and are increased by using higher acoustic powers, by higher concentrations of microbubbles and by close proximity to cells, especially when they microbubbles have been phagocytosed. There does not seem to be a lower threshold for these effects.

Similar effects have been demonstrated *in vivo*, either using clinical scanners or with similar pulsing and power conditions and clinical microbubble concentrations. In particular, rupture of the microvasculature and intestinal peticheae have been observed. Though it is difficult to extrapolate these observations to human conditions, presumably these effects can also occur in humans. Their clinical relevance is unclear because capillary haemorrhage is commonplace under minor everyday stresses, including in the feet due to walking and in the lungs due to coughing, suggesting that they should not be of great concern. The possibility of damage to the cerebral microcirculation has been studied in human transcranial Doppler examinations and no effect has been found [44].

Microbubbles in the blood increase the vulnerability of many mammalian tissues and organs to damage from lithotripter fields *in vivo*. The increased vulnerability can persist for hours and this forms the basis for the advice not to use US contrast materials for 24 hours before lithotripsy.

Overall, though more work needs to be done, this class of contrast agents is very well tolerated and the agents may be used in patients with renal, cardiac and hepatic failure without concern. The restriction to avoid the use of SonoVue in patients with ongoing angina is the only safety-related limitation to have emerged in a period when microbubble agents have been used safely to benefit many thousand patients.

Key Points

- The complex behaviour of microbubbles in the sound field leads to unique signatures that can be selectively displayed.
- Specific software can show the microbubble distribution alongside a conventional B-mode image in real-time.
- The use of low MIs minimises microbubble destruction and allows real-time observation for the duration of the microbubbles in blood, up to several minutes after injection.
- The exquisite sensitivity of the combination of microbubble-specific imaging modes and newer types of microbubble extends the abilities of ultrasound so that now the microcirculation can be studied as well as larger blood vessels.
- The use of microbubbles as tracers for ultrasound opens the way to functional studies.
- Ligands and large molecules can be attached to microbubbles, offering the possibility of targeted, molecular imaging and of drug and gene delivery using these tools.

References

1. Darge K, Troeger J, Duetting T et al (1999) Reflux in young patients: comparison of voiding US of the bladder and retrovesical space with echo enhancement versus voiding cystourethrography for diagnosis. Radiology 210:201-207
2. Degenhardt F (1996) Contrast Sonography in Gynaecology. Thieme, Stuttgart6
3. Dawson P, Cosgrove D, Grainger R (1999) Contrast Agents in Radiology. Isis Medical Press, Oxford
4. Cosgrove D, Blomley M, Jayaram V, Nihoyannopoulos P (1998) Echo-enhancing (Contrast) Agents. Ultrasound Quarterly 14:66-75
5. Dawson P, Cosgrove D, Grainger R (1999) Textbook of Contrast Media. Isis Medical Press, Oxford
6. de Jong N, Ten Cate F, Lancee C et al (1991) Principles and recent developments in ultrasound contrast agents. Ultrasonics 9:324-330
7. EFSUMB Study Group (2004) Guidelines for the use of contrast agents in ultrasound. Ultraschall in der Medizin 25:249-256
8. Cosgrove DO (2004) Advances in Contrast Agent Imaging. Eur Radiol 14[Suppl 8]:1-124
9. Gramiak R, Shah P (1968) Echocardiography of the aortic root. Invest Radiol 3:356-366
10. Schlief R (1991) Ultrasound contrast agents. Curr Opin Radiol 3:198-207
11. Rasor J, Tickner E (1984) Microbubble precursors and methods for their production and use. United States Patent. Apr 17
12. Blomley M, Cosgrove D, Albrecht T (1998) SAE in the liver. Radiology 224:124-134
13. Albrecht T, Blomley MJ, Cosgrove DO et al (1999) Non-invasive diagnosis of hepatic cirrhosis by transit-time analysis of an ultrasound contrast agent. Lancet 353:1579-1583
14. Lim A, Taylor-Robinson S, Patel et al (2005) Hepatic Vein Transit Times using a Microbubble Agent can Predict Disease Severity Non-invasively in Patients with Hepatitis C. Gut 24:128-133
15. Bernatik T, Becker D, Neureiter D et al (2004) Hepatic transit time of an echo enhancer: an indicator of metastatic spread to the liver. Eur J Gastroenterol Hepatol 16:313-317
16. Eckersley R, Chin C, Burns P (2005) Optimising phase and amplitude modulation schemes for imaging microbubble contrast agents at low acoustic power. Ultrasound Med Biol 31:213-219

16a. de Jong N, Cornet R et al (1994) Higher harmonics of vibrating gas-filled microspheres. 1. Simulations. Ultrasonics 32(6):447-453

17. Albrecht T, Blomley MJ, Heckemann RA et al (2000) Stimulated acoustic emissions with the ultrasound contrast medium levovist: a clinically useful contrast effect with liver-specific properties. Rofo Fortschr Geb Rontgenstr Neuen Bildgeb Verfahr 172:61-67
18. Burns PN (1996) Harmonic imaging with ultrasound contrast agents. Clin Radiol 51 Suppl 1:50-55
19. Burns PN, Wilson SR, Simpson DH (2000) Pulse inversion imaging of liver blood flow: improved method for characterizing focal masses with microbubble contrast. Invest Radiol 35:58-71
20. Hope-Simpson D, Burns P (1997) Pulse Inversion Doppler: a new method for detecting nonlinear echoes from microbubble contrast agents. IEEE Trans UFFC pp 1599-1600
21. Phillips P (2001) Contrast Pulse Sequences (CPS): Imaging nonlinear microbubbles. 2001 IEEE Ultrasonics Symposium
22. Phillips P, Gardner E (2004) Contrast Agent Detection and Quantification. Eur Radiol 14:4-10
23. Maier P, Zierler K (1954) On the theory of indicator dilution method for the measurement of blood flow and volume. J Appl Physiol 4:308-314
24. Blomley M, Jayaram V, Cosgrove D et al (1997) Linear dose response relationship with the US contrast agent BR1; a quantitative study in normal volunteers. Europ Radiol 7[Suppl]:S 69
25. Schwarz K, Bezante G, Chen X (1993) Quantitative echo-contrast concentration measurement by Doppler sonography. Ultrasound Med Biol 129:289-297
26. Blomley MJ, Albrecht T, Cosgrove DO, Bamber JC (1997) Can relative contrast agent concentration be measured in vivo with color Doppler US? Radiology 204:279-281
27. Capkun V, Eteroviv D (1985) A critical approach to gamma variate fit of radionuclide-angiography pulmonary histograms. Eur J Nucl Med 11:120-122
28. Eckersley, R, Cosgrove, D, Blomley, M, Hashimoto, H (1988) Functional imaging of tissue response to bolus injection of ultrasound contrast agent. Proc IEEE Ultrasonics Symposium 2:1779-1782
29. Wei K, Jayaweera AR, Firoozan S et al (1998) Quantification of myocardial blood flow with ultrasound-induced destruction of microbubbles administered as a constant venous infusion. Circulation 97:473-483
30. Seidel G, Meyer K, Metzler V et al (2002) Human cerebral perfusion analysis with ultrasound contrast agent constant infusion: a pilot study on healthy volunteers. Ultrasound Med Biol 28:183-189
31. Kishimoto N, Mori Y, Nishiue T et al (2003) Renal blood flow measurement with contrast-enhanced harmonic ultrasonography: evaluation of dopamine-induced changes in renal cortical perfusion in humans. Clin Nephrol 59:423-428
32. Klibanov AL, Hughes MS, Villanueva FS et al (1999) Targeting and ultrasound imaging of microbubble-based contrast agents. Magma 8:177-184
33. Liang HD, Blomley MJ (2003) The role of ultrasound in molecular imaging. Br J Radiol 76 Spec No 2:S140-150
34. Bayer E, Wilchek M (1980) The use of the avidin-biotin complex as a tool in molecular biology. Methods Biochem Anal 26:1-45
35. Savage M (1992) Avidin-Biotin Chemistry: A Handbook. Pierce Chemical Co, Rockford, IL
36. Schumann PA, Christiansen JP, Quigley RM et al (2003) Targeted-microbubble binding selectively to GPIIb IIIa receptors of platelet thrombi. Invest Radiol 37:587-593
37. Unger EC, Hersh E, Vannan M, McCreery T (2001) Gene delivery using ultrasound contrast agents. Echocardiography 18:355-361
38. Tachibana K, Tachibana S (1995) Albumin microbubble echo-contrast material as an enhancer for ultrasound accelerated thrombolysis. Circulation 92:1148-1150
39. Yang L, Shirakata Y, Tamai K et al (2005) Microbubble-enhanced ultrasound for gene transfer into living skin equivalents. J Dermatol Sci 40:105-114

40. Rott HD (1999) Safety of ultrasonic contrast agents. European Committee for Medical Ultrasound Safety. Eur J Ultrasound 9:195-197
41. ter Haar GR (2002) Ultrasonic contrast agents: safety considerations reviewed. Eur J Radiol 41:217-221
42. van Der Wouw PA, Brauns AC, Bailey SE et al (2000) Premature ventricular contractions during triggered imaging with ultrasound contrast. J Am Soc Echocardiogr 13:288-294
43. EFSUMB (2004) weo. www.efsumb.org.
44. Haggag KJ, Russell D, Walday P et al (1998) Air-filled ultrasound contrast agents do not damage the cerebral microvasculature or brain tissue in rats. Invest Radiol 33:129-135

SECTION II

Clinical Application of Contrast Ultrasound in Liver Diseases

II.1

Characterisation of Benign Focal Liver Lesions with Contrast-Enhanced Ultrasound (CEUS)

Christoph F. Dietrich

Introduction

Conventional B-mode ultrasound (US) allows for the definite diagnosis of common typical liver cysts by differences in echogenicity in comparison to the surrounding liver tissue using the following criteria: round, non-echogenic, smooth surface, sharp borders, lateral shadowing, posterior echo enhancement. Conventional B-mode US also allows for the definite diagnosis of calcifications due to their typical appearance: echo-rich with acoustic shadows [1].

Other focal liver lesions (FLL) are characterised sonographically, not only by analysis of differences in echogenicity from the surrounding liver tissue, but also by the detection of hyper- or hypovascularization (colour duplex US) and by changes occurring in inflow kinetics (enhancement) of contrast media. As a result of their double blood supply via both the portal vein and the hepatic artery, focal lesions in the liver often exhibit no sustained hyper- or hypoperfusion, but depending on the perfusion phase and the histology, present with a complex spatio-temporal picture of increased and reduced contrast-enhancement. Certain lesions display a characteristic vascular picture (e.g., wheel-spoke phenomenon in FNH) or a distinctive perfusion pattern (e.g., iris diaphragm phenomenon in haemangioma), allowing the lesions to be characterised. Unfortunately, contrast-enhancement does not always exhibit such typical and unique patterns. Multiple reviews and guidelines, as well as multicentre trials have been recently published using contrast-enhancing techniques [2-7].

The following chapter focuses on benign liver tumours and nodules, summarized in Table 1.

Table 1. Classification of liver tumours and nodular lesions (modified from [7a])

Cell of origin	Benign liver tumour or nodular lesion (in parenthesis malignant transformation)	Abbreviation
Hepatocyte	Hepatocellular adenoma (→ hepatocellular carcinoma)	HCA (HCC)
	Focal nodular hyperplasia (→ fibrolammelar hepatocellular carcinoma)	FNH (FLHCC)
	Nodular regenerative hyperplasia	NRH
	Partial nodular transformation	PNT
	Macroregenerative nodule	MRN
Bile duct epithelium	Bile duct adenoma (→ combined hepatocellular and cholangiocarcinoma)	BDA (HCC/CCC)
	Bile duct cystadenoma (→ cystadenocarcinoma)	BDCA (BDCACa)
	Bile duct adenofibroma	BDAF
Mixed liver and bile duct cell	Mesenchymal hamartoma (→ angiosarcoma)	
Endothelial cell	Haemangioma	Haem
	Infantile haemangioendothelioma	

Differentiation of Benign and Malignant Lesions

Characterization of a liver lesion begins once an abnormality is found. An imaging procedure that is used to detect liver masses should also enable the examiner to differentiate between benign and malignant lesions, since benign and malignant lesions have been reported to vary in their uptake during the portal-venous and liver specific late phase after injection of Levovist. Homogeneous parenchymal Levovist uptake in the portal-venous and liver specific late phase seems to be indicative of benign focal liver lesions [8-13]. We propose that the non-enhancing defects of malignant liver lesions, and also abscesses, might be explained by the lack of liver specific tissue, such as portal veins, sinusoids and reticulo-endothelial cells. The extent of late phase contrast uptake by a lesion is mainly determined by the degree of similarity of the lesion to normal liver parenchyma, resulting in false positive findings and misinterpretation in patients with abscesses, necrosis, scars, calcifications, cysts, and thrombosis. As conventional B-mode US can correctly diagnose cysts and calcifications, it is therefore mandatory to perform a baseline scan before using US contrast agents. The results of a previously published study show that contrast-enhanced phase inversion sonography may discriminate between benign liver specific tissue and non-liver specific tissue - mainly malignant focal liver lesions in the portal-venous and liver specific late phase (Tables 2, 3) [13].

Only a few false positive findings were observed, mainly due to abscesses or necrosis, and in two liver tumours. Of these, one was a case of old focal nodular hyperplasia with predominantly scar tissue, and one was a case of an inflammatory pseudo-tumour of the liver, which was definitively diagnosed only by surgical exploration. The difficulties in diagnosing inflammatory pseudo-tumour of the liver is in accordance with current literature [14].

Role of Contrast-Enhanced US in Clinical Practice

Contrast-enhanced US (CEUS) improves the detection rate of liver tumours in comparison to conventional B-mode US. CEUS was shown to be as effective as computed tomography (CT) and magnetic resonance imaging (MRI) in detecting neoplasia of the liver. We and others have obtained similar results when differentiating between benign and malignant lesions using

Table 2. Demographic profile and tumour size of patients with histologically proven liver tumours [13]

Characteristics	
Demography	
No (M/F)	80/94
Mean age (yr)+	52 ± 15 [7 - 80]
	Mean size [mm]+
Benign liver lesions (n = 95)	41 ± 24 [8-130]
Focal nodular hyperplasia (n = 36)	51 ± 18 [20-110]
Haemangioma (n = 31)	37 ± 31 [8-130]
Adenoma (n = 10)	40 ± 20 [15-80]
Abscess (n = 5)	40 ± 24 [10-80]
Microhamartomas (n = 4)	12 ± 2 [9-15]
Focal steatosis (n = 4)	32 ± 5 [25-38]
Nodular regenerative hyperplasia (n = 1)	40
Hyperregenerative nodule (n = 1)	35
Focal biliary cirrhosis (n = 1)	25
Bacillary angiomatosis (n = 1)	50
Inflammatory pseudotumour (n = 1)	40
Malignant liver lesions (n = 79)	40 ± 21 [7-120]
Metastatic liver tumour (n = 37)	33 ± 12 [10-75]
Hepatocellular carcinoma (n = 33)	42 ± 24 [7-120]
Cholangiocellular carcinoma (n = 4)	59 ± 42 [40-100]
Lymphoma (n = 4)	44 ± 17 [17-60]
Hemangioendotheliosarcoma (n = 1)	100

+Mean ± standard deviation [range]

Table 3. Contrast-enhancement in 95 patients with histologically proven benign liver tumours or lesions [13]

Liver tumour	Isoechoic contrast-enhancement
Benign liver lesions (n = 95)	88/95
Focal nodular hyperplasia (n = 36)	35/36
Haemangioma (n = 31)	31/31*
Adenoma (n = 10)	10/10
Abscess (n = 5)	0/5
Microhamartomas (n = 4)	4/4
Focal steatosis (n = 4)	4/4
Focal biliary cirrhosis (n = 1)	1/1
Bacillary angiomatosis (n = 1)	1/1
Nodular regenerative hyperplasia (n = 1)	1/1
Regenerative nodule (n = 1)	1/1
Inflammatory pseudotumour (n = 1)	0/1

*The vascular phase contrast-enhancement pattern of haemangiomas was variable. Characteristic was a progressive heterogeneous centripetal fill-in and considerable enhancement on liver specific late phase imaging, revealing diminished contrast to the surrounding liver parenchyma in all patients

SonoVue. Homogeneous uptake is indicative of benign focal liver lesions. The importance of this dual imaging approach (conventional B-mode US/contrast-enhanced ultrasonography) is highlighted by the recognition of the high prevalence of benign liver lesions in the adult population that do not require treatment. These include cysts, calcifications and most benign liver tumours. Therefore, correct characterisation by the ultrasonography as the primary imaging method is crucial for the further diagnostic, therapeutic and prognostic approaches.

Hepatic Tumour and Liver Nodule Characterisation

Liver Cyst

Conventional B-mode US

Liver cysts are a common sonographic finding. They are readily diagnosed using conventional B-mode US. The typical cysts are echo-free, round/oval, with well-defined borders with lateral shadowing and posterior echo-enhancement. Very early echinococcosis might be confused with atypical liver cysts.

Colour Doppler Imaging

Blood vessels have to be excluded by colour Doppler imaging ruling out arterio-portal-venous malformations with a cystic appearance.

Contrast-Enhanced US

Using CEUS, cysts show no contrast-enhancement at all. As they may be confused with metastases in CEUS, conventional B-mode US has to precede CEUS. CEUS is helpful in recognising echinococcosis at all stages.

Role of Contrast-Enhanced US in Clinical Practice

In clinical practice, CEUS has no role in routine diagnosis of cysts, since sensitive colour Doppler techniques differentiate between vascular abnormalities and typical and atypical liver cysts in almost all cases. CEUS can be helpful, however, in the differentiation of neoplastic nodules in atypical liver cysts, which is a very rare condition.

Haemangioma

Conventional B-mode US

Most haemangiomas demonstrate typical sonomorphological features in conventional B-mode, including less than 3 cm in diameter, lobulated with a well-defined outline, located next to liver vessels, demonstrating an echo-rich texture and sometimes posterior acoustic enhancement due to blood filled capillaries (Table 4).

Table 4. Typical haemangioma, diagnostic criteria

B-mode Criteria
Less than 3 cm in diameter
Echo-rich structure
Homogeneous interior
Round or slightly oval shape
Smooth outline
Absence of any halo sign
Possible detection of feeding and draining vessel
Absence of any signs of invasive growth
Dorsal through-enhancement

Colour Doppler Imaging

Although haemangiomas are highly vascularised masses, from the histo-pathological point of view they consist essentially of a large number of capillary-sized vessels and so, even with the use of high-end machines, conventional colour Doppler US often detects little or no blood flow inside haemangiomas. This is due to the fact that the blood flow velocity in the capillary haemangiomas is too slow. The supplying and draining vessels ('feedings vessels') may be visualised (depending on the US system's peformance) (Table 5).

Table 5. Sonographic findings in 100 patients with haemangioma

Characteristics	
Mean size [cm]	3 cm ± 3 cm
Echogenicity	
Echo-rich	90 (90%)
Isoechoic or echo-poor	10 (10%)
Vascularity using colour Doppler imaging	
No intra-lesional vessels	92 (92%)
Intra-lesional vessels (hypervascular)	8 (8%)
Peripheral nodular enhancement	
Using Levovist	25%
Using SonoVue	> 75%
Complete iris diaphragm phenomenon within 60 seconds	>10%
Complete iris diaphragm phenomenon within 3 minutes	*

*depending on the technique and US machine used

Contrast-Enhanced US

Tumour enhancement characteristics differ depending on the contrast medium and technique used (intermittent scanning versus continuous real-time technique). Haemangioma characterisation using Levovist reveals arterial fill-in within 1 minute in up to 10% of patients histologically demonstrating arterio-portal-venous shunts (so-called 'shunt haemangioma'). Contrast-enhancement using Levovist showed peripheral nodular contrast-enhancement in about 25% of patients. In contrast, the typical CEUS sign of haemangioma using SonoVue is peripheral nodular contrast-enhancement, observed in more than 75% of patients, focussing on the tumour periphery (Fig. 1). There is a significant learning curve not to confuse a small thrombosed haemangioma with a metastasis. Centripetal fill-in is the second typical sign sparing thrombosed areas and calcifications. The iris diaphragm phenomenon known from angio-CT as caused by centripetal perfusion of a haemangioma, is only visible by repeated imaging of the same region, which is easy to perform using SonoVue but difficult using Levovist due to bubble destruction. Depending on the size of the haemangioma, the typical 'filling-in' of contrast medium from the periphery towards the centre can take several minutes in CT, but is constantly observed to occur faster in CEUS. The kinetics are variable, and in the case of haemangiomas with abundant arterio-portal-venous shunts, the process can last less than a minute or even only a few seconds (Fig. 2). Therefore, imaging in the first 60 seconds is of utmost importance in characterising haemangiomas by CEUS, demonstrating the superiority of SonoVue in comparison to Levovist in that a continuous real-time technique may be performed.

Using echo signal enhancers, the iris diaphragm phenomenon is ideally also detectable with contrast-enhanced power Doppler US. Injection of the signal enhancer often produces strong artefacts, in particular 'blooming' - a gush of colour coding after administration of the agent. Since the effect is intensified by movement of the surrounding structures, exact imaging of the agent's flow into a haemangioma cannot be achieved in the vicinity of the diaphragm and in the left liver lobe (artefacts due to the action of the heart). In the phase-inversion technique, any artefacts appearing after the injection of the signal enhancer can be avoided, or at least considerably reduced. Unfortunately, even with this typical representation of perfusion, confusion with liver metastases from gastrointestinal carcinomas is possible, potentially leading to a wrong diagnosis. An examination in the liver specific late phase with Levovist may be useful in such situations (5-10%), since in the late phase metastases exhibit a sharp contrast to normal liver tissue, while in the case of haemangiomas, the contrast relative to the surrounding tissue decreases. There are many reports in the literature characterising liver haemangioma, but results so far are inconsistent [3-6, 8-11, 15-31].

Role of Contrast-Enhanced US in Clinical Practice

CEUS has markedly improved the correct diagnosis of haemangioma, which is possible in about 95% of patients. Difficult differential diagnosis includes shunt haemangioma in the cirrhotic liver, which might be confused with hepatocellular adenoma or carcinoma. A thrombosed haemangioma might be confused with a metas-

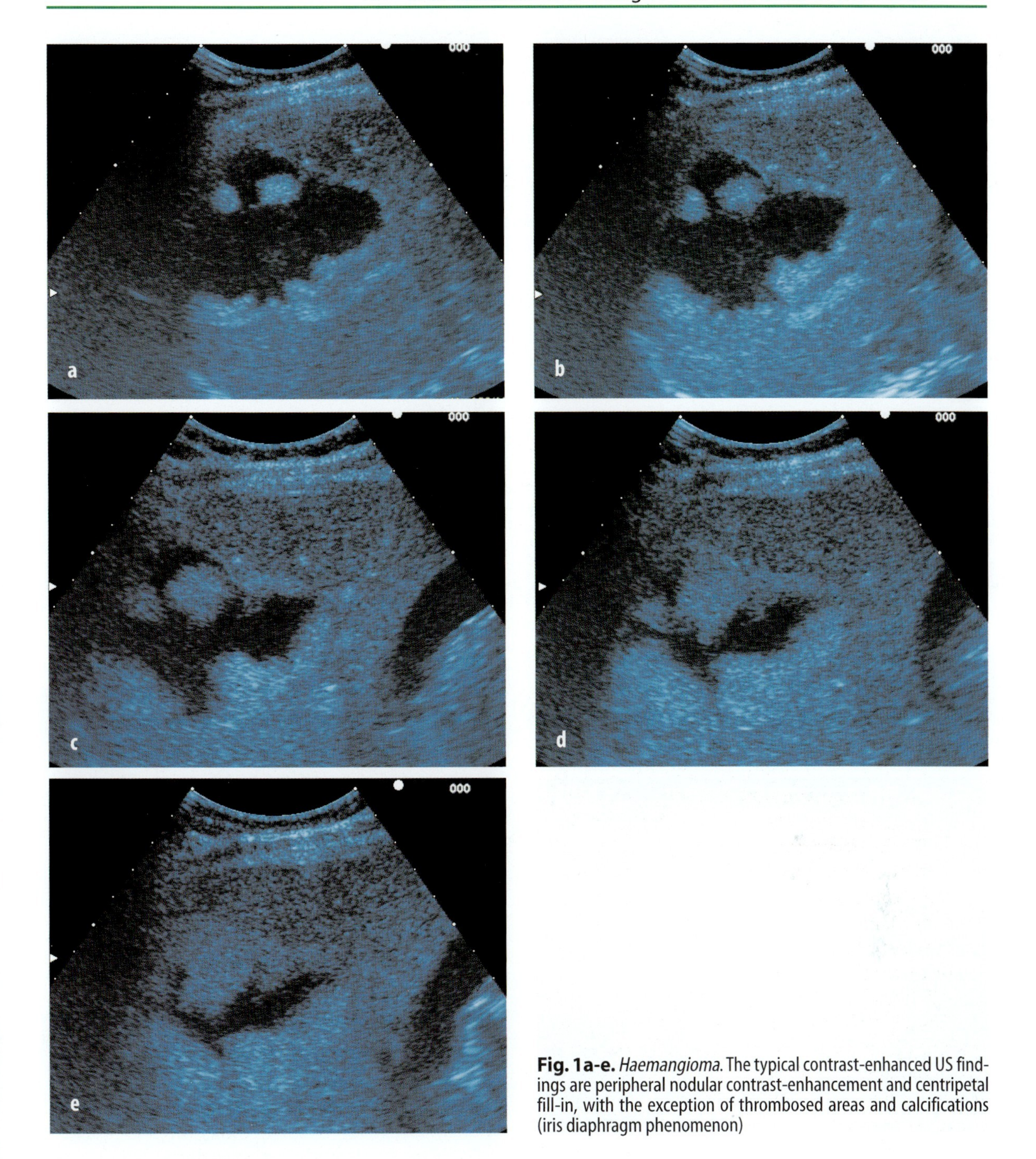

Fig. 1a-e. *Haemangioma.* The typical contrast-enhanced US findings are peripheral nodular contrast-enhancement and centripetal fill-in, with the exception of thrombosed areas and calcifications (iris diaphragm phenomenon)

tasis by demonstrating contrast sparing in the portal-venous phase.

Focal Nodular Hyperplasia (FNH)

Focal nodular hyperplasia (FNH) and the important differential diagnosis of hepatocellular adenoma (HCA) are two benign, mostly incidentally-discovered hepatic neoplasias, which occur predominantly in young and middle-aged women. Differentiation is essential because of different therapeutic approaches: HCA is an indication for surgery because of the risk of haemorrhage and potential malignant transformation, while FNH can be managed conservatively. However, until recently the non-invasive differentiation of especially atypical FNH from HCA and other benign or malignant neoplasias has remained challenging, with no satisfactory tests apart from histological examination of a liver biopsy sample. Histological features of FNH are controversially discussed in the literature. In contrast to a recent report in three patients demonstrating no portal veins [32],

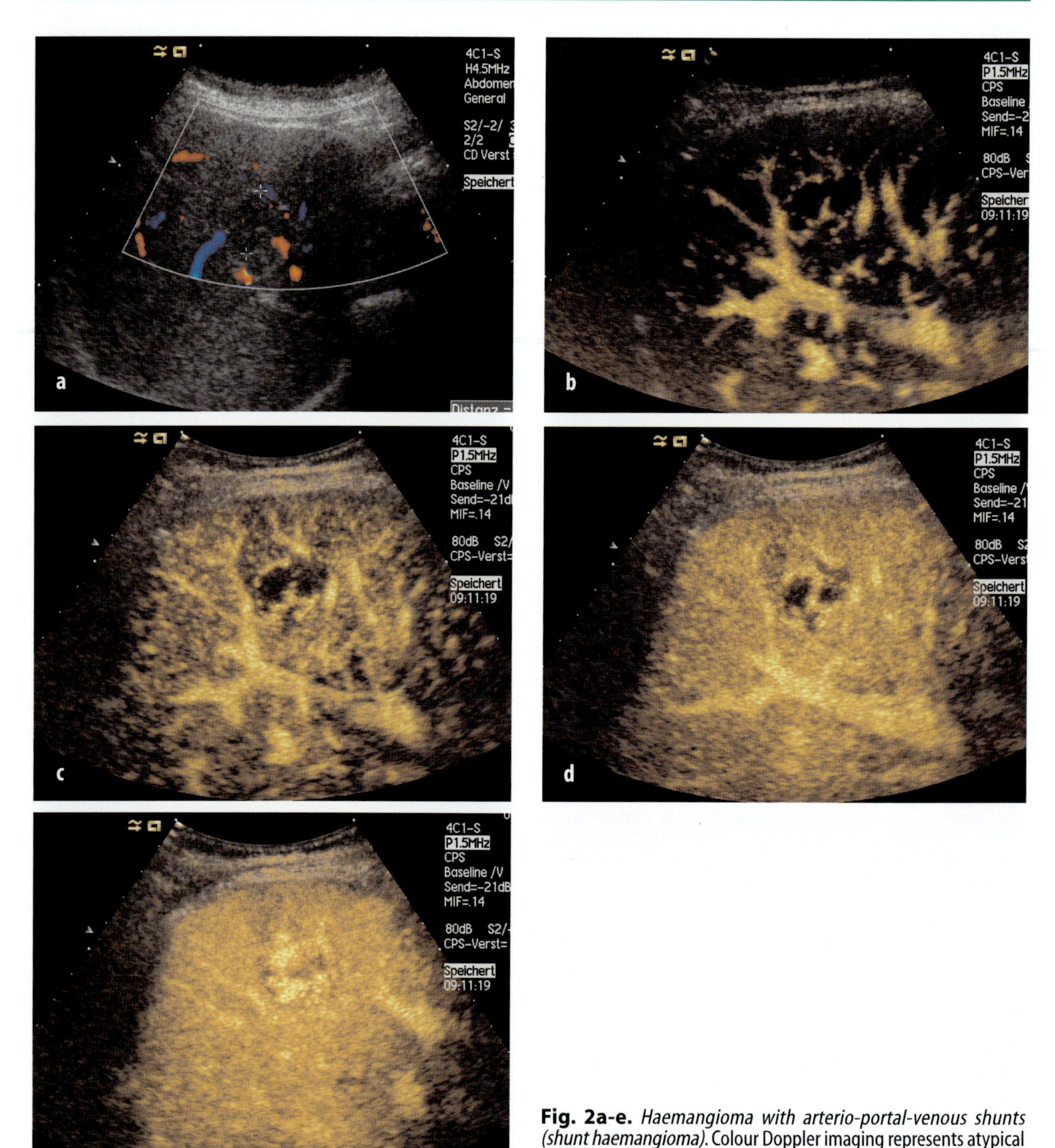

Fig. 2a-e. *Haemangioma with arterio-portal-venous shunts (shunt haemangioma).* Colour Doppler imaging represents atypical liver lesion (**a**). The typical contrast-enhanced US finding is centripetal fill-in within seconds (**b-e**)

most reports describe (arterio-portal-venous) vascular abnormalities [33, 34], but there are still some controversies [29]. Scoazec et al. report that the extracellular matrix is similar to that of portal tracts [35]. Kondo et al. report that in FNH nodules, severe anomaly of portal tracts including portal veins and hepatic arterial branches can be observed [33]. In addition, congenital absence of portal veins has been reported in few patients, mainly children. The cited literature has been recently summarised [36].

Helical CT and MR imaging do provide some useful information for the diagnosis of FNH, especially when the lesion depicts typical features, such as a central scar and uniform hypervascularity. Typical features are only reported in about 50% of patients. In a series of 305 FNHs studied macroscopically, a central scar could be found only in about 50% of cases [34].

Conventional B-mode US

FNH is typically an isoechoic tumour of variable size, with a central scar and calcifications (50-80% of patients).

Colour Doppler Imaging

Typically, colour Doppler imaging reveals an (arterially) hypervascularized tumour (in more than 90% of patients) with characteristic (para-) central arterial blood supply. In many patients, increased blood flow compared with the surrounding liver tissue can be detected even in colour duplex mode, causing a so-called wheel-spoke phenomenon. This hyperperfusion that can be recognised in native imaging is by no means obligatory and is reported only in about 50-70% of patients. It could also be shown that inter-observer reliability in recognising the wheel-spoke appearance is very low.

Contrast-Enhanced US

In a contrast-enhanced examination, FNH typically appears as a hyperperfused tumour-like lesion relative to the surrounding liver tissue in the early arterial phase. This hyperperfusion is easily visible during continuous scanning with a low mechanical index (MI), comparing the contrast-enhancement of the lesion with the surrounding hepatic arteries. Depending on the patient's cardiac output, some 8 to 20 seconds after injection of the echo-signal enhancer into the cubital vein, there is a rapid take-up of the substance, with demonstration of the arterial vascular pattern and enhancement from the (para)centre outwards. During the portal-venous phase, FNH is isoechogenic with the portal vein, and later with the liver parenchyma (Figs. 3, 4).

Forty patients with histologically proven FNH (n=30) or HCA (n=10) were included in a prospective study evaluating tumour characteristics. The pattern of tumours was described as hypoechoic, isoechoic, or hyperechoic when compared to the surrounding liver tissue, and tumour vascularity was classified as hypervascular, isovascular, or hypovascular by power Doppler sonography. The internal vascular architecture was also recorded. 4 g of Levovist (400 mg/ml) was given intravenously and the liver was scanned using phase inversion ultrasonography for the first 30 seconds, followed by intermittent scanning. The following parameters for imaging after Levovist were used: mechanical index 1.6, power 100%, gain 20 dB, and 10-14 frames/sec.

In all 40 patients enhancement of the hepatic artery and portal vein was observed. In 29 of 30 patients with FNH, the contrast pattern revealed pronounced arterial and portal-venous/sinusoidal enhancement. Only one patient with FNH lacked portal-venous/sinusoidal enhancement, possibly due to extensive, histologically-documented fibrosis. Using Levovist, homogeneous enhancement was detected during the hepatic arterial phase in all ten patients with HCA, preceding enhancement of normal liver parenchyma. In contrast to patients with FNH, no enhancement was seen in HCA during the hepatic portal-venous/sinusoidal phase, with isoechoic or slight hypoechoic appearance in the parenchymal and sinusoidal late phase. Sonographic findings of this study are summarized in Table 6. Some of the pa-

Table 6. Patient characteristics and sonographic findings in 40 patients with histologically proven FNH and hepatocellular adenoma examined with Levovist (Data not yet published)

	FNH	HCA
Number	30	10
Male/Female	4 / 26	1 / 9
Age [years]	40 ± 12 [18 - 64]	41 ± 14 [23 - 70]
Size of lesion [mm]	52 ± 18 [26 - 110]	40 ± 20 [15 – 80]
Conventional B-mode ultrasonography		
Echo texture		
Hypoechoic	10*	3*
Isoechoic	19	6
Hyperechoic	1	1**
Central scar	14	2
Colour/Power Doppler Imaging		
Hypervasular	29	8
Radial vascular architecture	10	0
Contrast-enhanced ultrasonography		
Arterial phase enhancement	30	10
portal-venous phase enhancement	29	0

*all in a sonographically bright liver; **in a patient with glycogen storage disease

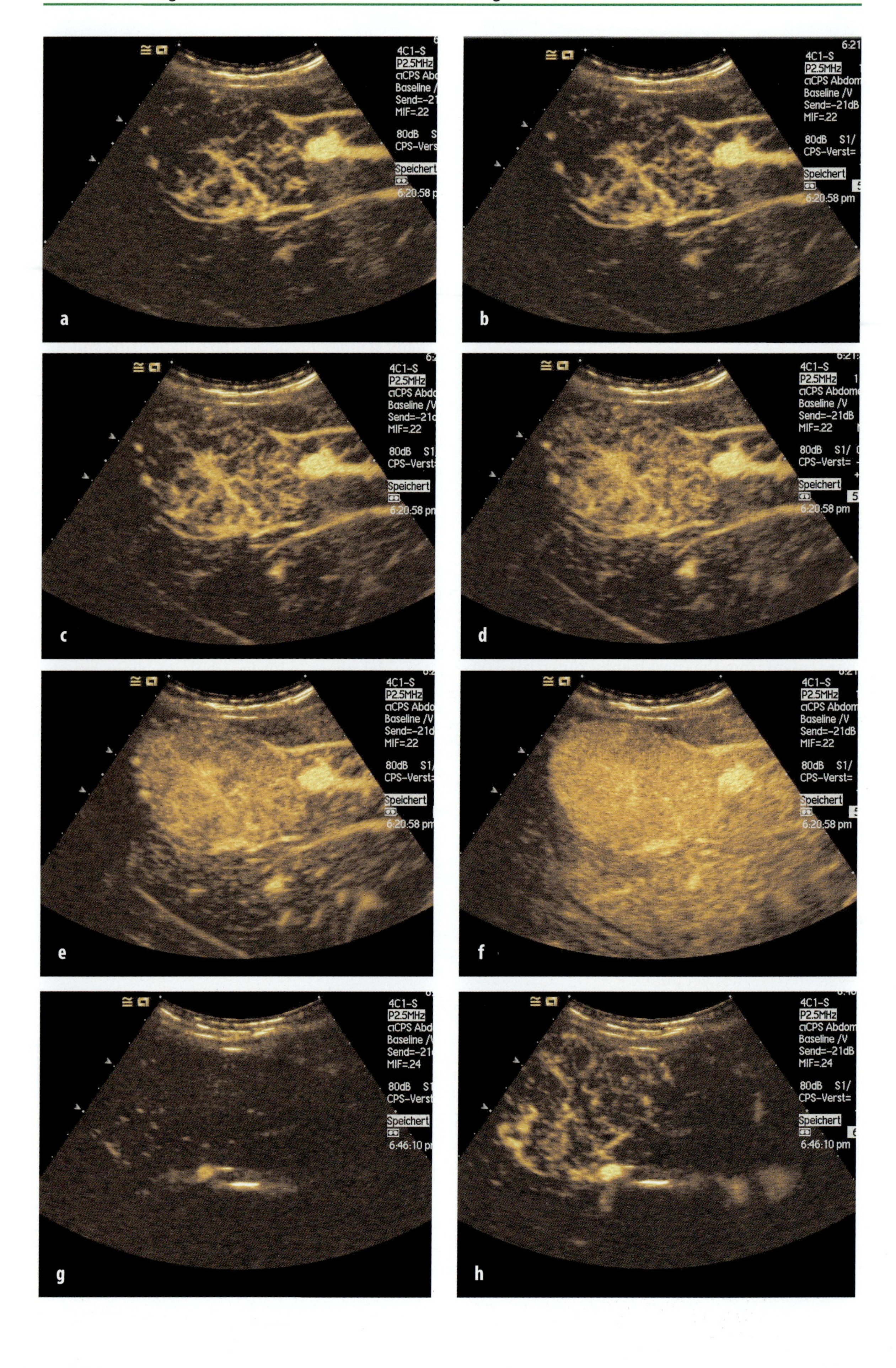
4C1-S
P2.5MHz
Baseline /V
Send=-21dB
MIF=.22
80dB S1/
CPS-Verst=
Speichert
6:20:58 pm
MIF=.24
6:46:10 pm
a
b
c
d
e
f
g
h

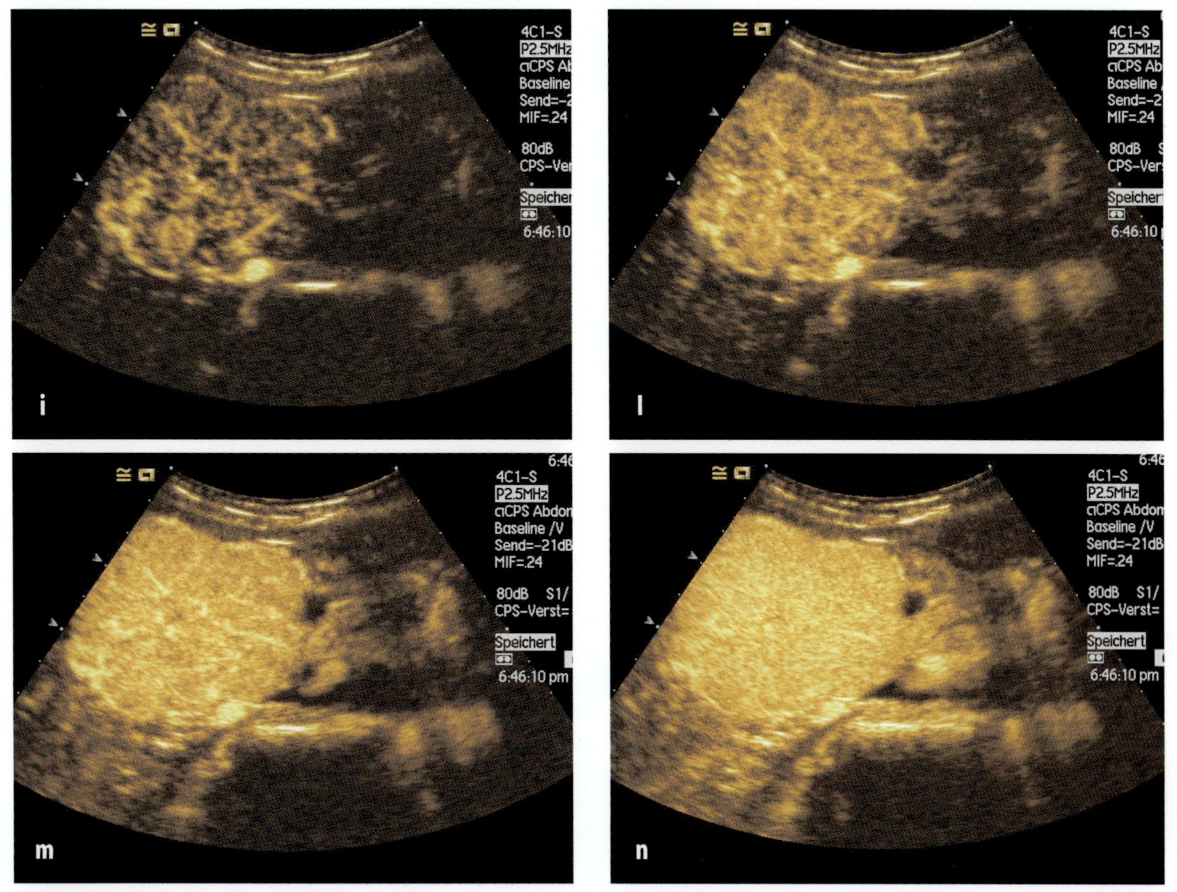

Fig. 3a-n. FNH in the early arterial phase appears typically as a hyperperfused structure relative to the surrounding liver tissue. During the portal-venous phase, FNH is isoechogenic with the portal vein, and later with the parenchyma. In the following sequences the same tumour is displayed, focussing on the central artery (**a-f**) and slightly beside the typical central artery revealing confusing vascular architecture (**g-n**) demonstrating the need to focus 'on the right place at the right time'

tients were also examined after intravenous application of 4.8 ml of SonoVue using phase inversion ultrasonography. Comparing Levovist and SonoVue during the arterial and portal-venous/sinusoidal phase, there was a better visualisation of hepatic vessels with SonoVue in all patients examined (data not yet published).

Recently, a study was published using SonoVue to characterise histologically proven FNH (n=24) or HCA (n=8). In a pre-study phase in ten consecutive patients the onset of hepatic arterial enhancement was observed to commence 8-22 seconds after injection and the early onset of portal-venous began 12-30 seconds after injection. Phase inversion ultrasonography was used before biopsy, using the following imaging parameters: MI 0.2-0.3, power 3%, gain 52-60 dB, and 10-14 frames/sec. The liver was scanned continuously for up to 5 minutes. Using this approach, contrast-enhancing tumour characteristics were evaluated during the hepatic arterial and early portal-venous phase, comparing the contrast-enhancement to the enhancing hepatic artery and portal vein branches (Table 7) [36].

Role of Contrast-Enhanced US in Clinical Practice

The examination of the hepatic arterial and portal-venous/sinusoidal phase by contrast-enhanced phase inversion ultrasonography allows the reliable differentiation of FNH from HCA. This important finding could be explained by the lack of portal veins in contrast to FNH, which presents (atypical) portal veins in many, but not all patients.

Hepatocellular Adenoma (HCA)

Conventional B-mode US

In B-mode US of an otherwise normal liver, an adenoma, like FNH, is usually isoechogenic with the surrounding liver tissue. An adenoma can be

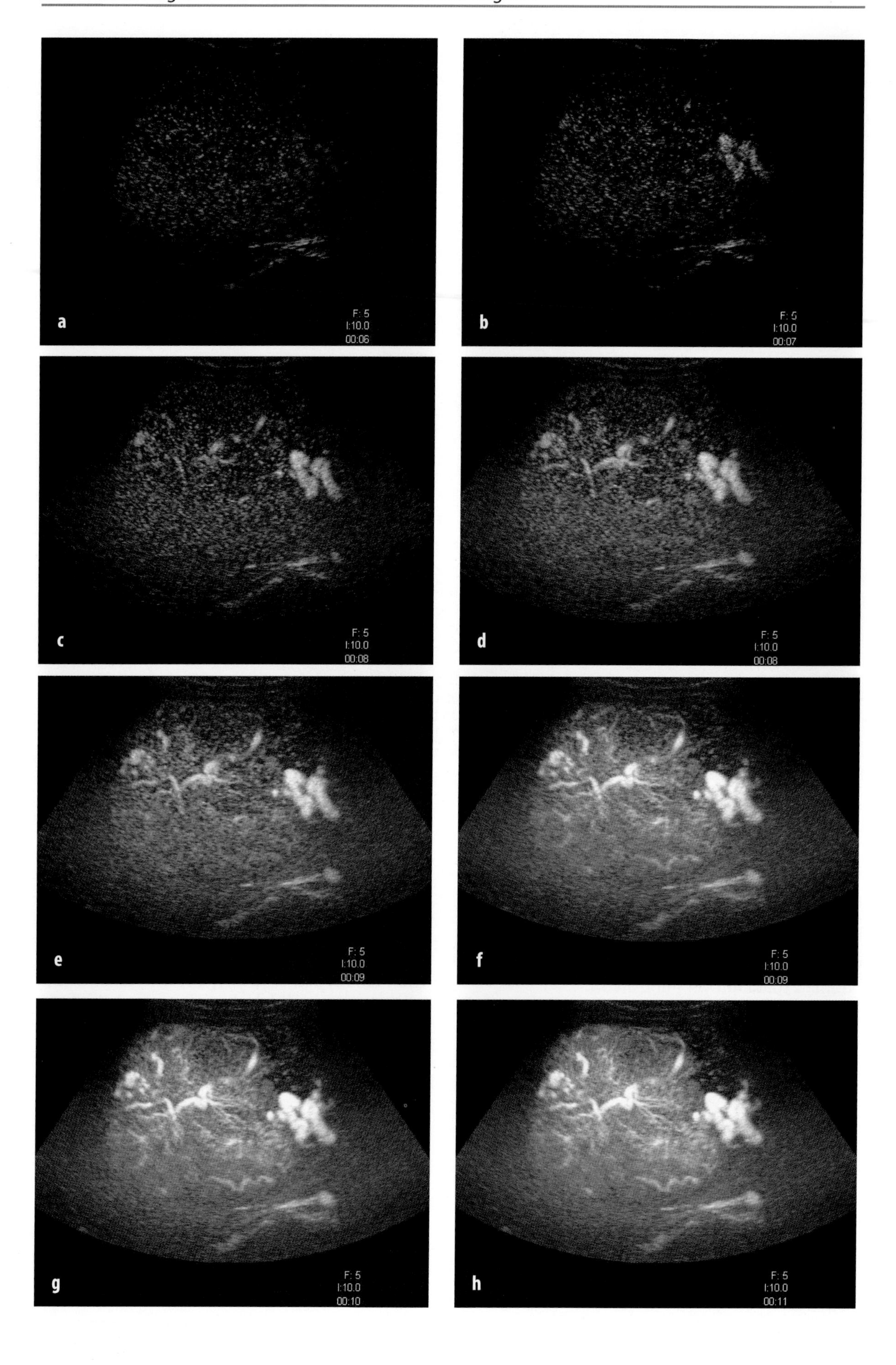
a
F: 5
I:10.0
00:06
b
F: 5
I:10.0
00:07
c
F: 5
I:10.0
00:08
d
F: 5
I:10.0
00:08
e
F: 5
I:10.0
00:09
f
F: 5
I:10.0
00:09
g
F: 5
I:10.0
00:10
h
F: 5
I:10.0
00:11

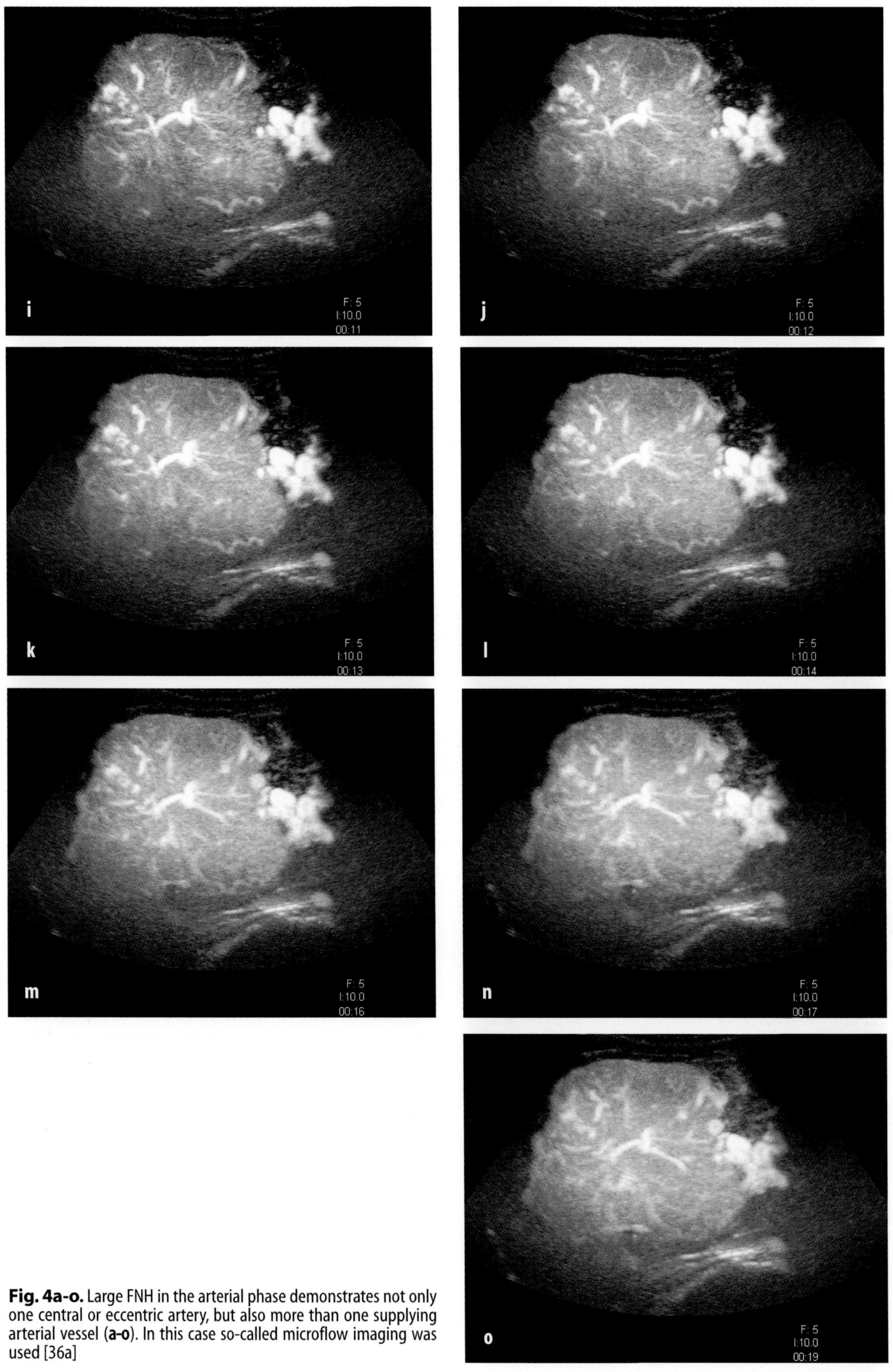

Fig. 4a-o. Large FNH in the arterial phase demonstrates not only one central or eccentric artery, but also more than one supplying arterial vessel (**a-o**). In this case so-called microflow imaging was used [36a]

Table 7. Patient characteristics and sonographic findings in 32 patients with histologically proven FNH and hepatocellular adenoma examined with SonoVue (modified from [36])

	FNH	HCA
Number	24	8
Male/Female	2 / 22	0 / 8
Age [years]	37 ± 10 [18 - 64]	37 ± 10 [23 – 47]
Size of lesion [mm]	55 ± 21 [26 - 110]	32 ± 15 [15 – 55]
Conventional B-mode ultrasonography		
Echo texture		
Hypoechoic	7*	4*
Isoechoic	16	4
Hyperechoic	1	
Central scar	10	0
Colour/Power Doppler Imaging		
Hypervasular	23	8
Radial vascular architecture	10	0
Contrast-enhanced ultrasonography		
Arterial phase enhancement	24	8
(Early) portal-venous phase enhancement	23	0

*all in a sonographically bright liver

very difficult to differentiate from the surrounding liver tissue because of this lack of echogenicity. In a fatty liver, adenomas may be poorly echogenic, whereas in patients with storage diseases (e.g. glycogenosis or Niemann-Pick disease) adenomas may even give stronger echoes [37]. As in the case of FNH, a rounded contour or a vascular impression may indicate a tumour poorly discernible from liver parenchyma. There are no other typical criteria in B-mode US.

Colour Doppler Imaging

According to the available data there are still no standardised criteria for the differentiation of adenomas from other hepatic masses based on perfusion pattern. The typical wheel-spoke structure with a central vascular supply and a central scar, which is seen in FNH is absent in adenoma, although calcifications are observed depending on size. Like FNH, an adenoma exhibits arterial hypervascularity (predominantly marginal). However, this vascular pattern can also be encountered in hepatocellular carcinomas and hyperperfused metastases, and is therefore not pathognomonic.

Contrast-Enhanced US

Contrast-enhanced phase inversion US was recently assessed in patients with histologically proven focal nodular hyperplasia or hepatocellular adenoma. It has to be taken into account that histologically, no portal veins (and in addition, no bile ducts) are present in adenomas. CEUS demonstrated pronounced arterial and portal-venous enhancement in all but one patient with FNH. In contrast, after homogeneous enhancement during hepatic arterial phase (8-25 seconds after the injection), no enhancement during hepatic portal-venous phase was detected in any patients with HCA [36] (Figs. 5, 6).

Role of Contrast-Enhanced US in Clinical Practice

Differentiation of focal nodular hyperplasia and hepatocellular adenoma is essential because of different therapeutic implications. However, establishing a correct diagnosis non-invasively has been reported to be difficult. Contrast-enhanced US improves characterisation and differentiation of FNH and HCA. In addition, we could recently show that small adenomas may be overlooked in CT and MRI scans, especially if no images are taken during the arterial phase.

Bile Duct Adenoma (Cholangiocellular Adenoma)

Contrast-enhanced US using Levovist in high dosage and concentration (4 g at 400 mg/ml) analyzing only the liver specific phase, or SonoVue analyzing the late portal-venous/sinusoidal phase

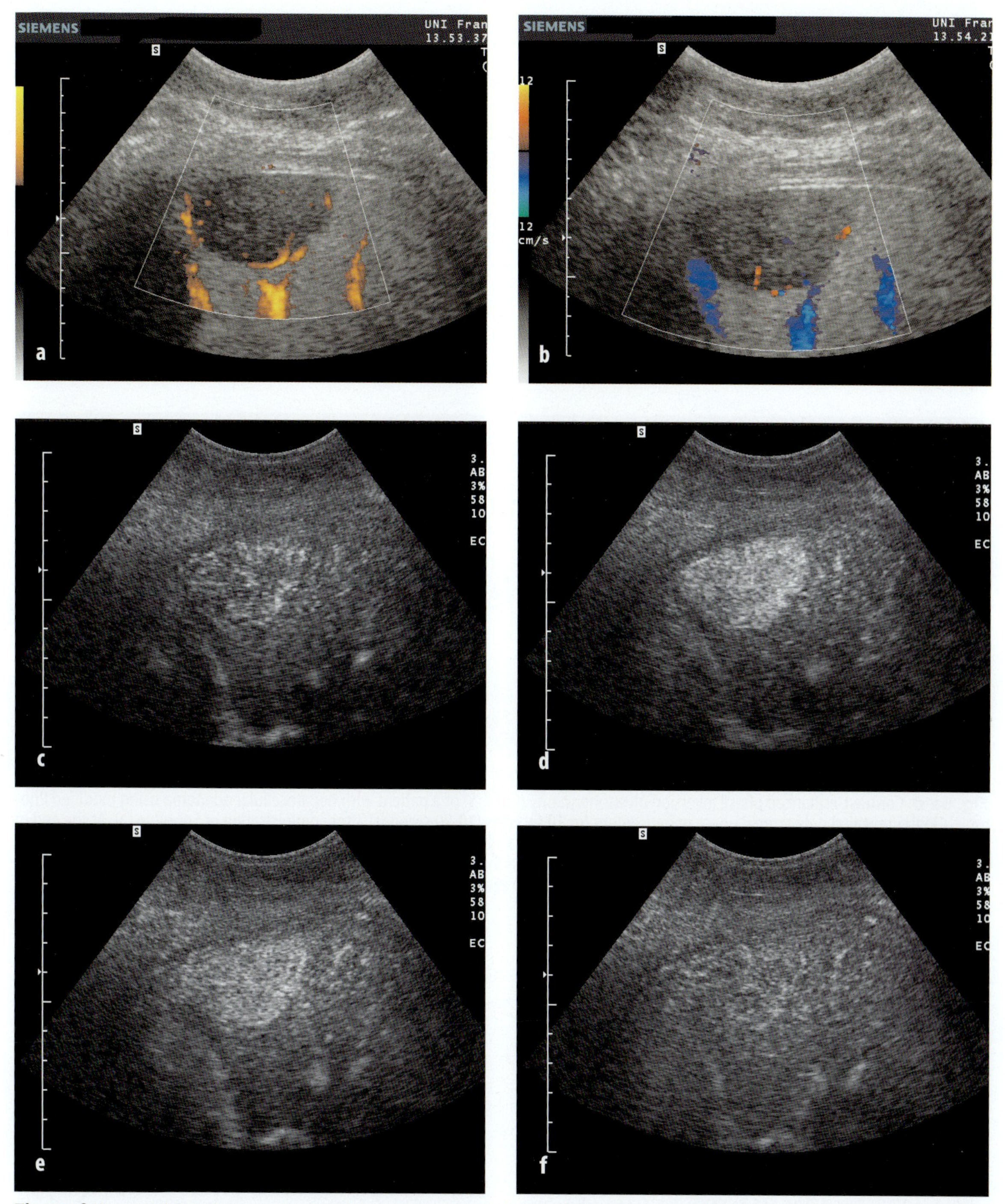

Fig. 5a-f. Hepatocellular adenoma. Hepatocellular adenoma is typically isoechoic to the surrounding liver tissue but might be hypoechoic in fatty liver disease. Power Doppler and colour Doppler imaging demonstrate peripheral vessels (**a, b**). CEUS reveals typical arterial but no portal-venous enhancement (**c-d**, arterial phase; **e**, portal-venous phase)

may differentiate between most benign and malignant liver tumours [13]. It was recently shown that, using contrast-enhanced US techniques, benign liver tumours may also mimic malignancy. Bile duct adenoma (BDA) is a benign liver tumour, typically located subcapsularly and demonstrating lack of a portal-venous phase. Large bile duct adenomas, (also called cholangiocellular adenomas, if larger than 10 mm), lack liver specific tissue. In a recently published abstract all three observed lesions more than 10 mm were hypervascular in the arterial phase. In the portal-venous/sinusoidal phase all lesions were prominently hypovascular, taken as a sign of malignancy [38].

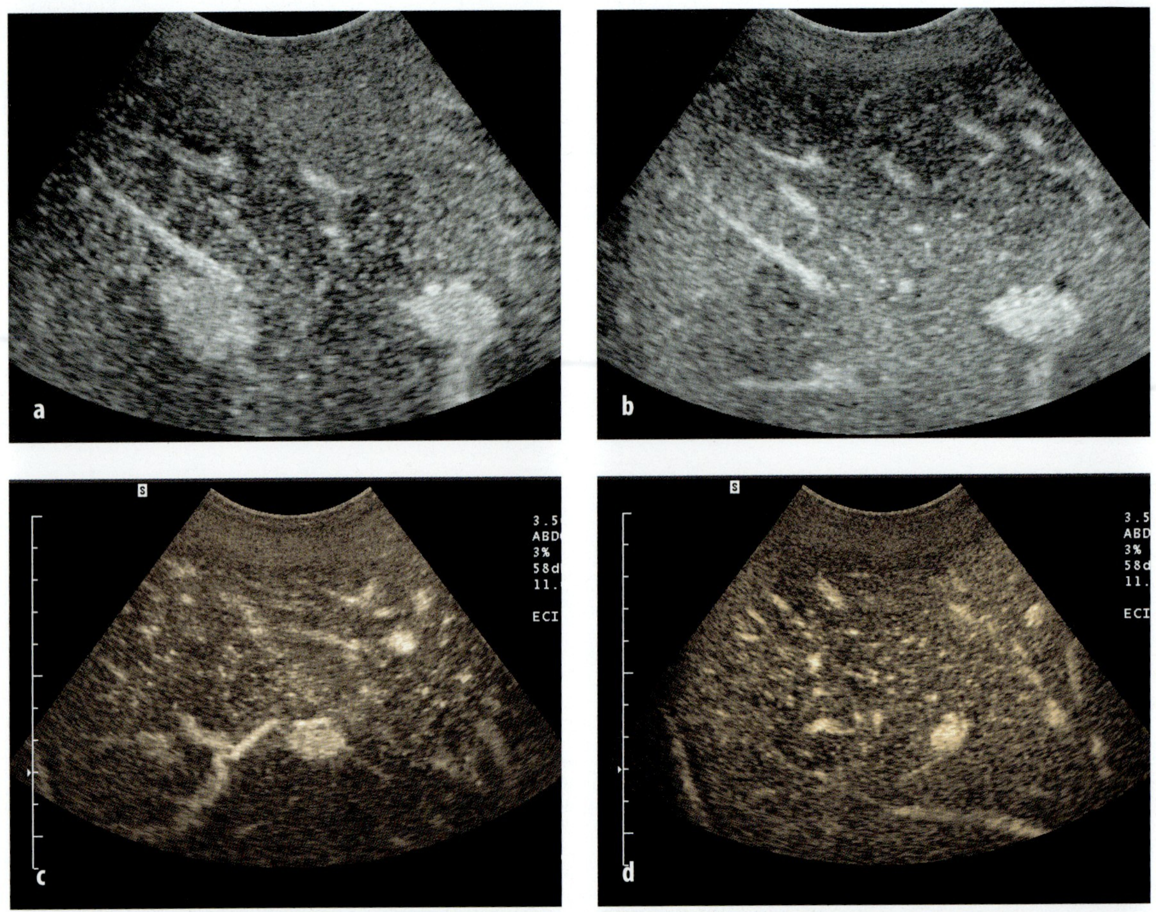

Fig. 6a-d. Contrast-enhanced phase inversion ultrasonography (CEPIUS) of a patient with hepatocellular adenoma using modified Photopic. CEPIUS revealed only arterial phase enhancement for 10 seconds (10-20 seconds) after administration of SonoVue (**a**). At the end of the arterial phase (< 25 seconds after administration of SonoVue), a slightly hypoechoic liver tumour was detected by contrast-enhanced phase inversion ultrasonography and no portal-venous sinusoidal enhancement was observed (**b**). The same patient was examined after stem cell transplantation due to acute leukaemia. Tumour size decreased but enhancement characteristics did not change, as shown in **c** and **d**

Focal Fatty Lesion (Regional Focal Fatty Infiltration)

Fatty infiltration was generally considered to be a diffuse process involving the entire liver. Since Brawer and Scott identified focal hepatic fatty infiltration at autopsy and in imaging studies in 1980, focal hepatic fatty infiltration has been widely discussed [39-41]. Diffuse fatty changes of the liver were recognized on CT examination soon after the introduction of CT technology. Focal fatty changes of the liver were subsequently described as histological and radiological entities soon after. It is well known that diffuse hepatic fatty infiltration may occur in association with many conditions such as alcoholism, diabetes mellitus, obesity, intravenous hyperalimentation, malnutrition, pregnancy, Cushing's syndrome, corticosteroid medication, hepatitis, porphyria, hepatotoxic drugs, congestive heart failure and many others, like Kwashiorkor syndrome, Wilson's disease or intestinal bypass.

Bright focal areas in the liver hilum occur in more than 40% of inflammatory bowel disease patients on corticosteroid medication. In our experience, hyperechoic lesions may be observed 3 weeks after corticosteroid intake (more than 10 mg prednisolone per day), and usually resolve within 3 months of corticosteroid therapy cessation. This phenomenon occurs as frequently in inflammatory bowel disease (IBD) patients and as intensely as in patients with autoimmune disease and longstanding corticosteroid therapy. The histological nature of these corticosteroid-derived lesions is not yet clear. Different amounts or types (large, small vacuoles) of fat deposition are likely, because a change of appearance over time can be observed. Haemangiomas may mimic such lesions, but not all bright lesions in the liver are haemangiomas. In 20 unselected corpses, four showed similar bright echogenic lesions in the liver hilum, but the histology differed remarkably (two with fibrous tissue, one with fatty infiltration and one with haemangioma). It is well known that the vascular supply of the hilar region in liver segment IV differs from the perfusion of liver tissue adjacent to the gallbladder. This could give a possible explanation for different reactions of liver parenchyma to fatty infiltration. Although well-documented, the underlying mechanism is still unknown. Changes in arterio-portal-venous perfusion have been suggested. In patients with focal fatty lesions, we observed centrally located arterial blood supply and direct venous drainage from and into the liver hilum; in contrast, portal-venous perfusion varies [39-41].

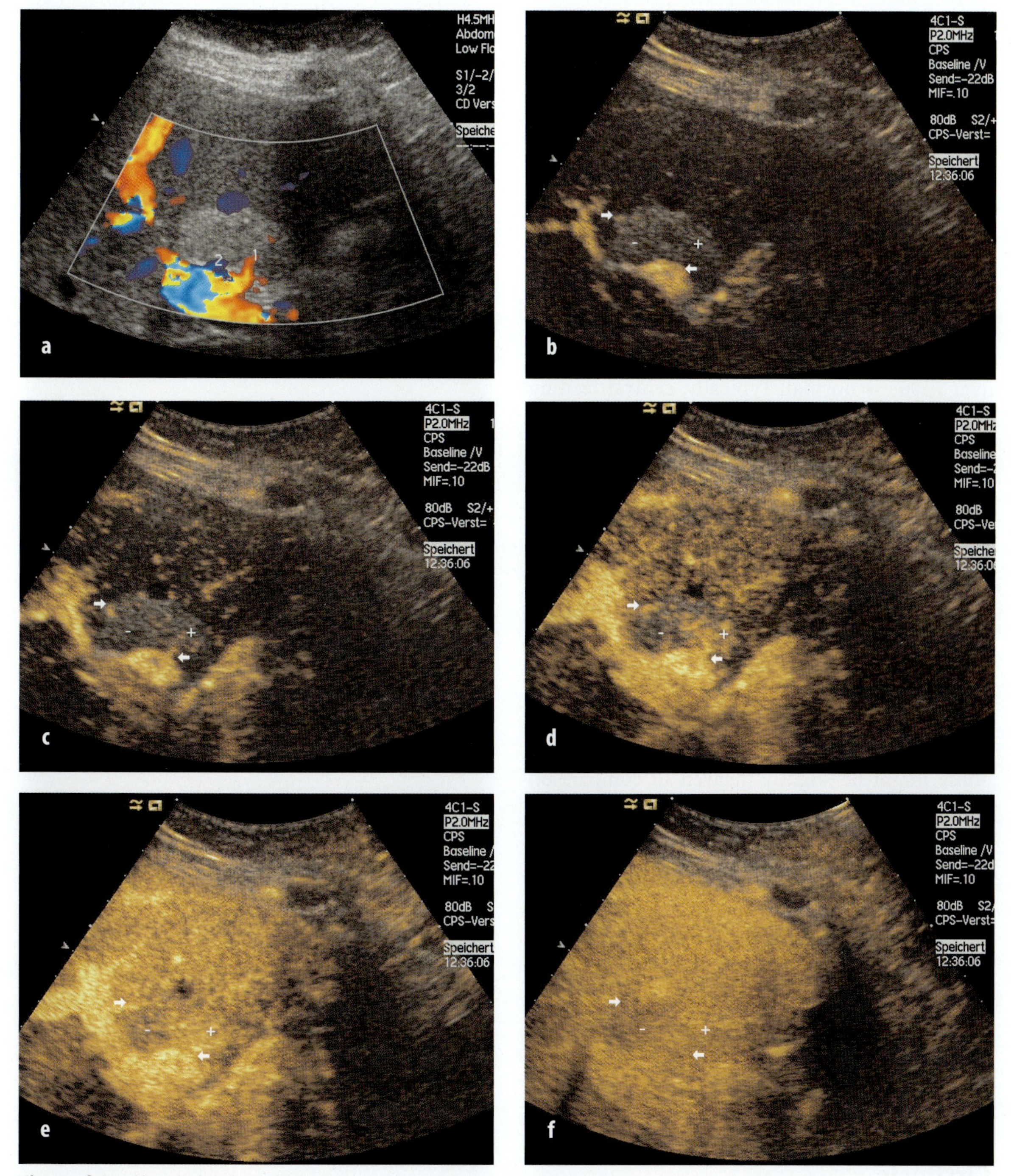

Fig. 7a-f. *Focal hyperechoic lesion in the quadrate lobe adjacent to liver hilum, which was found to be fatty infiltration.* Using conventional colour Doppler ultrasound, arterial and venous draining vessels are visualised (**a**). The contrast-enhancement pattern is also displayed. Notice a hypoenhancing hypoechoic part of the lesion ('-') vessel supplied via the liver parenchyma (left upper part) and an arterial hyperenhancing hyperechoic part, vessel supplied via the liver hilus (right lower part of the images) (**b-f**)

Conventional B-mode US

Fatty infiltration may affect the liver diffusely or focally, but it does not usually cause any mass effect or displace vessels. Sonographically, hepatic fatty infiltration appears as segmental or lobular areas of brighter echogenicity, in contrast to the echogenicity of the normal liver parenchyma. A central, peri-hilar location in segment IV or V is typical; other locations are rarely involved.

An oval-shaped hypoechoic lesion in the liver hilum is always related to fatty liver and could represent normal liver tissue surrounded by diffuse fatty infiltration of the liver. A hypoechoic lesion in the liver hilum without signs of expansion seems to be a relevant sign of fatty liver and should not be confused with mass lesions. The typical relationship to fatty liver, the typical location and shape are helpful in differential diagnosis.

Colour Doppler Imaging

In colour Doppler US, both focal fatty degeneration and its absence appear normal; neither hyper- nor hypoperfusion is apparent, since the liver tissue is normal. Typically, central feeding and draining vessels may be detected in a high percentage of patients, demonstrating the pathogenetic mechanism of different vascularisation of the liver hilum.

Contrast-Enhanced US

In the arterial and venous phase, the supplying and draining vessels of the liver hilum can be imaged. In the enhanced echo signal sequence, different fatty degeneration regions are imaged like normal liver tissue in the capillary and portal-venous phase. Therefore, in the portal-venous phase these lesions are indistinguishable from background. Enhancement in the arterial phase might be slightly delayed in comparison with the surrounding liver parenchyma (Fig. 7).

Role of Contrast-Enhanced US in Clinical Practice

Focal fatty changes in the liver may simulate mass lesions, thus focal hepatic lesions might be mistaken for hepatic neoplasm at US. This is important to know when it comes to a differential diagnosis, especially in patients with underlying malignant disease. Contrast-enhanced US is helpful to rule out malignant infiltration.

Benign Liver Lesions in Liver Cirrhosis

Benign liver lesions in liver cirrhosis have the same occurrence rate as in patients without parenchymal liver disease, with the exception of FNH, which is difficult to prove in liver cirrhosis. Recently, 100 consecutive patients (80 male, 20 female, 62 ± 12 (31-90) years) with histologically proven hepatocellular carcinoma at time of diagnosis were investigated. Sonographic evaluation of the entire liver was possible in 88% of cases. In 25 patients (25%), additional focal lesions were found (8 hepatocellular adenoma, 8 atypical haemangioma, 5 regenerative nodules, 4 cysts larger than 10 mm). Apart from cysts, all additional liver tumours were histologically proven and without severe complications (e.g., haemorrhage, severe pain, or perforation). Cirrhosis of the liver was confirmed in 91 of 100 patients (91%), while 9 patients (9%) had no cirrhosis. Patients characteristics are summarized in Table 8. Therefore, biopsy and histology is crucial before extended liver surgery [23]. The problem of hypovascular hepatocellular carcinoma has been recently addressed [42].

Table 8. Patientscharacteristics of 100 patients with histologically proven hepatocellular carcinoma [13]

Characteristics	n
Aetiology or associated illness	
Viral hepatitis B/C	52
Alcohol consumption	25
Autoimmune hepatitis	2
Primary biliary cirrhosis	1
Primary sclerosing cholangitis	1
Hemochromatosis	7
Glycogenosis v. Gierke	1
Unknown origin	10
Liver cirrhosis	
Histologically proven	91
Child-Pugh Score A	44
Child-Pugh Score B	36
Child-Pugh Score C	11
Histologically unproven (excluded)	9
Patients with additional liver tumour	*25*
Adenoma	8
Hemangioma	8
Regenerative nodules	5
Cysts larger than 10 mm	4
Alpha-fetoprotein	
< 15 ng/ml	31
> 15 ng/ml	69

n = number of patients

3D Contrast-Enhanced US

Recent advances in computer technology have supported the development of new systems with motion detection methods and image registration algorithms making it possible to acquire 3D data without position sensors, before and after administration of contrast-enhancing agents. The so-called *freehand 3D method* is a multistep procedure (data acquisition, correlation algorithms with segmentation, and quantification) based on correlation algorithms, including the display of the 3D image without position sensors. As a basic requirement for correct 3D data acquisition, the transducer must be moved at a constant speed. The examination technique with 3D acquisition before and after iv injection of SonoVue was possible in almost all patients. Ensemble contrast imaging with low mechanical index revealed excellent enhancement of the arterial, portal-venous and venous vessels of the liver in all patients with liver tumours. The enhancement was strongest and homogeneous at a band of approximately 8 cm around the level of the focal zone and the enhancement of the liver parenchyma persisted for between five and ten minutes under continuous scanning conditions.

The method is limited by motion artifacts due to both the operator and the patient under examination. When sampling moving organs and structures (e.g., heart, peristaltic bowel, breathing), the reconstructed 3D image can lack detail. As with all new methods, a certain training factor has to be taken into account, since a steady and targeted transducer manipulation is the prerequisite for optimal image documentation in a 3D procedure [43, 44].

Role of 3D Contrast-Enhanced US in Clinical Practice

The hypothetical advantages and disadvantages of 3D US technology include clearer visualisation of anatomy and topography, visualisation of the extension of changes into surrounding tissue with special emphasis on the reconstructed coronary plane, measurement of volumes (also non-symmetrical) or pathologic changes, improved diagnoses (quality of results) through analysis of the third plane, higher quality of results through imaging the surrounding structures with landmarks (quality management), improved examination quality through planning and performing an optimised image acquisition and image documentation, improved acceptance by the referring physician through clearer visualisation and therefore fewer follow-up examinations, and demonstration of findings with reference to any desired scan plane (e.g., as part of the daily findings discussion).

Rare Entities

In many other focal liver lesions, contrast-enhanced US is helpful for characterisation and diagnosis, e.g., abscesses, hematoma, hamartoma, angioma of the liver [45], nodular regenerative hyperplasia [46], bile duct adenoma (cholangiocellular adenoma), echinococcosis, granuloma, tuberculosis, sarcoidosis, sickle cell anaemia with liver infarct, bartonellosis [47], pseudoaneurysm of hepatic arteries [48], nodules in Wilson's disease, Peliosis, inflammatory pseudotumour of the liver [14], cholangiofibroma and other entities, which have been recently published [44].

Abscess

The patient's medical history and physical examination (febrile temperature, signs of sepsis) are most helpful in differentiation from necrotic metastases.

Conventional B-mode US

Phlegmonous inflammation and abscesses demonstrate variable and sometimes confusing B-mode images that change over time. The initial phlegmonous inflammation is often isoechogenic in comparison to the surrounding liver parenchyma and is sometimes difficult to recognise. In older (chronic) abscesses, hypervascularity of the nodule border might be confused with pseudotumour of the liver, even histologically. Small disseminate candida abscesses might be confused with lymphoma or circumscribed hemophagocytosis (especially in the young). Puncture and drainage (if necessary) are the diagnostic and therapeutic implications. Abscesses up to 5 cm might be drained in one procedure, whereas larger abscesses need to be treated over days.

Colour Doppler Imaging

The initial phlegmonous inflammation is often hypervascular in comparison to the surrounding liver parenchyma, but is difficult to recognize. Hypervascularitiy of the nodule border is typical in older (chronic) abscesses.

Contrast-Enhanced US

In typical cases, CEUS shows sharply delineated hypervascularity demonstrating the pseudocapsule and no gas bubbles inside the lesion (Fig. 8).

Role of Contrast-Enhanced US in Clinical Practice

The role of CEUS in clinical practice has not yet been determined. CEUS was helpful in clinically uncertain cases with similar results as those

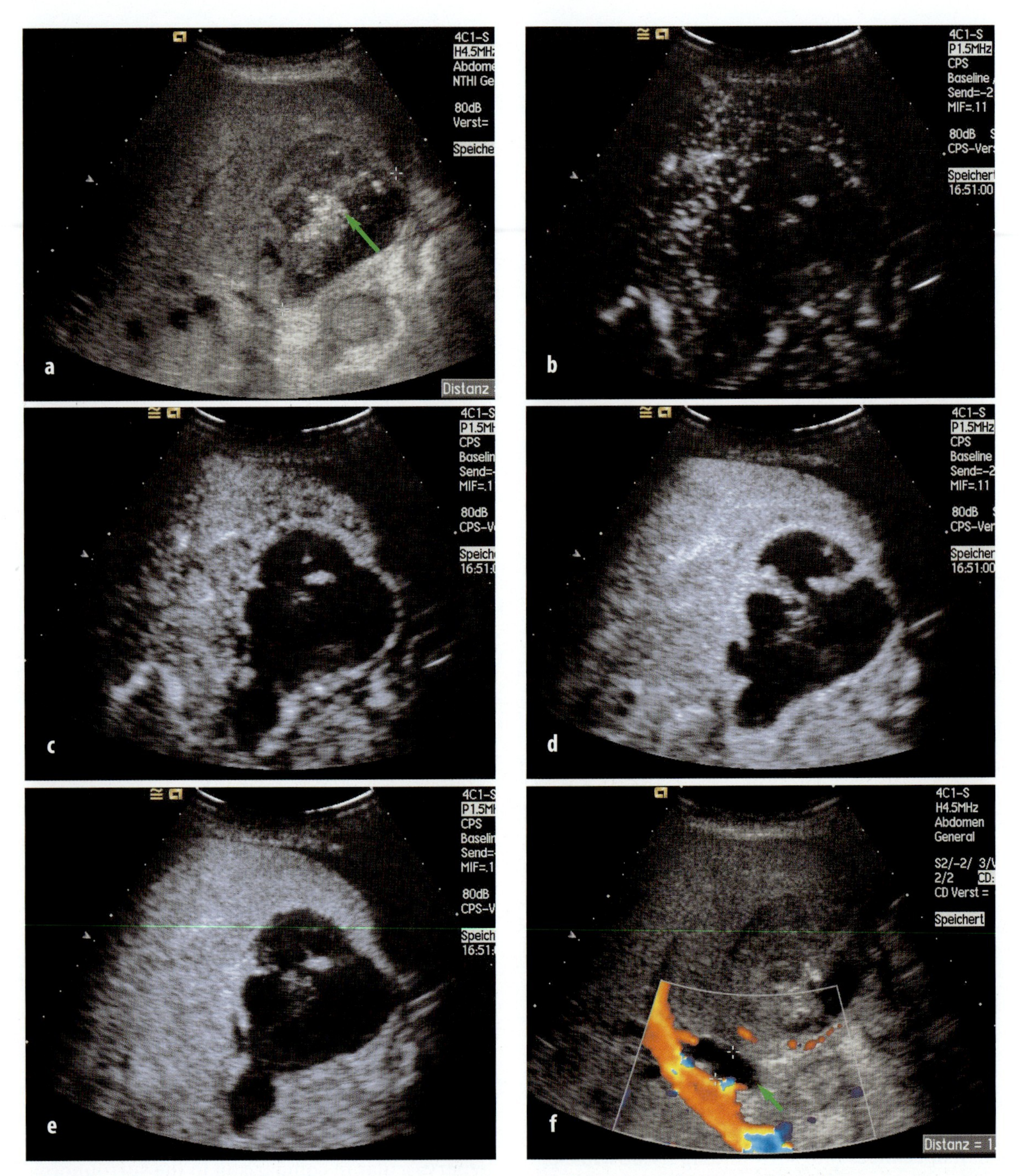

Fig. 8a-f. Liver abscess. Typical liver abscesses demonstrating air inside the lesion (**a**, *arrow*). Using SonoVue, enhanced US abscesses reveal no signal enhancement at all depending on the stage of abscess but reveal hyperperfusion at the abscess border (**b–e**). The cause (choledocholithiasis) is also marked (**f**, *arrow*)

shown for CT. Until now there are no large studies using this technique.

Haematoma

Haematoma can be clinically diagnosed in most cases. Spontanously evolving and painful haematoma is typical of amyloidosis of the liver.

Conventional B-mode US

B-mode image depends on the stage of haematoma. The very early haematoma is hyperechoic, while later stages are iso- or mostly hypoechoic. Change in morphology is therefore typical for haematoma.

Colour Doppler Imaging

Colour Doppler imaging demonstrates no flow pattern.

Contrast-Enhanced US

CEUS is helpful in defining circumscribed versus diffuse infiltrating haematoma.

Role of Contrast-Enhanced US in Clinical Practice

The role of CEUS in the diagnosis of haematoma in clinical practice has not yet been determined. CEUS might be helpful in clinically uncertain cases with similar results as those shown for CT.

Nodular Regenerative Hyperplasia (NRH)

Nodular regenerative hyperplasia of the liver (NRH) is a rare pathological finding, typically associated with haematological or autoimmune disease. The main clinical symptom is portal hypertension without underlying liver cirrhosis. A retrospective study of 2500 autopsies showed a prevalence of 2.6% for NRH. Furthermore, in 10.2% of those autopsy cases, variable degrees of nodular transformation were found. NRH itself consists of multiple hepatic nodules resulting from peri-portal hepatocyte regeneration with surrounding atrophy. Typically, fibrous septa between the nodules are missing. The pathogenesis remains unknown, although some authors suggested that NRH may be a secondary and nonspecific tissue adaptation to heterogeneous perfusion. Histological assessment of the liver is necessary for diagnosis, because the nodular appearance of the hepatic surface may otherwise be difficult to differentiate from cirrhosis or hepatic metastases. The prognosis of NRH depends on the development and severity of portal hypertension, which often requires only pharmacological treatment. Development of NRH without any underlying disease is typically characterised by liver failure and a poor clinical outcome.

Conventional B-mode US

Ultrasonography typically shows multiple (unspecific) hepatic nodules, which are suggestive of multilocular hepatocellular carcinoma or metastatic disease of the liver.

Colour Doppler Imaging

Signs of portal hypertension and the more rare Budd-Chiari syndrome should be carefully sought.

Contrast-Enhanced US

CEUS is helpful in defining circumscribed versus diffuse infiltrating nodular regenerative hyperplasia.

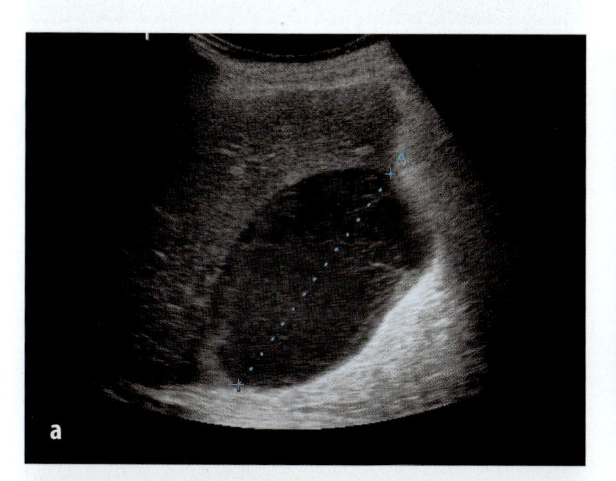

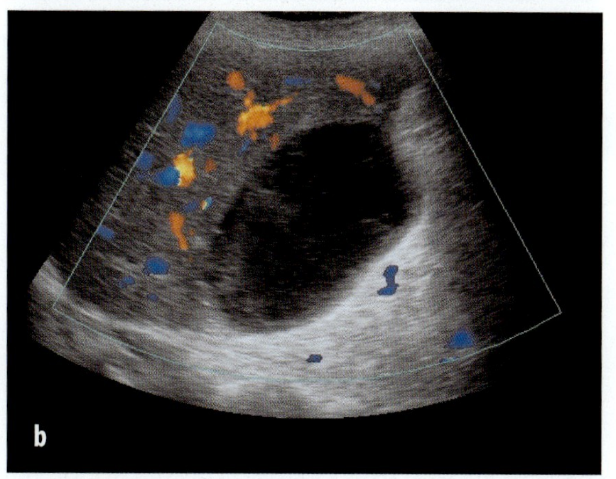

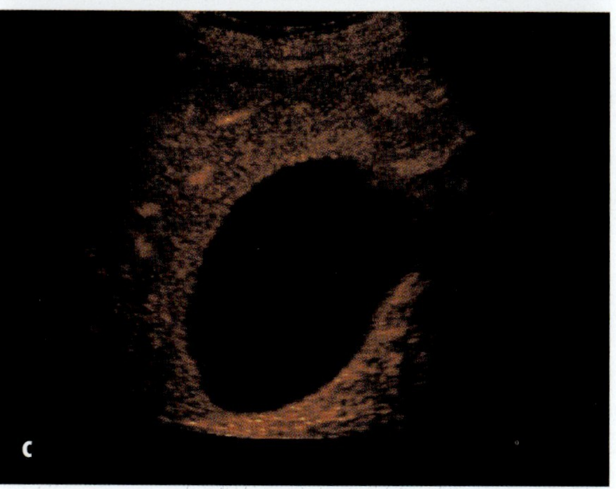

Fig. 9a-d. Haematoma, demonstrating no flow characteristics using B-mode (**a**), colour Doppler imaging (**b**) and CEUS (**c**)

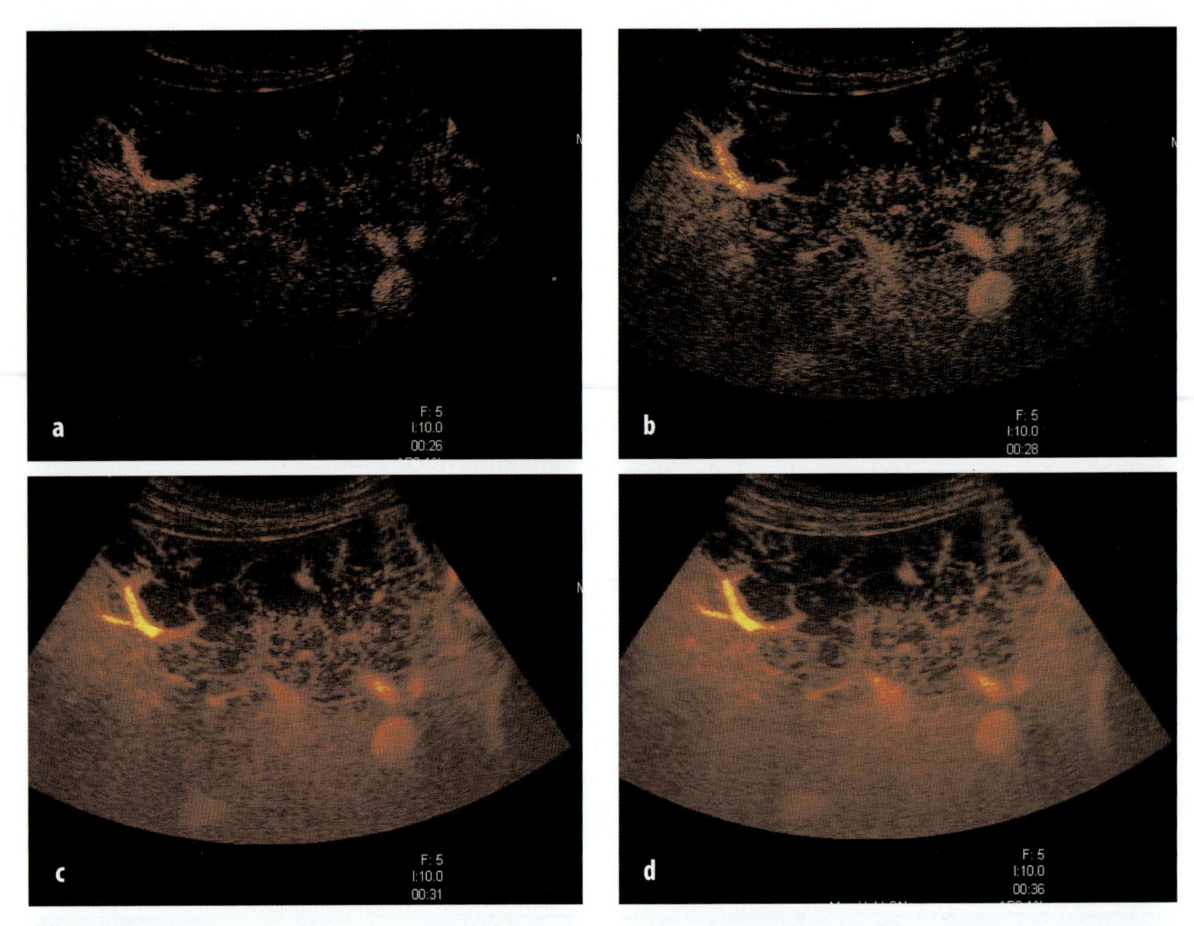

Fig. 10a-d. Liver infarct in a patient with hepatocellular carcinoma after transarterial chemoembolisation using microflow technique

Role of Contrast-Enhanced US in Clinical Practice

The role of CEUS in clinical practice has not yet been determined in patients with NRH. It was shown that CEUS-guided puncture is helpful in identifying the right puncture site.

Key Points

- Benign liver tumours are more frequent than generally assumed. This is also true in patients with liver cirrhosis (prevalence of more than 5%).
- In patients without diffuse parenchymal disease, the differentiation of benign and malignant liver lesions up to 50 mm and, therefore, typical behaviour without regressive changes, is possible in more than 95% of patients using CEUS analysing the portal-venous/sinusoidal phase.
- The contrast pattern of typical FNH is characterised by arterial and portal-venous enhancement.
- The contrast pattern of adenomas less than 50 mm in size is characterised by a homogenous arterial, but a lack of portal-venous enhancement.
- The contrast pattern of haemangioma is characterised by peripheral nodular contrast-enhancement and centripetal fill in non-thrombosed tumours.

References

1. Linhart P, Bonhof JA, Baque PE, Pering C (1998) [Ultrasound in diagnosis of benign and malignant liver tumors.] Zentralbl Chir 123:119-123
2. Albrecht T, Blomley M, Bolondi L et al (2004) Guidelines for the use of contrast agents in ultrasound. Ultraschall Med 25:249-256
3. Leen E (2001) The role of contrast-enhanced ultrasound in the characterisation of focal liver lesions. Eur Radiol 11:E27-E34
4. Dietrich CF, Kratzer W, Strobel D et al (2006) Assessment of metastatic liver disease in patients with primary extrahepatic tumours by contrast-enhanced sonography versus CT and MRI. WJG, (in press)
5. Dietrich CF (2004) Characterisation of focal liver lesions with contrast-enhanced ultrasonography. Eur J Radiol 51:S9-17
6. Schuessler G, Ignee A, Hirche T, Dietrich CF (2003) [Improved detection and characterisation of liver tumors with echo-enhanced ultrasound.] Z Gastroenterol 41:1167-1176
7. Dietrich DF, Becker D (2002) Signalverstärkte Lebersonographie zur verbesserten Detektion und Charakterisierung von Leberraumforderungen. Dt Aerzteblatt 24:1666-1672

7a. Schener PJ, Lefkowitch JH (2000) Liver Biopsy Interpretation, 6th edn. WB Saunders, p 191

8. Strunk H, Borner N, Stuckmann G et al. (2005) [Contrast-enhanced "Low MI Real-Time" phase-inversion sonography to differentiate between malignant and benign focal liver lesions.] Rofo 177:1394-1404
9. von Herbay A, Vogt C, Willers R, Haussinger D (2004) Real-time imaging with the sonographic contrast agent SonoVue: differentiation between benign and malignant hepatic lesions. J Ultrasound Med 23:1557-1568
10. von Herbay A, Vogt C, Haussinger D (2004) Differentiation between benign and malignant hepatic lesions: utility of color stimulated acoustic emission with the microbubble contrast agent Levovist. J Ultrasound Med 23:207-215
11. von Herbay A, Vogt C, Haussinger D (2002) Pulse inversion sonography in the early phase of the sonographic contrast agent Levovist: differentiation between benign and malignant focal liver lesions. J Ultrasound Med 21:1191-1200
12. von Herbay A, Vogt C, Haussinger D (2002) Late-phase pulse-inversion sonography using the contrast agent Levovist: differentiation between benign and malignant focal lesions of the liver. AJR Am J Roentgenol 179:1273-1279
13. Dietrich CF, Ignee A, Trojan J et al (2004) Improved characterisation of histologically proven liver tumours by contrast-enhanced ultrasonography during the portal-venous and specific late phase of SHU 508A. Gut 53:401-405
14. Schuessler G, Fellbaum C, Fauth F et al (2005) Der inflammatorische Pseudotumor - eine schwierige Differzialdignose. Ultraschall Med in press
15. Albrecht T, Blomley MJ (2001) Characteristics of hepatic hemangiomas at contrast-enhanced harmonic US. Radiology 220:269-270
16. Bartolotta TV, Midiri M, Quaia E et al (2005) Liver haemangiomas undetermined at grey-scale ultrasound: contrast-enhancement patterns with SonoVue and pulse-inversion US. Eur Radiol 15(4):685-693
17. Brannigan M, Burns PN, Wilson SR (2004) Blood flow patterns in focal liver lesions at microbubble-enhanced US. Radiographics 24:921-935
18. Bryant TH, Blomley MJ, Albrecht T et al (2004) Improved characterization of liver lesions with liver-phase uptake of liver-specific microbubbles: prospective multicenter study. Radiology 232:799-809
19. Burns PN, Wilson SR, Simpson DH (2000) Pulse inversion imaging of liver blood flow: improved method for characterizing focal masses with microbubble contrast. Invest Radiol 35:58-71
20. Dill-Macky MJ, Burns PN, Khalili K, Wilson SR (2002) Focal hepatic masses: enhancement patterns with SH U 508A and pulse-inversion US. Radiology 222:95-102
21. Harvey CJ, Albrecht T (2001) Ultrasound of focal liver lesions. Eur Radiol 11:1578-1593
22. Hohmann J, Skrok J, Puls R, Albrecht T (2003) [Characterization of focal liver lesions with contrast-enhanced low MI real time ultrasound and SonoVue.] Rofo 175:835-843
23. Ignee A, Weiper D, Schuessler G et al (2005) Sonographic characterisation of hepatocellular carcinoma at time of diagnosis. Z Gastroenterol 43:289-294
24. Quaia E, Stacul F, Gaiani S et al (2004) Comparison of diagnostic performance of unenhanced vs SonoVue - enhanced ultrasonography in focal liver lesions characterization. The experience of three Italian centers. Radiol Med 108:71-81
25. Strobel D, Raeker S, Martus P et al (2003) Phase inversion harmonic imaging versus contrast-enhanced power Doppler sonography for the characterization of focal liver lesions. Int J Colorectal Dis 18:63-72
26. Strobel D, Hoefer A, Martus P et al (2001) Dynamic contrast-enhanced power Doppler sonography improves the differential diagnosis of liver lesions. Int J Colorectal Dis 16:247-256
27. Strobel D, Krodel U, Martus P et al (2000) Clinical evaluation of contrast-enhanced color Doppler sonography in the differential diagnosis of liver tumors. J Clin Ultrasound 28:1-13
28. Tranquart F, Bleuzen A, Kissel A (2004) [Value of combined conventional and contrast-enhanced sonography in the evaluation of hepatic disorders.] J Radiol 85:755-762
29. Wanless IR, Mawdsley C, Adams R (1985) On the pathogenesis of focal nodular hyperplasia of the liver. Hepatology 5:1194-1200
30. Wilson SR, Burns PN (2001) Liver mass evaluation with ultrasound: the impact of microbubble contrast agents and pulse inversion imaging. Semin Liver Dis 21:147-159
31. Wilson SR, Burns PN, Muradali D et al (2000) Harmonic hepatic US with microbubble contrast agent: initial experience showing improved characterization of hemangioma, hepatocellular carcinoma, and metastasis. Radiology 215:153-161
32. Fukukura Y, Nakashima O, Kusaba A et al (1998)

Angioarchitecture and blood circulation in focal nodular hyperplasia of the liver. J Hepatol 29:470-475
33. Kondo F, Nagao T, Sato T et al (1998) Etiological analysis of focal nodular hyperplasia of the liver, with emphasis on similar abnormal vasculatures to nodular regenerative hyperplasia and idiopathic portal hypertension. Pathol Res Pract 194:487-495
34. Nguyen BN, Flejou JF, Terris B et al (1999) Focal nodular hyperplasia of the liver: a comprehensive pathologic study of 305 lesions and recognition of new histologic forms. Am J Surg Pathol 23:1441-1454
35. Scoazec JY, Flejou JF, d'Errico A et al (1995) Focal nodular hyperplasia of the liver: composition of the extracellular matrix and expression of cell-cell and cell-matrix adhesion molecules. Hum Pathol 26:1114-1125
36. Dietrich CF, Schuessler G, Trojan J et al (2005) Differentiation of focal nodular hyperplasia and hepatocellular adenoma by contrast-enhanced ultrasound. Br J Radiol 78:704-707
36a. Dietrich CF (2005) Tumour characterization using Micro Flow Imaging. Toshiba Vision 7
37. Gossmann J, Scheuermann EH, Frilling A et al (2001) Multiple adenomas and hepatocellular carcinoma in a renal transplant patient with glycogen storage disease type 1a (von Gierke disease). Transplantation 72:343-344
38. Ignee A, Schuessler G, Schlottmann K et al (2005) Benign liver tumors mimicking malignancy using contrast-enhanced ultrasound. Ultraschall Med 26
39. Dietrich CF, Wehrmann T, Zeuzem S et al (1999) [Analysis of hepatic echo patterns in chronic hepatitis C.] Ultraschall Med 20:9-14
40. Dietrich CF, Schall H, Kirchner J et al (1997) Sonographic detection of focal changes in the liver hilus in patients receiving corticosteroid therapy. Z Gastroenterol 35:1051-1057
41. Dietrich CF, Lee JH, Gottschalk R et al (1998) Hepatic and portal vein flow pattern in correlation with intrahepatic fat deposition and liver histology in patients with chronic hepatitis C. AJR Am J Roentgenol 171:437-443
42. Bolondi L, Gaiani S, Celli N et al (2005) Characterization of small nodules in cirrhosis by assessment of vascularity: the problem of hypovascular hepatocellular carcinoma. Hepatology 42:27-34
43. Dietrich CF (2002) [3D real time contrast-enhanced ultrasonography,a new technique.] Rofo 174:160-163
44. Dietrich CF, Ignee A, Frey H (2005) contrast-enhanced endoscopic ultrasound with low mechanical index, a new technique. Z Gastroenterol 43:1219-1223
45. Rickes S, Wermke T, Ocran K et al (2002) [Contrast behaviour of a angiomyolipoma of the liver at echo-enhanced power-Doppler sonography.] Ultraschall Med 23:338-340
46. Faust D, Fellbaum C, Zeuzem S, Dietrich CF (2003) Nodular regenerative hyperplasia of the liver: a rare differential diagnosis of cholestasis with response to ursodeoxycholic acid. Z Gastroenterol 41:255-258
47. Braden B, Helm B, Fabian T, Dietrich CF (2000) [Bacillary angiomatosis of the liver, a suspected ultrasound diagnosis?] Z Gastroenterol 38:785-789
48. Braden B, Thalhammer A, Schwarz W, Dietrich CF (2002) Bleeding complications from hepatic mucoidal aneurysmata: value of color duplex sonography after liver transplantation. Liver Transpl 8:636-638

II.2

Characterisation of Hepatocellular Carcinoma in Cirrhosis

Carlos Nicolau and Concepcio Bru

Introduction

Hepatocellular carcinoma (HCC) is the most common primary malignancy of the liver, and the fifth most common solid tumour in the world [1]. In Sub-Saharan areas and south-east Asia, the prevalence of HCC is high, while in Mediterranean areas it is medium, and in northern Europe and North America it is considered to be low. However, the incidence of HCC is increasing in economically developed areas, including Europe and the United States, probably related to the spread of the hepatitis C virus. Most HCC occur in the setting of cirrhosis, being especially attributed to hepatitis C and B. Other factors such as alcohol, aflatoxin, and other chronic liver diseases, such as primary biliary cirrhosis, are responsible for a low percentage of patients with HCC. Finally, in less than 5% of the HCC patients, the underlying liver is normal.

Clinically, HCC mimics the symptoms of the underlying liver disease, being difficult to diagnose on a clinical basis. When the tumour progresses, complications such as infiltration of biliary structures, tumoural thrombosis of the portal vein, and bone and/or lung metastases may be presented. In these cases, jaundice, enlarged liver, refractory ascites, non-bacterial diarrhoea, abdominal pain or pain related to bone metastases, and paraneoplasic neurologic symptoms may suggest the presence of HCC in a patient with cirrhosis. Unfortunately, when clinical manifestations of HCC are present, none of the existing therapies are usually effective to cure or to stop the progression of the disease.

Early detection of HCC is critical to achieve effective treatment and prolong survival [2, 3], thus, several protocols including imaging modalities have been described to identify small HCCs. Imaging screening of patients with cirrhosis may be performed with ultrasound (US), computed tomography (CT) or magnetic resonance imaging (MRI), but US is recommended for surveillance, due to its greater acceptance by patients, low cost, lack of irradiation and high level of detection. In Europe, patients with chronic liver disease usually take part in a surveillance program that includes US study and alpha-fetoprotein (AFP) determination every six months [4], as recommended by the European Association for the Study of the Liver (EASL). However, there is a lack of evidence regarding the utility of performing a study every four to six months, or every 12 months, for early detection. The trend is to perform US every six months and the determination of AFP or other tumoural markers depends on the protocol of each hospital. AFP has been useful in screening of large populations, because of its high specificity, but its use in early detection is not effective due to its low sensitivity. In fact, the levels of AFP correlate well with tumour volume, and nowadays, it is mainly used to confirm the diagnosis of known focal hepatic lesion with suspicion of HCC, or in the follow-up of patients with previous HCC.

In the surveillance of cirrhotic patients, small focal liver lesions are usually HCCs or cirrhotic macronodules, which include regenerative and dysplastic nodules. However, other lesions such as haemangiomas and cholangiocarcinomas may also appear in less than 5% of cases, and an accurate differential diagnosis is mandatory.

Hepatocarcinogenesis is considered a multistep process characterised by the development of a spectrum of nodules from benign regenerating nodules and dysplastic nodules (DN), to overt malignant HCC. Dysplastic nodules, which may have different grades of differentiation, may be considered premalignant lesions that represent the step prior to the development of HCC.

Morphological differentiation of well-differentiated early-stage HCCs and DNs is often difficult, and the differential diagnosis between the two lesions remains controversial. Thus, many of the early HCCs diagnosed in Japan tend to be interpreted as high-grade DNs in Western countries [5]. During this process of hepatocarcinogenesis, there is a haemodynamic change that is the basis for the understanding of the usefulness of imaging techniques in the diagnosis of HCC. This change consists in an increase in arterial blood supply and a subsequent decrease in portal blood flow, with the detection of this arterial blood supply the key to the diagnosis of HCC. In this progressive pathway, the vascular supply of regenerative nodules is similar to the liver parenchyma [6]. The vascular supply of DNs is more complex compared to surrounding cirrhotic parenchyma. Dysplastic nodules show a degree of capillarisation intermediate to that of regenerative nodules and that of HCC, and high-grade DNs may contain unpaired arteries, which are isolated arteries unaccompanied by bile ducts. In addition, sinusoidal capillarisation or neovascularisation is evident, as well as a loss of capillary properties. The development of HCC is characterised by arterial hypervascularisation. Thus, a reduction of both portal vein and normal hepatic artery branches, with a progressive increase in abnormal hepatic arteries are considered histologic features of malignant transformation [6]. However, it remains unclear which DNs progresses to HCC, since some DNs remain stable and others may even regress completely [7]. Borzio et al. found that the risk of developing HCC is higher in patients with high-grade DN, especially in those cases associated with extranodular large cell dysplasia [7]. In that study, only 31% of the macronodules transformed into HCC, while most stabilised or disappeared. However, on analysing the subgroup of high-grade DNs, 63% transformed into HCC during the follow-up, suggesting that they are the true precursors of HCC. There is no knowledge concerning the factors that may influence this transformation. However, time, and the oncogenic background have been described as the most important factors.

When a focal liver lesion is detected in a screening protocol, histologic analysis has been considered the gold standard for a definite diagnosis of HCC. However, liver biopsy may give false negative results and contraindications, such as the presence of important ascites and coagulopathy, and also have potential complications, such as a risk of bleeding and tumour seeding [8]. Nowadays, it is accepted that the diagnosis of HCC in a patient with liver cirrhosis can be based on clinical, laboratory and imaging techniques with an accuracy of up to 99% [9]. In 2000, a group of experts from the EASL provided a guideline for the diagnosis of HCC [4]. This guideline recommends an US follow-up for new nodules smaller than 1 cm detected by US in the surveillance screening, and the use of needle biopsy for new nodules between 1 and 2 cm. However, if the detected lesion is larger than 2 cm, the diagnosis can be achieved non-invasively if two coincident imaging techniques find the characteristic arterial vascularisation of the HCC, with arterial enhancement and wash-out in the portal phase. If the focal hepatic lesion shows uncharacteristic features on imaging, a fine needle biopsy is recommended, especially if the patient requires transplantation because of suspicion of HCC.

Baseline Ultrasound

Worldwide, US is the imaging technique of choice as a screening test for the diagnosis of HCC in patients with chronic liver disease [10, 11], due to its widespread availability, absence of adverse effects, lack of invasiveness, and cost. The accuracy of US for the detection of HCC in the cirrhotic liver varies widely, ranging from 20.5% to 96% [12], and the sensitivity of US in detecting small HCCs continues to improve due to the advances in US technology, including multi-frequency transducers and harmonic imaging. In this latter technique, the US beamformer transmits at fundamental frequency and receives at least twice that frequency. The returning harmonic echo is lower in signal intensity, but the signal is higher in contrast resolution and contains fewer artefacts, resulting in superior image quality over fundamental imaging [13]. Thus, harmonic imaging increases the lesion conspicuity, allowing a higher detection of nodules, as was described in a study performed in cirrhotic patients [14]. In screening programs, the detection of a small focal lesion in the context of liver cirrhosis is HCC in more than 50% of the cases and the other frequently found lesions are cirrhotic macronodules, which include regenerative and dysplastic nodules. However, HCC may present a variable appearance on baseline US, reflecting the variable pathologic characteristics of this tumour, and there is an overlap in the US features of HCC and other hepatic lesions. In addition, cirrhotic livers have alterations in echogenicity or echostructure due to the presence of structural changes such as steatosis or fibrosis, making definite diagnosis more difficult. The US imaging of a HCC is related to its own evolution and probably to the homogeneity of the tumour (steatoses, necrosis or fibrosis may alter the image). One of the most frequent shapes of HCC on conventional US is a sharply demarcated hypoechogenic lesion with a smooth boundary. However, HCC can show an irregular or blurred margin that indicates the presence of extranodular growth or a poorly demarcated nodular type. Most small HCCs are more frequently hypoechoic [15, 16]. In a recent study, Kim et al. [16] described the US patterns of 42 small HCCs (less than 2 cm), and found that 66% were hypoechoic, 5% isoechoic, 14% hyperechoic and 14% mixed echoic. The increase in echogenicity detected in some small HCC has mainly been related to the presence of fatty changes [17]. When they grow, most hypoechoic HCCs tend to be isoechoic and then heterogeneous in a pattern that has been described as a mosaic pattern [15]. This mosaic pattern is characterised by the presence of some areas of different echogenicity that have been related to the degree of differentiation and to the presence of fatty transformation, and on occasion, this pattern has a nodule-in-nodule appearance [18]. This fact is most often seen in cases of HCC with fatty change, with a hyperechoic appearance by US showing a distinct hypoechoic nodule inside.

In clinical practice, HCC cannot be reliably distinguished based on US findings and every new solid lesion found in a cirrhotic setting should be considered as a potential HCC unless a different diagnosis can be proved. After the detection of a nodule on US screening, a reasonable protocol would be to perform a US follow-up every three months if the nodule is smaller than 1 cm, and await changes in its size. On the contrary, if the nodule is larger than 1 cm, a biopsy or other imaging techniques are recommended in order to detect arterial hypervascularisation. US Doppler modalities increase the accuracy of US for the characterisation of HCCs because they allow the detection of increased arterial flow, but the value of Doppler US is dependent on tumour size, with a low sensitivity in small HCC. Color Doppler and power Doppler give qualitative information of the flow, whereas pulsed Doppler can obtain a quantitative evaluation. Moreover, Duplex scanning provides the possibility of simultaneously recording a B-mode image with a pulsed signal, and triplex scanning adds colour or power Doppler to the former possibilities. With colour or power Doppler, intratumoural color signals reflecting arterial hypervascularisation are detected, but Doppler US has the advantage of detecting the characteristic arterial flow that differentiates HCC from benign lesions, such as regenerating nodules that only have portal vascularisation. With the advancement of Doppler techniques associated with US imaging, different groups have attempted to identify the hypervascularisation of HCC. Abnormal arterial structures inside the nodules were detected with pulsed Doppler, but the sensitivity of 85% was limited to tumours exceeding 3 cm in size. With the introduction of colour and power Doppler, the sensitivity increased [19] and abnormal flow was detected in lesions smaller than 2 cm. However, the good results obtained in the study were only related to tumours located at less than 10 cm in depth. Results obtained in studies on the usefulness of Doppler US in the detection of arterial blood supply to HCC showed a detection rate of around 80% [19-20]. In a recent study, Kumada et al. [21] detected Doppler US signals in 37 out of 45 HCCs (82.2%) with a lower detection of the intratumoural flow signals in HCCs smaller than 15 mm. In this study, the authors also found that the types of blood flow supply detected by Doppler US correlated with the degree of HCC differentiation. Moderately and poorly differentiated HCCs had afferent pulsatile flow without continuous afferent flow, while well-differentiated HCCs had continuous afferent flow. Intratumoural vessels with a high resistive index and high pulsatility index have been reported to be predictive of malignancy [22]. In addition, some studies have evaluated different parameters of the Doppler register, such as the maximum velocity and the pulsatility index in order to differentiate between benign and malignant hypervascular nodules [23, 24]. In the study by Fracanzani et al. [24], the mean peak resistive index and pulsatility index were significantly lower in DN than in HCC. However, technical difficulties are present with the use of all Doppler techniques, mainly when evaluating the left lobe, especially in the proximity of the heart, and when evaluating the deepest part of the liver [21].

Contrast Ultrasound Features

Advances in US technology and the development of a new generation of contrast agents have improved the clinical applications of US. Nowadays, contrast-enhanced US (CEUS) provides high quality and detailed vascular information in real-time, and it can be used for the detection and characterisation of the vascularity of nodules detected in cirrhotic patients, with a very good sensitivity to detect weak flow in small vessels. One of the most important technical developments is the capacity to obtain harmonic imaging, that suppresses the fundamental linear echoes from the tissue, whereas the non-linear echoes reflected from the microbubbles remain, producing the US signal. Moreover, manufacturers of US equipment are attempting to solve some limitations of the technique, such as the severe suppression of background grey-scale signal, inferior image resolution, lower frame rate and microbubble destruction. New techniques use a low mechanical index, allowing real-time evaluation of the contrast agent enhancement. Recently developed technology, such as CPS from Acuson, also processes the fundamental non-linear signals generated by US contrast agents that are stronger than the harmonic signal, thereby increasing the specificity of microbubble-to-tissue. The combination of second-generation US contrast agents such as SonoVue with these new specific microbubble techniques using a low mechanical index allows evaluation of the dynamic enhancement of the blood supply of a liver nodule during the various phases of contrast agent circulation (arterial, portal and late phase), similar to that which occurs with helical CT or MRI.

Before the appearance of US contrast agents, multiphasic contrast-enhanced CT and MRI after the administration of contrast agents were widely used as accurate diagnostic techniques for patients with cirrhosis and suspicion of HCC [25, 26]. Detection and analysis of the degree and pattern of tumoural vascularisation were the most important signs for differential diagnosis. Nowadays, CEUS also allows the detection of vascularisation with several advantages. It is a simple, safe and cost-saving alternative to other imaging modalities. It has very few contraindications: it does not irradiate and can be used in patients with renal insufficiency. Moreover, small doses of contrast agent (a few millilitres) are sufficient to detect arterial enhancement, and real-time evaluation is able to detect slowly enhancing HCCs, which with CT could be interpreted as hypoenhancing lesions when using an early arterial phase. Limitations of CEUS are the same as baseline US, and involve difficulties in studying subcapsular nodules or nodules in obese patients, and patients with quick breathing or with severe steatosis.

The most common feature of HCC using CEUS is the presence of early, intense and homogeneous intratumoural enhancement (Fig. 1). In some cases, the enhancement is inhomogeneous,

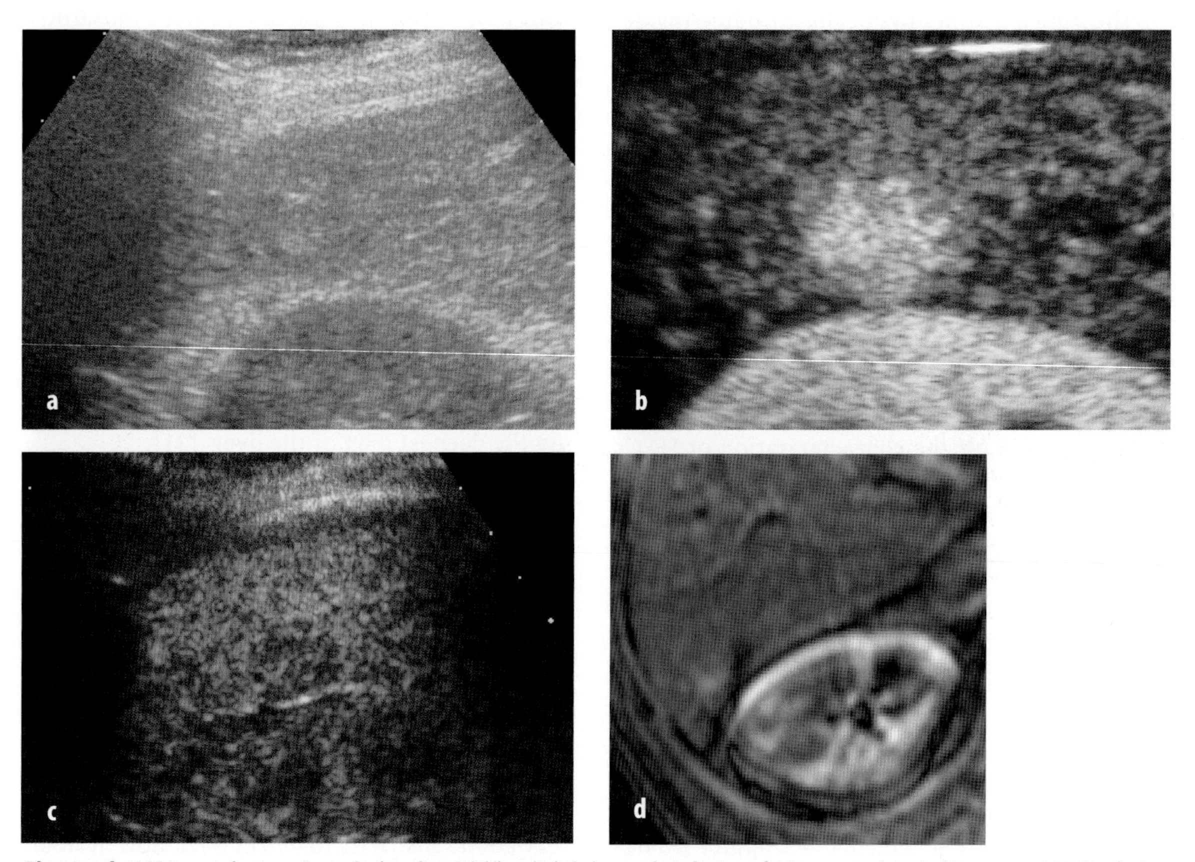

Fig. 1a-d. *HCC in a cirrhotic patient.* On baseline US (**a**) a slightly hypoechoic lesion of 1.5 cm was detected in segment VI. The lesion shows homogeneous enhancement in the arterial phase (**b**). After the peak of enhancement there is a wash-out and in the late phase (**c**) the lesion is slightly hypoechoic. T1-weighted MR imaging after the administration of gadolinium shows the hyperenhancing mass in segment VI (**d**)

especially in tumours with internal necrotic areas or fat degeneration (Fig. 2). These areas show poor or a complete lack of enhancement in comparison with the strong and homogeneous enhancement of the remainder of the HCC. In very few cases with extensive necrotic changes, only peripheral arterial enhancement is detected without central enhancement (Fig. 3). The nutritious artery is often visualised as an arterial vessel that reaches the lesion, and real-time evaluation is able to detect peripheral vessels encircling and internally penetrating the tumour with a distribution which is known as the basket pattern, representing a fine blood-flow network surrounding the tumour nodule. In addition, multiple small tumour vessels flowing into the tumour and irregular internal vessels can be identified and are also characteristic findings of HCC.

After the arterial hyperenhancement, HCC shows 'wash-out', a term defining the hypoenhancement in the portal and delayed phase in a tumour that hyperenhanced in the arterial phase (Fig. 2). In most cases, the wash-out of HCC is slower than in other malignant lesions such as metastases. Thus, most hypervascular metastases become hypoechoic in late arterial phase, while the wash-out of HCC is more progressive-appearing during the portal phase. After the portal phase, most HCC are hypoechoic. However, some HCC remain isoechoic in the late phase, especially those that are well-differentiated or small in size (Fig. 4) [27]. The degree of late phase enhancement by a nodule is determined by the degree of similarity of the nodule to the normal liver parenchyma, and some HCC conserve sinusoids as the normal liver parenchyma.

Thus, in the setting of cirrhosis, the finding of a hyperenhancing lesion in the arterial phase and hypoenhancing in the venous phase using CEUS, is highly specific for HCC and allows differentiation with the most frequently found nodules. Macroregenerating nodules usually have a hypoechoic or isoechoic appearance in the arterial phase, followed by an isoechoic appearance in the portal and late phases [28, 29] (Fig. 5). Thus, in the US follow-up of a previously confirmed macroregenerating nodule, the detection of arterial hypervascularisation reflects transformation into an HCC (Fig. 6).

Several studies have demonstrated the high accuracy of CEUS using Doppler US or gray-scale imaging, in the detection of the arte-

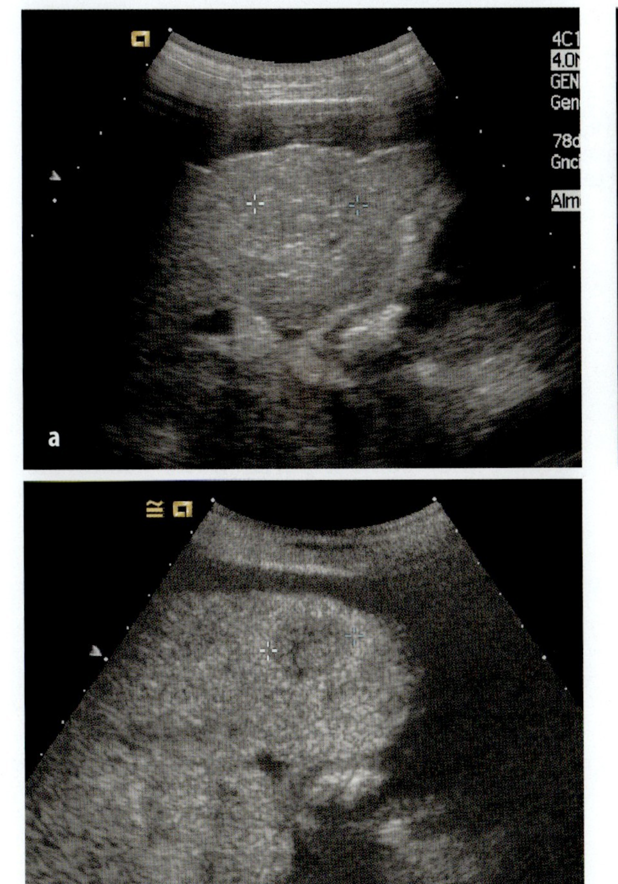

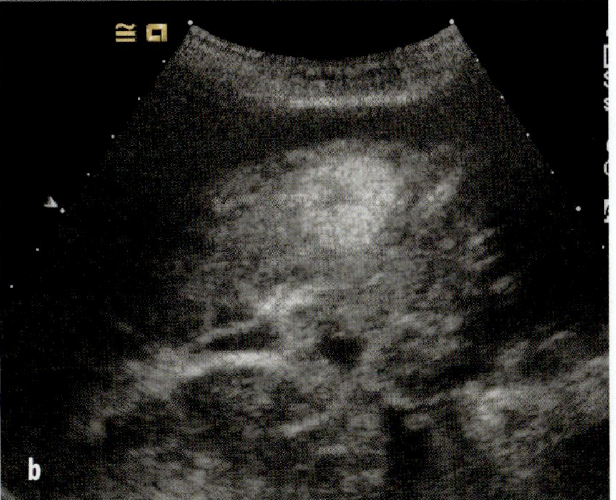

Fig. 2a-c. *HCC in a cirrhotic patient.* This lesion of 2.3 cm was hypoechoic on baseline US (**a**) and shows an almost homogeneous enhancement in the arterial phase with a small non-enhancing hypoechoic area (**b**). The HCC shows a uniform hypoechogenicity in the late phase (**c**)

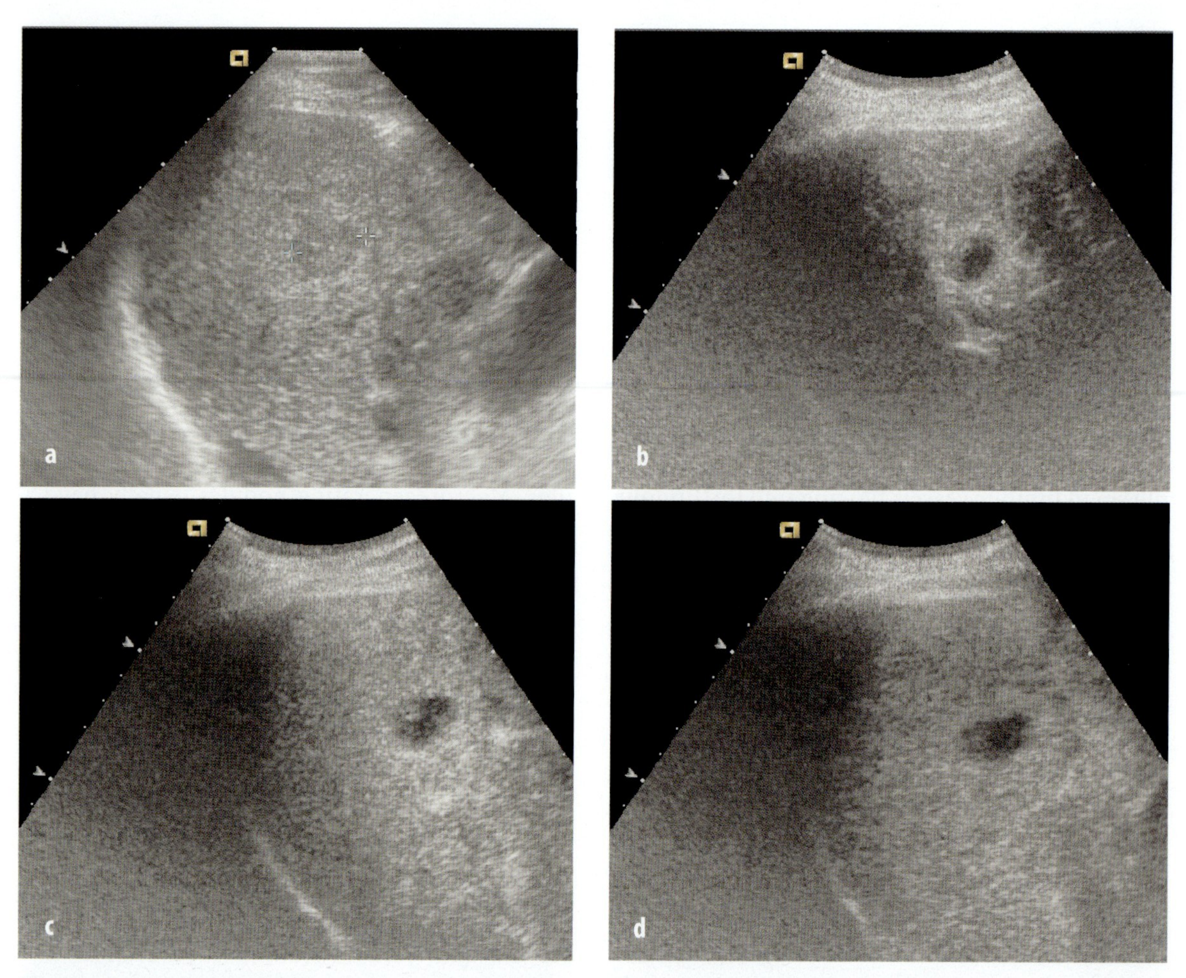

Fig. 3a-d. *HCC with extensive necrotic changes.* On baseline US, a hypoechoic lesion of 2.4 cm was detected (**a**). On contrast-enhanced US, the lesion displayed strong peripheral rim enhancement in the arterial phase (**b**). Portal-venous phase imaging (**c**) shows fading of the rim enhancement, with the centre of the lesion remaining without enhancement. In late phase (**d**) the lesion also remained as a hypoechoic enhancement defect

rial enhancement of HCC, even in nodules smaller than 2 cm [24, 30-32]. With the use of contrast-enhanced Doppler US, Fracanzani et al. [24] detected an increase of 35% in the detection of vascularisation in HCCs after the administration of contrast agent (from 60% (12/20) of HCCs with unenhanced color Doppler US to 95% (19/20) of HCCs with contrast-enhanced colour Doppler US), with the same sensitivity when compared with spiral CT. Other reports with power Doppler US showed similar results, with marked enhancement of tumour vascularity after the administration of contrast agent [31, 33]. Results have also been extremely good using contrast-enhanced US in gray-scale imaging [27, 31, 32]. With the use of CEUS, few HCC remain undetected due to the absence of arterial enhancement. This limitation has been quantified in several studies [27, 31, 32, 34], but the sensitivity of CEUS for the detection of arterial hypervascularisation is the same as other imaging techniques such as CT or MRI, and has been correlated with the degree of HCC differentiation [35]. Overt HCC receives an exclusive arterial blood supply, but most early well-differentiated HCCs also receive a portal blood supply, because they contain portal tracts within the tumour. Thus, some of these early small HCCs do not show hypervascularity. In a study performed by Kumada et al. [21], the type of vascularisation by Doppler US correlated with angiography-assisted CT and pathological findings. Well-differentiated HCCs showed decreased arterial blood supply without decreased portal blood supply, or an insufficient development of arterial tumour vessels [4]. In contrast, moderately or poorly differentiated HCCs showed an increased arterial blood supply with decreased portal blood supply. Thus, with imaging modalities such as CEUS, CT or MRI with contrast agents, or angiography, a subset of well-differentiated HCCs have a nearly normal vascular profile [27,

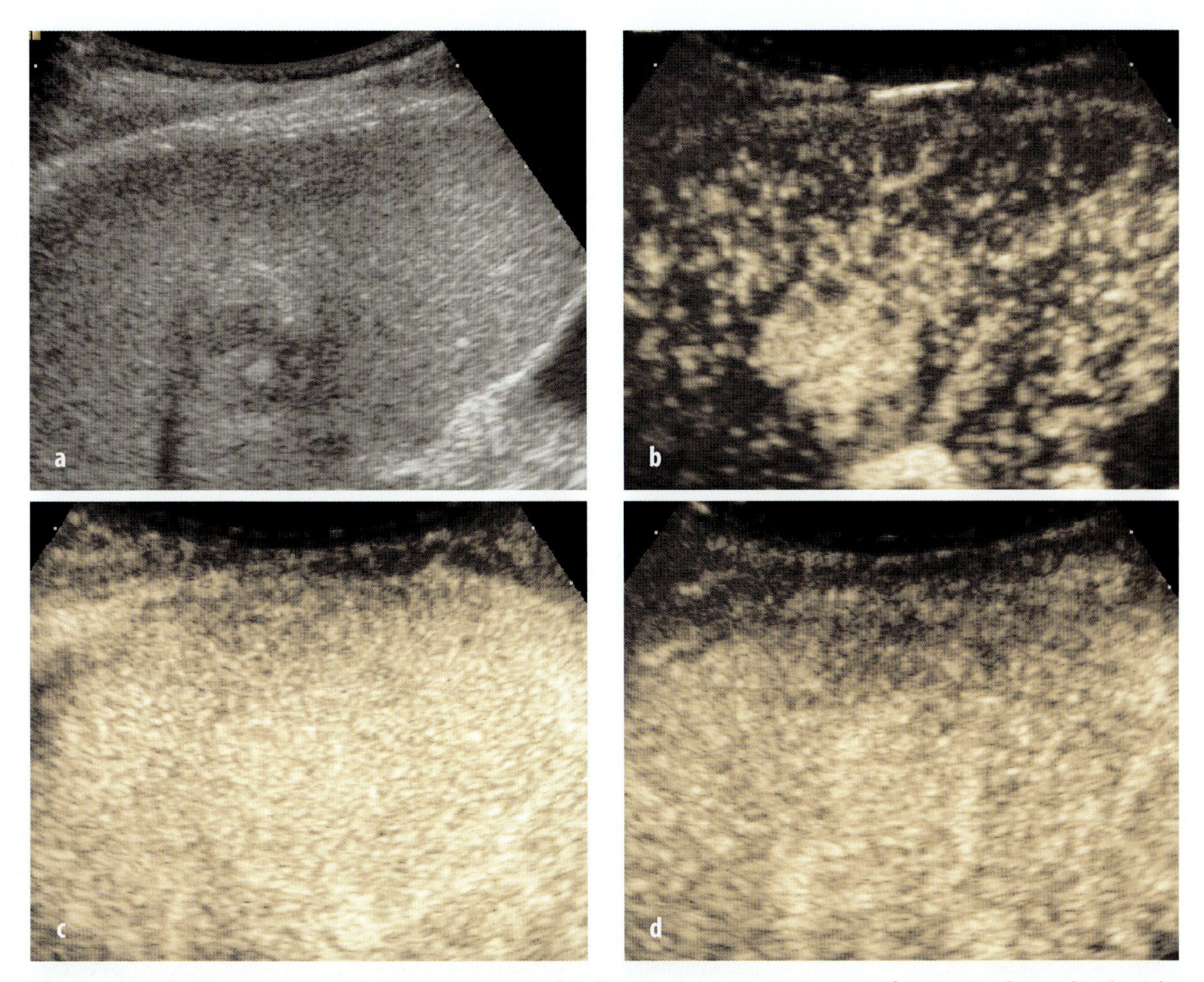

Fig. 4a-d. *Well-differentiated HCC in a cirrhotic patient.* On baseline US a heterogeneous tumour of 2.6 cm was detected in the right hepatic lobe. **a** After the administration of contrast agent, the lesion showed intense and homogeneous enhancement in the arterial phase (**b**). The HCC became isoechoic with respect to the surrounding liver in the portal phase (**c**), remaining undetectable in the late phase due to its isoechogenicity with respect to the liver parenchyma (**d**)

36] and this is usually found in small HCC. In this regard, Giorgio et al. and Gaiani et al. [31, 32] found a decrease in sensitivity in the detection of selective arterial enhancement, depending on the tumour size and degree of differentiation. Giorgio et al. found a sensitivity of 53.6% and Gaiani et al. of 83.3% in nodules 2 cm or less, with sensitivity of 91.3% and 94.5%, respectively, in nodules 2 cm or greater. We obtained a high sensitivity in nodules less than 2 cm (95.2%), which was higher than the sensitivity achieved in these studies, but most of our lesions (91%) were greater than 1 cm in size. More recently, Bolondi et al. [34] found that 17% of HCC between 1 to 2 cm were hypovascular, whereas none of the HCC larger than 2 cm were hypovascular.

HCC must be differentiated from benign lesions such as haemangiomas, hypervacular DN and pseudonodules related to arterio-portal shunts, which may mimic HCC due to the presence of homogeneous arterial enhancement. This diagnostic problem is more accentuated in nodules smaller than 2 cm. Most haemangiomas larger than 2 cm that are incidentally found in a cirrhotic patient show a very specific peripheral nodular enhancement in the arterial phase that can be differentiated from the homogeneous enhancement of HCC. However, pathognomonic nodular enhancement is frequently absent in small haemangiomas, as has been described using CT [37] (Table 1). In a study comparing pre-transplant HCC diagnosis to explant histology, Hayashi et al. [38] reported that 33% of enhancing tumours diagnosed by imaging techniques were not HCC, whereas 63% of misdiagnosed tumours were arterially-enhancing lesions less than 2 cm. However, the incidence of enhancing lesions or pseudolesions is higher in CT and MRI than in US because most vascular abnormalities can be discarded using US.

The differential diagnosis with these hyper-

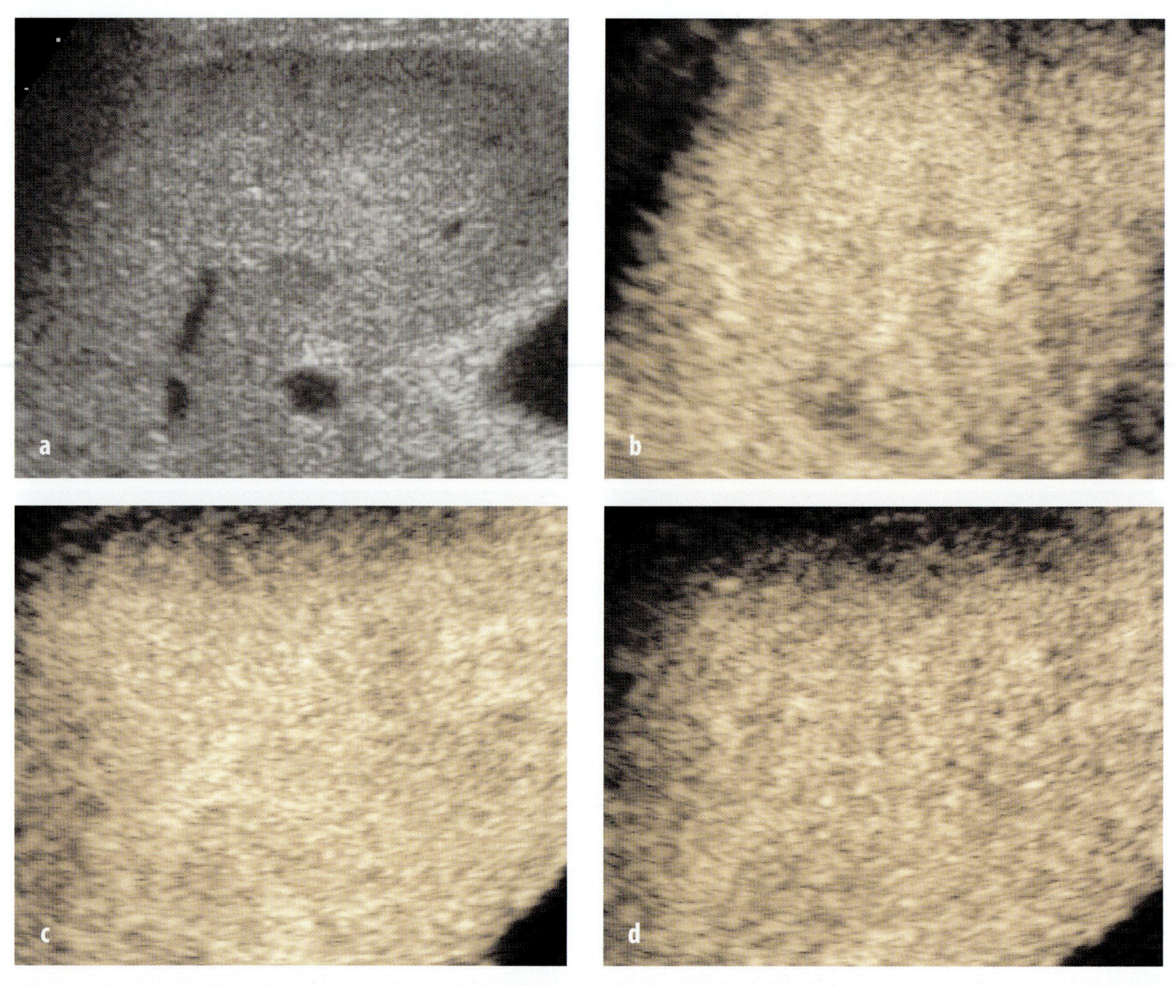

Fig. 5a-d. *Regenerating nodule in a cirrhotic patient.* On baseline US a hypoechoic lesion of 1.2 cm was detected in segment V (**a**). On contrast-enhanced US, the lesion did not show enhancement in the arterial phase (**b**), being isoechoic with respect to the surrounding liver in the portal (**c**) and late phases (**d**). Diagnosis was confirmed by fine needle biopsy and a follow-up US at 12 months

enhancing lesions in the arterial phase can be performed by the evaluation of the enhancement in the late phase as has been remarked by the European Federation of Societies for Ultrasound in Medicine and Biology (EFSUMB) [39]. This society held a special consensus conference in January, 2004 to present guidelines for the use of US contrast agents, including the characterisation of focal liver lesions. The presence of a washout in the portal phase with hypovascularity in the equilibrium phase contributes to improve the specificity of the technique, because benign lesions enhance at least with the same intensity of the normal liver in the late phase. This fact is in concordance with other studies using CT and MRI. Marrero et al. [40] found that the presence of a delayed hypointensity of an arterially enhancing lesion using dynamic gadolinium-enhanced MRI was the most important independent predictor for a diagnosis of HCC, regardless of tumour size. However, late phase contrast scanning in cirrhotic patients is more difficult to evaluate than in non-cirrhotic livers [29, 41]. Haemodynamic changes with hyperdynamic circulation and shunting may make parenchymal enhancement in the late phase in cirrhotic patients appear heterogeneous and less intense than in normal livers, making evaluation difficult. In a recent study, we evaluated the accuracy of the late phase of SonoVue for the differentiation between benign and malignant tumours [29]. We obtained 93.6% of accuracy in non-cirrhotic patients, whereas the accuracy of the late phase in cirrhotic patients was 75.2%. This lower accuracy was due to the presence of 29.3% of isoechoic HCC in the late phase. The presence of a significant number of isoechoic HCCs in the delayed phase has been described in previous studies [27, 28], but other authors have described a very low incidence of isoechoic HCC in the delayed phase using Levovist or SonoVue [42]. In a study by Dietrich et al. [41] using the late phase

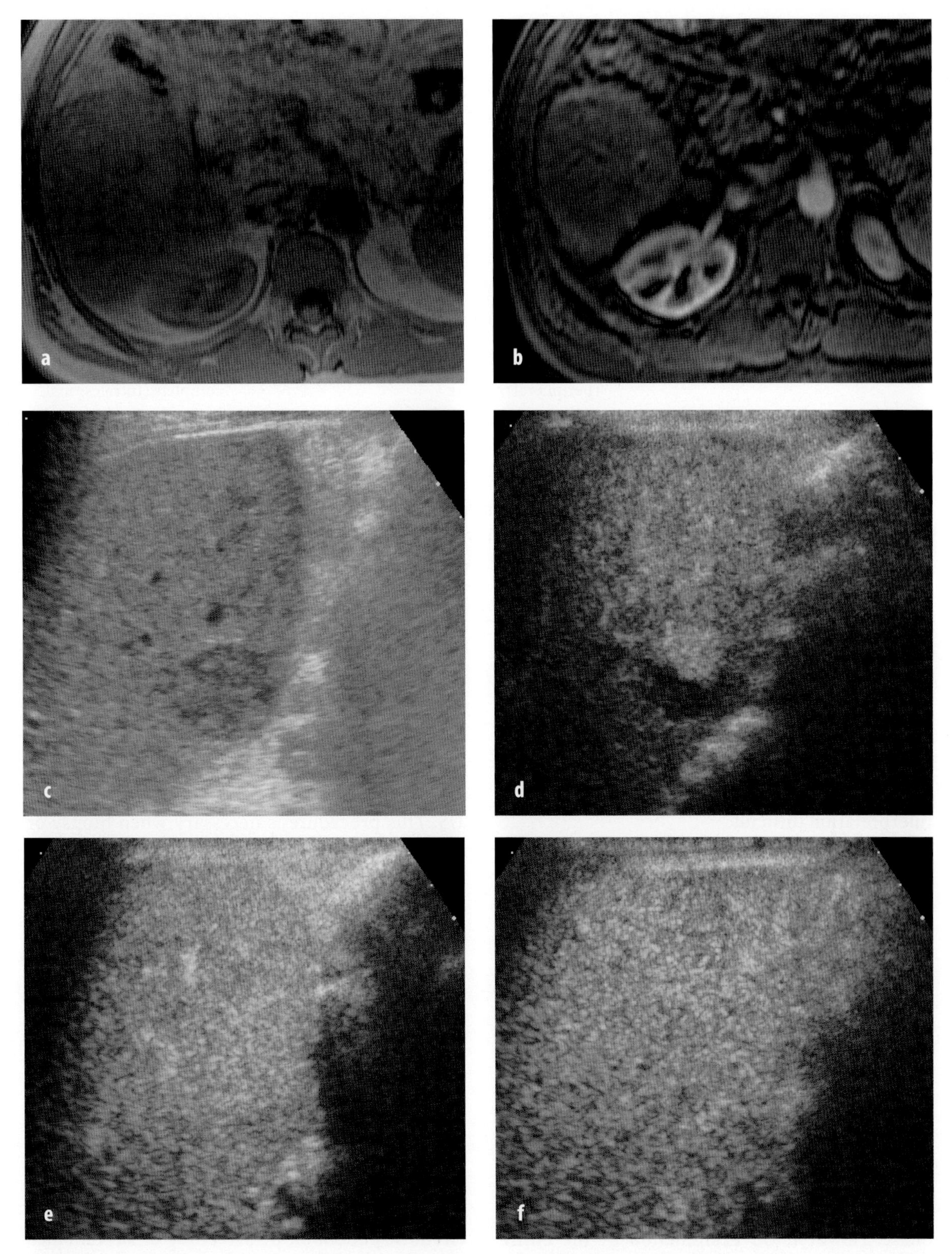

Fig. 6a-f. *Transition from a dysplastic nodule to well-differentiated HCC.* On MRI imaging, a lesion of 2 cm was diagnosed as a dysplastic nodule. The lesion was hyperintense in a T1-weighted image (**a**) and in a T2-weighted image, without enhancement in the arterial phase after the administration of Gadolinium (**b**). Three months later, a follow-up US was performed demonstrating tumor growth to 2.3 cm (**c**), thus contrast-enhanced US was also performed. After the administration of SonoVue, the posterior part of the lesion showed absence of enhancement in the arterial phase, but there was nodular enhancement in the anterior part of the tumor, suggesting the presence of a foci of HCC inside the dysplastic nodule (**d**). The whole lesion became isoechoic in the portal (**e**) and late phases (**f**). A fine needle biopsy of the enhancing area was performed, confirming the presence of a well-differentiated HCC

Table 1. Summary of contrast-enhanced US findings of the nodules most frequently found in cirrhotic patients in the arterial, portal and late phases

	Arterial	Portal	Late phase
Hepatocellular carcinoma	Hyperechoic	Isoechoic	Hypoechoic
			Isoechoic (30%, especially in small and well-differentiated HCC)
Regenerating and dysplastic nodules	Iso- or hypoechoic	Isoechoic	Isoechoic
Haemangiomas	Hyperechoic (peripheral nodular enhancement)	Centripetal filling	Isoechoic if filling is complete (Intralesional hypoechoic areas in 50%)
	Homogeneous hyperechoic in 20% of small haemangiomas	Hyper- or Isoechoic	Hyper- or Isoechoic
Cholangiocarcinoma	Hypoechoic Hyperechoic (15%)	Iso- or hypoechoic	Hypoechoic

of Levovist, 100% HCCs were hypoechoic in the late phase. However, these authors remarked that 39.3% of HCC had variable and less impressive signal voids in the setting of heterogeneous enhancement of the liver parenchyma, making interpretation difficult.

Role of Contrast Ultrasound in Clinical Practice

Detection of Hepatic Lesions in Cirrhotic Patients

US has a limited sensitivity for the detection of small nodules in the setting of cirrhotic patients, especially if nodules are isoechoic or subcapsular. The use of contrast-enhanced US in the detection of invisible nodules on baseline US relies on the detection of arterial hypervascularisation or the detection of the hypoechogenicity with respect to the liver parenchyma in the late phase. However, US examination of the entire liver is almost impossible in the arterial phase, because it only lasts 20-30 seconds. Thus, multiple doses of contrast agent would be necessary to screen all the liver parenchyma. Moreover, evaluation of the late phase is difficult because the appearance of HCC in the late phase is variable with several isoechoic HCC. Moreover, enhancement of the liver parenchyma is inhomogeneous due to the alterations of cirrhotic microvascularisation. Thus, in our institution, we use CEUS to identify lesions suspicious of HCC detected using CT or MRI that are invisible on baseline US. This procedure is necessary when biopsy or percutaneous treatment of a HCC is considered and the nodule is not detected on US. CEUS study focused on the segment in which the tumour has been detected with the other imaging technique usually helps to detect arterial enhancement (Fig. 7).

Characterisation of Liver Lesions

Characterisation of hepatic lesions is, at present, the main application of CEUS, together with the evaluation of responses to percutaneous treatment. Several studies have demonstrated the usefulness of CEUS in the diagnosis of HCC and the characterisation of cirrhotic nodules. Previously, when a new nodule is detected in a cirrhotic patient on US screening or surveillance programs, a follow-up every three months was recommended if the nodule was smaller than 1 cm, but nowadays it is preferable to administer a US contrast agent to detect the arterial enhancement that is the key to the diagnosis of HCC. If the enhancement pattern is characteristic (hypervascular in the arterial phase and hypoe-

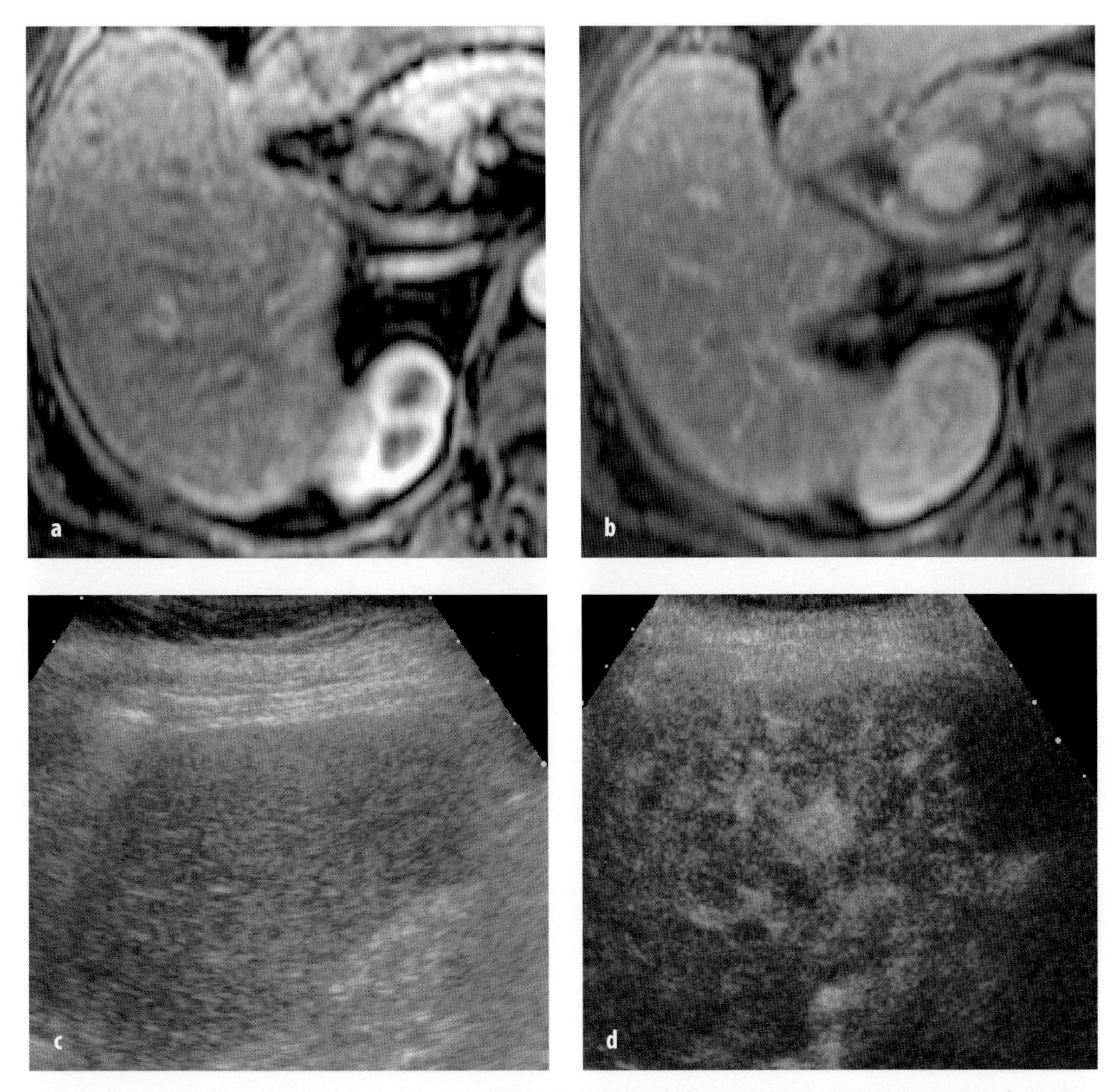

Fig. 7a-d. *Detection of an undetectable HCC.* This small HCC was detected in an MRI study and sent to the US department for percutaneous treatment. T1-weighted MR imaging before (**a**) and after the administration of gadolinium (**b**) showed a small lesion in segment VI (1.5 cm) with peripheral enhancement during the arterial phase. On baseline US (**c**), there was no evidence of focal hepatic lesions in this segment. After the administration of SonoVue (**d**), nodular enhancement in arterial phase allowed the detection of the tumour

choic in the late phase), CT and MRI are used to complete the staging before treatment. If the enhancement pattern is not characteristic, but shows arterial hypervascularity and the lesion is smaller than 2 cm, biopsy is recommended. If it is larger than 2 cm a MRI may be the most useful technique for characterising the nodule. Moreover, as a negative biopsy does not exclude the diagnosis of HCC [6], close follow-up is recommended in patients with a focal lesion with negative HCC biopsy to detect any change in size that may require another biopsy.

Other Applications

US Staging of HCC

Accurate staging is crucial to determine the best treatment for HCC, and also influences the prognosis of the patient. Staging depends on tumour size, the number and location of lesions, the presence of satellite nodules and biliary extension, and vascular and extrahepatic invasion. Evaluation of satellite nodules can usually be performed because most satellite foci are very near the primary tumour. However, CEUS cannot replace other imaging techniques such as CT or MRI for evaluating all of the liver parenchyma to discard additional nodules and extrahepatic invasion. One of the utilities of CEUS is the assessment of vascular invasion that represents an enormous change in therapeutic possibilities. Thrombosis in the portal vein can be visualised as a solid mass inside the tumour. Characterisation of the thrombi can be easily performed with CEUS. Fine-needle aspiration biopsy is safe and sensitive for establishing whether portal vein thrombosis is benign or malignant [43], and the presence of arterial vascularisation inside the tumour using Doppler techniques is a highly specific sign of malignancy [44]. In some cases, especially in patients with only a thrombus in a small or peripheral segment of the portal vein, evaluation with colour Doppler is not useful. With the use of contrast agents, the detection of enhancement in the arterial phase inside the tumoural thrombus allows its differentiation from a non-tumoural thrombus (Fig. 8).

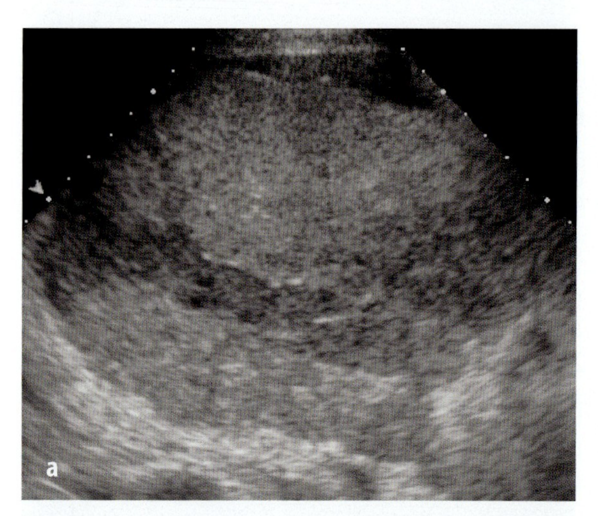

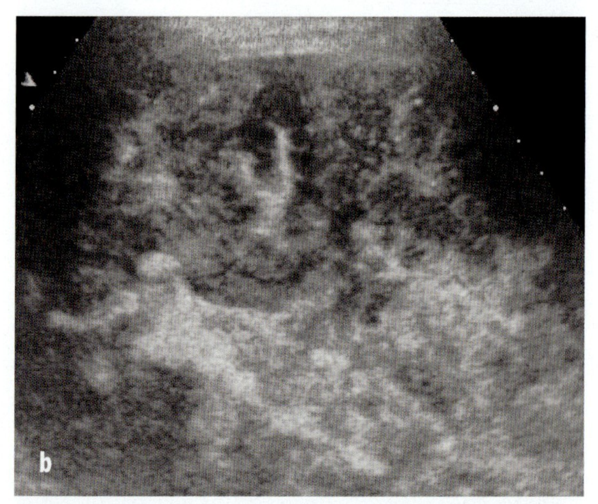

Fig. 8a, b. *Malignant portal thrombus in a cirrhotic patient.* An expanded right portal vein was detected on baseline US (**a**). In the early arterial phase there was a clear intrathrombus enhancement that is typical of the presence of tumor inside the thrombus (**b**). The suspicion was confirmed with fine needle aspiration

Key Points

- Arterial neovascularisation of HCC is the key to differentiate it from other liver tumours.
- Contrast-enhanced ultrasound is indicated for detection of the vascularisation of suspected or known lesions in patients with chronic liver disease or cirrhosis.
- Using contrast-enhanced ultrasound, the finding of a hyperenhancing lesion in the arterial phase and hypoenhancing in the venous phase is highly specific for HCC in the cirrhotic setting.

References

1. Parkin DM, Pisani P, Ferlay J (1990) Estimates of the worldwide incidence of 25 major cancers in 1990. Int J Cancer 80:827-841
2. Taura N, Hamasaki K, Nakao K et al (2005) Clinical benefits of hepatocellular carcinoma surveillance: A single-center, hospital-based study. Oncol Rep 14:999-1003
3. Sala M, Llovet JM, Vilana R et al (2004) Initial response to percutaneous ablation predicts survival in patients with hepatocellular carcinoma. Hepatology 40:1352-1360

4. Bruix J, Sherman M, Llovet JM et al (2001) Clinical management of hepatocellular carcinoma. Conclusions of the Barcelona-2000 EASL conference. European Association for the Study of the Liver. J. Hepatol. 35:421-430
5. Kojiro M, Roskams T (2005) Early hepatocellular carcinoma and dysplastic nodules. Semin Liver Dis 25:133-142
6. Roncalli M, Roz E, Coggi G et al (1999)The vascular profile of regenerative and dysplastic nodules of the cirrhotic liver: implications for diagnosis and classification. Hepatology 30: 1174-1178
7. Borzio M, Fargion S, Borzio F et al (2003) Impact of large regenerative, low grade and high grade dysplastic nodules in hepatocellular carcinoma development. J Hepatol 39:208-214
8. Terjung B, Lemnitzer I, Dumoulin FL et al (2003) Bleeding complications after percutaneous liver biopsy. An analysis of risk factors. Digestion 67:138-145
9. Torzilli G, Minagawa M, Takayama T et al (1999) Accurate preoperative evaluation of liver mass lesions without fine-needle biopsy. Hepatology 30:889-893
10. Zoli M, Magalotti D, Bianchi G et al (1996) Efficacy of a surveillance program for early detection of hepatocellular carcinoma. Cancer 78:977-985
11. Oka H, Yamamoto S, Kuroki T et al (1990) Prospective study of early detection of hepatocellular carcinoma in patients with cirrhosis. Hepatology 12:680-687
12. Bennett GL, Krinsky GA, Abitbol RJ et al (2002) Sonographic detection of hepatocellular carcinoma and dysplastic nodules in cirrhosis: correlation of pretransplantation sonography and liver explant pathology in 200 patients. AJR Am J Roentgenol 179:75-80
13. Shapiro RS, Wagreich J, Parsons RB et al (1998) Tissue harmonic imaging sonography: evaluation of image quality compared with conventional sonography. AJR Am J Roentgenol. 171:1203-1206
14. Tanaka S, Oshikawa O, Sasaki T et al (2000) Evaluation of tissue harmonic imaging for the diagnosis of focal liver lesions. Ultrasound Med Biol 26:183-187
15. Sheu JC, Chen DS, Sung JL et al (1985) Hepatocellular carcinoma: US evolution in the early stage. Radiology 155:463-467
16. Kim KA, Lee WJ, Lim HK et al (2003) Small hepatocellular carcinoma: ultrasonographic findings and histopathologic correlation. Clin Imaging 27:340-345
17. Ogata R, Majima Y, Tateishi Y et al (2000) Bright loop appearance; a characteristic ultrasonography sign of early hepatocellular carcinoma. Oncol Rep 7:1293-1298
18. Bru C, Maroto A, Bruix J et al (1989) Diagnostic accuracy of fine-needle aspiration biopsy in patients with hepatocellular carcinoma. Dig Dis Sci 34:1765-1769
19. Lencioni R, Pinto F, Armillotta N, Bartolozzi C (1996) Assessment of tumor vascularity in hepatocellular carcinoma: comparison of power Doppler US and color Doppler US. Radiology 201:353-358
20. Koito K, Namieno T, Morita K (1998) Differential diagnosis of small hepatocellular carcinoma and adenomatous hyperplasia with power Doppler sonography. AJR Am J Roentgenol 170:157-161
21. Kumada T, Nakano S, Toyoda H et al (2004) Assessment of tumor hemodynamics in small hepatocellular carcinoma: comparison of Doppler ultrasonography, angiography-assisted computed tomography, and pathological findings. Liver Int 24:425-431
22. Gaiani S, Volpe L, Piscaglia F, Bolondi L (2001) Vascularity of liver tumours and recent advances in doppler ultrasound. J Hepatol 34:474-482
23. Kudo M, Tochio H, Zhou P (2004) Differentiation of hepatic tumors by color Doppler imaging: role of the maximum velocity and the pulsatility index of the intratumoral blood flow signal. Intervirology 47:154-161
24. Fracanzani AL, Burdick L, Borzio M et al (2001) Contrast-enhanced Doppler ultrasonography in the diagnosis of hepatocellular carcinoma and premalignant lesions in patients with cirrhosis. Hepatology 34:1109-1112
25. Valls C, Cos M, Figueras J et al (2004) Pretransplantation diagnosis and staging of hepatocellular carcinoma in patients with cirrhosis: value of dual-phase helical CT. AJR Am J Roentgenol 182:1011-1017
26. Yamashita Y, Mitsuzaki K, Yi T et al (1996) Small hepatocellular carcinoma in patients with chronic liver damage: prospective comparison of detection with dynamic MR imaging and helical CT of the whole liver. Radiology 200:79-84
27. Nicolau C, Catala V, Vilana R et al (2004) Evaluation of hepatocellular carcinoma using SonoVue, a second generation ultrasound contrast agent: correlation with cellular differentiation. Eur Radiol 14:1092-1099
28. Quaia E, Calliada F, Bertolotto M et al (2004) Characterization of focal liver lesions with contrast-specific US modes and a sulfur hexafluoride-filled microbubble contrast agent: diagnostic performance and confidence. Radiology 232:420-430
29. Nicolau C, Vilana R, Catala V et al (2006) The importance of the evaluation of all vascular phases on contrast-enhanced sonography in the differentiation of benign from malignant focal liver lesions. AJR Am J Roentgenol 186(1):158-167
30. Vilana R, Llovet JM, Bianchi L et al (2003) Contrast-enhanced power Doppler sonography and helical computed tomography for assessment of vascularity of small hepatocellular carcinomas before and after percutaneous ablation. J Clin Ultrasound 31:119-128
31. Giorgio A, Ferraioli G, Tarantino L et al (2004) Contrast-enhanced sonographic appearance of hepatocellular carcinoma in patients with cirrhosis: comparison with contrast-enhanced helical CT appearance. AJR Am J Roentgenol 183:1319-1326
32. Gaiani S, Celli N, Piscaglia F et al (2004) Usefulness of contrast-enhanced perfusional sonography in the assessment of hepatocellular carcinoma hypervascular at spiral computed tomography. J Hepatol 41:421-426
33. Choi BI, Kim TK, Han JK et al (2000) Vascularity of hepatocellular carcinoma: assessment with contrast-enhanced second-harmonic versus conventional power Doppler US. Radiology 214:381-386
34. Bolondi L, Gaiani S, Celli N et al (2005) Characterization of small nodules in cirrhosis by assessment of vascularity: the problem of hypovascular hepatocellular carcinoma. Hepatology 42:27-34
35. Matsui O (2004) Imaging of multistep human hepatocarcinogenesis by CT during intra-arterial contrast injection. Intervirology 47:271-276
36. Takayasu K, Muramatsu Y, Furukawa H et al (1995)

Early hepatocellular carcinoma: appearance at CT during arterial portography and CT arteriography with pathologic correlation. Radiology 194:101-105
37. Kim T, Federle MP, Baron RL et al (2001) Discrimination of small hepatic hemangiomas from hypervascular malignant tumors smaller than 3 cm with three-phase helical CT. Radiology 219:699-706
38. Hayashi PH, Trotter JF, Forman L et al (2004) Impact of pretransplant diagnosis of hepatocellular carcinoma on cadveric liver allocation in the era of MELD. Liver Transpl 10:42-48
39. Albrecht T, Blomley M, Bolondi L et al (2004) Guidelines for the use of contrast agents in ultrasound. January 2004. Ultraschall Med 25:249-256
40. Marrero JA, Hussain HK, Nghiem HV et al (2005) Improving the prediction of hepatocellular carcinoma in cirrhotic patients with an arterially-enhancing liver mass. Liver Transpl 11:281-289
41. Dietrich CF, Ignee A, Trojan J et al (2004) Improved characterisation of histologically proven liver tumours by contrast-enhanced ultrasonography during the portal-venous and specific late phase of SHU 508A. Gut 53:401-405
42. von Herbay A, Vogt C, Willers R, Haussinger D (2004)Real-time imaging with the sonographic contrast agent SonoVue: differentiation between benign and malignant hepatic lesions. J Ultrasound Med 23:1557-1568
43. Vilana R, Bru C, Bruix J et al (1993) Fine-needle aspiration biopsy of portal vein thrombus: value in detecting malignant thrombosis. AJR Am J Roentgenol 160:1285-1287
44. Dodd GD III, Memel DS, Baron RL et al (1995) Portal vein thrombosis in patients with cirrhosis: does sonographic detection of intrathrombus flow allow differentiation of benign and malignant thrombus? AJR Am J Roentgenol 165:573-577

II.3

Detection and Characterisation of Liver Metastases

Thomas Albrecht

Introduction

Both benign and malignant focal liver lesions are very common, and staging of the liver for metastases in cancer patients is one of the most frequent tasks of every day radiological practise.

The most common malignant liver lesions are metastases from other organs: 25 to 50% of patients with known solid malignant tumours have hepatic metastases at the time of diagnosis, with decreasing frequency of metastases in colon, gastric, pancreatic, breast and lung cancer [1]. On the other hand, the prevalence of solid benign liver tumours has been reported to be more than 20% in autopsy series [1, 2] and thus in patients with malignancy, 25-50% of lesions under 2 cm in size are benign [3, 4]. The most frequent benign lesion is haemangioma, which has a prevalence of 7-21% [2, 5], followed by focal nodular hyperplasia (FNH) with a prevalence of up to 3% [2, 6]. Adenomas are much rarer than FNH (by a factor of approximately 50) and they usually occur in female patients with a history of sex hormone medication. Other relatively rare benign lesions are pyogenic, parasitic or fungal abscesses. Areas of focal fatty change or focal fatty sparing are very common; they do not represent true lesions but may appear as pseudo-tumours on ultrasound (US) and are thus easily confused with real tumours such as metastases. Pseudo-tumours are particularly common in patients undergoing chemotherapy and their tendency to vary in extent and location over time can pose problems for serial imaging of tumour patients.

From the above, it is obvious that liver imaging of cancer patients requires an imaging modality that is not only provides highly sensitive detection, but also reliable characterisation of lesions, thus allowing differentiation of malignant from benign tumours. This is particularly important since almost all benign lesions, as well as non-end-stage metastases, are typically asymptomatic, and blood tests are non-specific.

Accurate and timely detection of hepatic metastases is very important because of their far-reaching therapeutic and prognostic implications. Especially through the recent improvements in liver resection and local ablation of metastases from colo-rectal and some other primary carcinomas, liver imaging has become more demanding. Accurate assessment of number, size and segmental location of metastases is required to identify patients that are suitable for surgical or interventional therapy, for treatment planning and for follow-up imaging under chemotherapy.

In the past, US had an important but somewhat limited role in liver imaging of cancer patients. Although commonly the first and most widespread modality used, its detection rate was inferior to that of computed tomography (CT) and magnetic resonance imaging (MRI), and its ability to differentiate metastases from other focal liver lesions was often limited. With the advent of US contrast agents (USCA) and new contrast-specific imaging techniques in the last few years, contrast-enhanced US (CEUS) has become a powerful tool, which has significantly changed the role of US for liver imaging in cancer patients.

Conventional Ultrasound

B-mode Features of Metastases

The ability of US to detect a focal liver lesion depends on a number of factors: echogenicity, size, location, and mass effect. The two most important factors are liver-to-lesion contrast and spatial resolution: even small strongly hyper- or hypoechoic lesions are easily detected (Fig. 1a). Conversely, isoechoic masses are usually missed and must be larger in order to be detected. Mass effect is important for the detection of isoechoic lesions. It manifests as deviation or invasion of the intrahepatic vasculature and/or bulges in the liver contour.

The echo patterns of metastases are numerous (Fig. 1), but some patterns are said to be associated with certain primary tumours (Table 1). US appearances of metastases may vary within a given patient as well as over time, and particularly following chemotherapy. Most metastases are round and have well-defined margins. Hypoechoic metastases are more common (approximately 65%) than hyper- or isoechoic

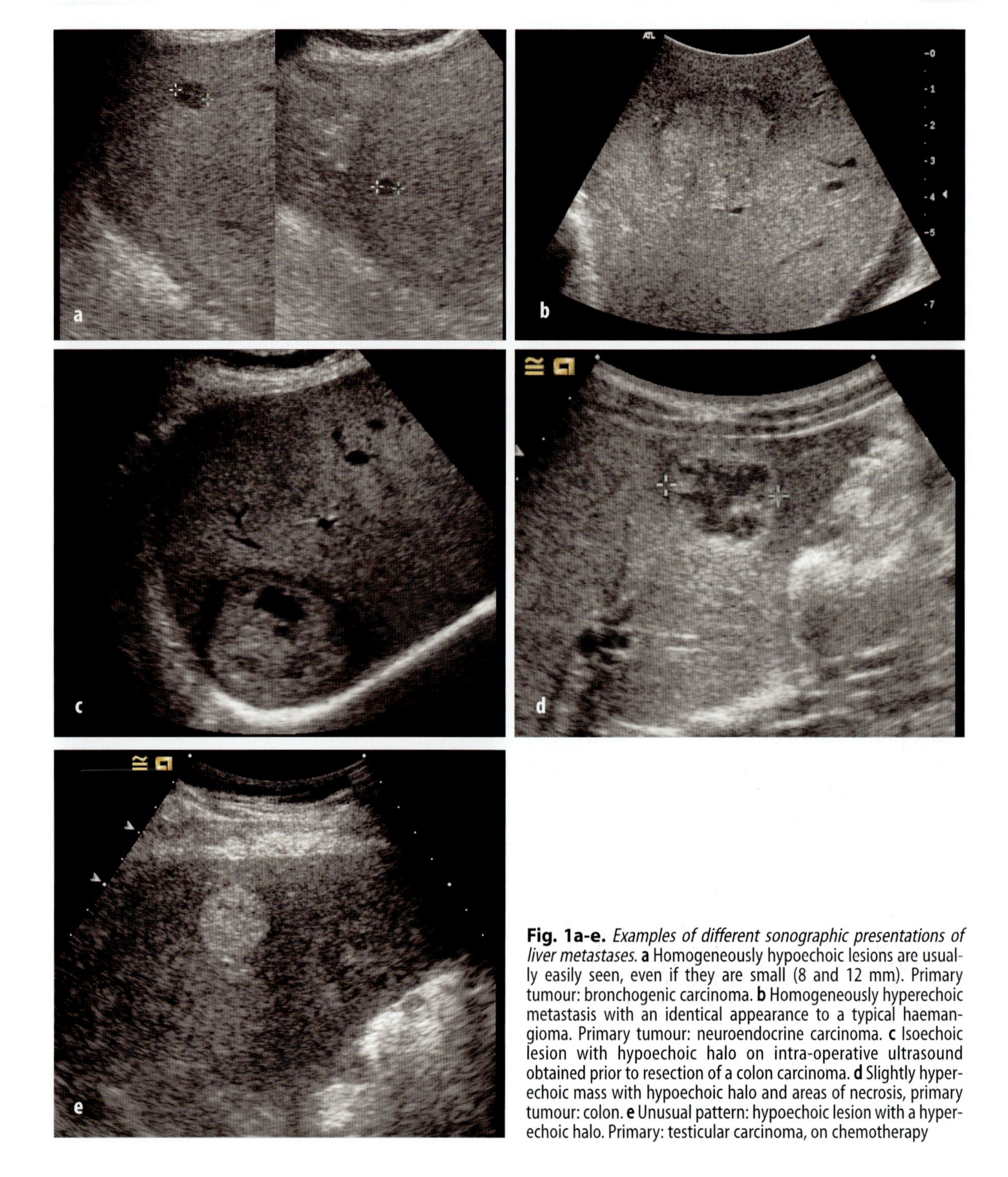

Fig. 1a-e. *Examples of different sonographic presentations of liver metastases.* **a** Homogeneously hypoechoic lesions are usually easily seen, even if they are small (8 and 12 mm). Primary tumour: bronchogenic carcinoma. **b** Homogeneously hyperechoic metastasis with an identical appearance to a typical haemangioma. Primary tumour: neuroendocrine carcinoma. **c** Isoechoic lesion with hypoechoic halo on intra-operative ultrasound obtained prior to resection of a colon carcinoma. **d** Slightly hyperechoic mass with hypoechoic halo and areas of necrosis, primary tumour: colon. **e** Unusual pattern: hypoechoic lesion with a hyperechoic halo. Primary: testicular carcinoma, on chemotherapy

Table 1. Common sonographic patterns of hepatic metastases from various primary malignancies. Note that any primary tumour may produce liver metastases with any of the patterns named

Hyporeflective (most common)
Breast
Lung
Lymphoma
Pancreas
Hyper-reflective
Colon
Neuroendocrine carcinoma
Renal cell
Choriocarcinoma
Target pattern ("halo")
Most commonly lung, colon
Occurs in all others
Calcified
Common: (treated) mucinous adenocarcinoma of colon, stomach, ovary
Rare: osteosarcoma, chondrosarcoma
Cystic
Ovary, pancreas, colon
Sarcoma
Squamous cell carcinoma
Infiltrative
Breast
Lung
Pancreas
Thyroid
Malignant melanoma

metastases. A hypoechoic halo is seen surrounding the lesions in 40% of cases [7], and is most often associated with iso- or hyperechoic metastases. The cause of the halo is controversial. It is not pathognomonic of metastases as it may also be seen in hepatocellular carcinoma (HHC), fungal abscess, adenoma and, less commonly, in FNH and haemangioma. Cystic areas indicative of necrosis may occur. Calcified metastases are sometimes seen in patients with mucinous adenocarcinoma of the gastrointestinal tract, and are more common after chemotherapy.

Multiple lesions in a patient with a known primary malignancy are highly suggestive of metastases. Multiple metastases may show as several individual lesions or as diffuse infiltration, producing the "moth-eaten" appearance of a heterogeneous liver, combined with definite or questionable individual lesions (Fig. 2).

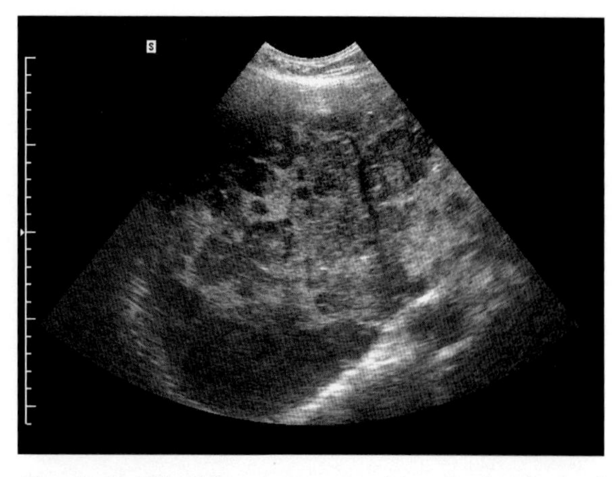

Fig. 2. Multiple/diffuse metastases giving the "moth-eaten" appearance

Doppler Imaging

For growth, liver malignancies require a neovascular supply. However, Doppler techniques are often limited in their ability to image the vascularity of metastases and other lesions since the flow signals are too low (small vessels with relatively slow flow). Power Doppler is slightly superior to conventional colour Doppler in this respect. Doppler typically shows no or some peripheral vascularity in hypovascular metastases, while hypervascular deposits may show vessels throughout the lesion (Figs. 3a, 3b). Both these patterns are also common in other focal liver lesions. The addition of Doppler is of limited value in differentiating metastases from other lesions, it has no added value for detection. Doppler can be useful to differentiate metastases from FNH (Fig. 3c) and focal fatty change/infiltration, as discussed below.

Differential Diagnosis

The differential diagnosis of metastases is wide, and includes any focal lesion that may be encountered in the liver. Generally speaking, any histologic type of lesion seen on B-mode US can mimic metastasis and vice versa. Only common lesions will be discussed here. Primary malignant lesions such as hepatocellular carcinoma and peripheral cholangiocarcinoma (CCC) cannot be differentiated from metastases based on lesion appearances alone. However, unifocal primary malignant tumours tend to present as large single tumours, which is less common in metastases. HCC usually occurs in patients with cirrhosis, and large HCC may form a tumour thrombus within the portal vein. Both of these

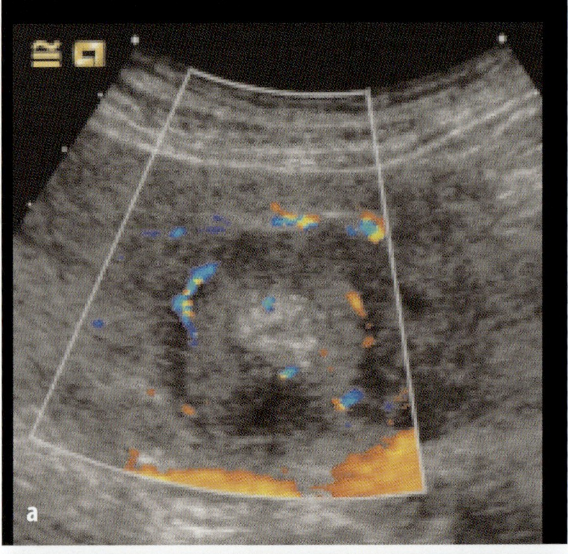

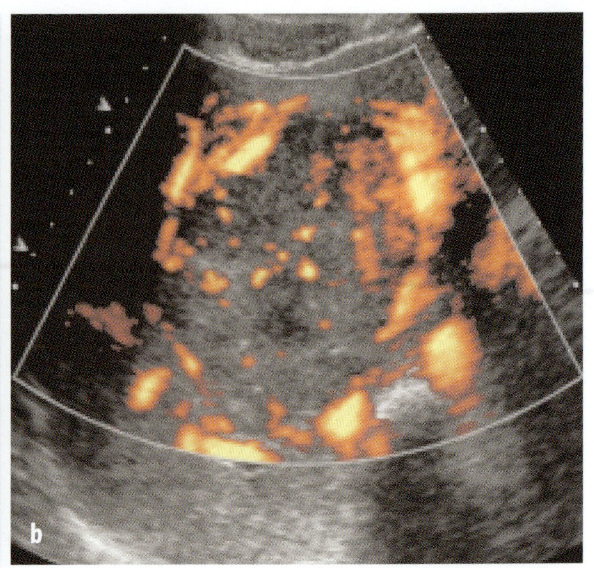

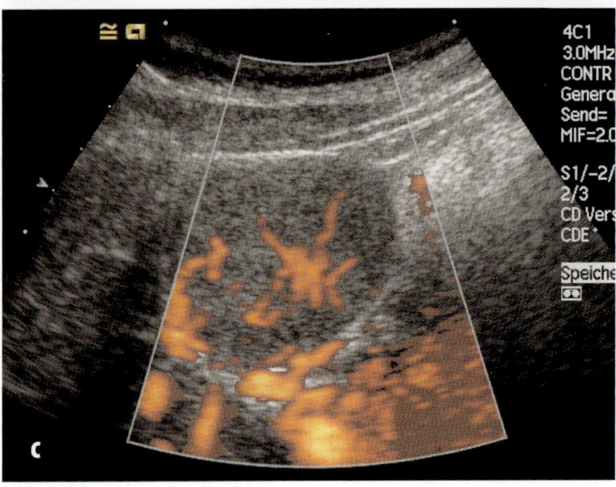

Fig. 3a-c. *Colour/power Doppler appearances of metastases versus FNH.* **a** Colour Doppler of a hypovascular metastasis from bronchogenic carcinoma showing peripheral rim vascularity of the lesion and only a few colour dots within the lesion. **b** Power Doppler of a hypervascular metastasis from malignant melanoma shows stronger rim enhancement and multiple small vessels almost evenly distributed throughout the lesion. **c** Power Doppler of FNH shows the characteristic "spoke-wheel pattern" of a central feeding artery branching and radiating centrifugally towards the periphery of the lesion

presentations are important differential diagnostic clues. (Peripheral) CCC more frequently causes (segmental) biliary obstruction than other malignant tumours. Multifocal HCC and CCC are not uncommon and may be indistinguishable from multiple metastases.

The two most common benign solid lesions – haemangioma and FNH – often have quite typical appearances, which are helpful for their diagnosis. The commonest sonographic appearance of *haemangioma* (60-70%) is a homogeneously hyperechoic lesion less than 3 cm in size. Not infrequently, these tumours show posterior acoustic enhancement, which is a very valuable differential diagnostic criterion (Fig. 4a). Atypical features are commoner in larger haemangiomas and include hypoechoic lesions (Fig. 4b), heterogeneous echogenicity with hypoechoic areas due to necrosis, haemorrhage, partial thrombosis or scarring. Calcification may also occur. A significant proportion of atypical haemangiomas have an echogenic periphery and a hypoechoic centre. Atypical haemangiomas are often indistinguishable from metastases (Fig. 4a). Despite its vascular nature, the blood flow within a haemangioma is too slow to be detected by Doppler modes.

FNH is typically homogeneously isoechoic and it is therefore often overlooked, especially when small. Its visualisation depends on mass effect, with displacement of normal vessels and a slightly different (coarser) echo pattern than the surrounding parenchyma. FNH may also be slightly hyper- or hypoechoic compared to normal liver. In large FNH (≥ 4-5 cm), a hypoechoic central scar may be visible, and colour Doppler often shows a spoke-wheel arterial pattern of vessels radiating from the centre to the periphery (Fig. 3c). While large FNHs are often easily diagnosed based on their almost isoechoic texture, the central scar, and the spoke-wheel pattern, small FNHs often lack these typical features and are easily confused with metastases, especially in young women with breast cancer (Fig. 5).

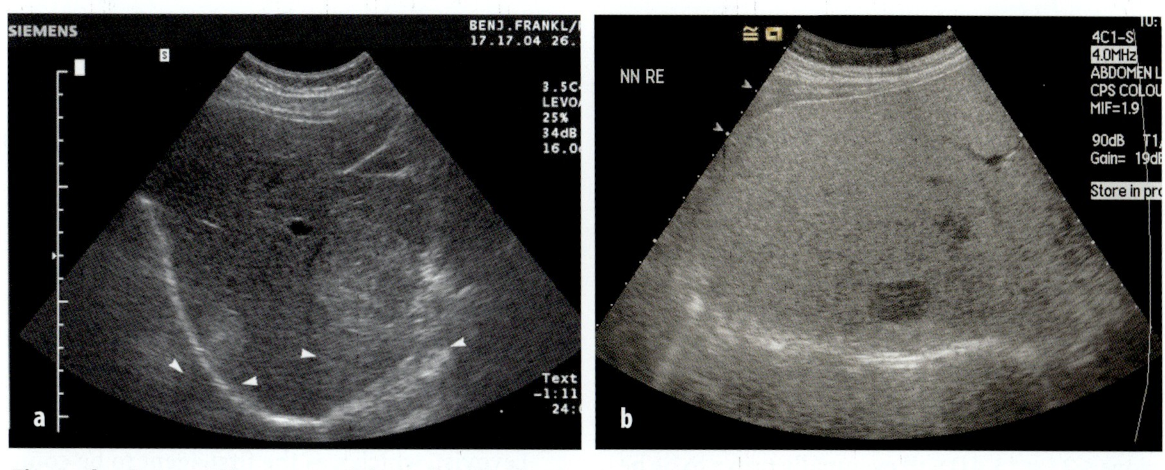

Fig. 4a, b. a Two typical homogeneously hyperechoic haemangiomas with posterior enhancement *(arrowheads)*. **b** Atypical hypoechoic haemangioma in a patient with a fatty liver and carcinoma of the prostate. The lesion is indistinguishable from a metastasis (cf. Fig. 1a)

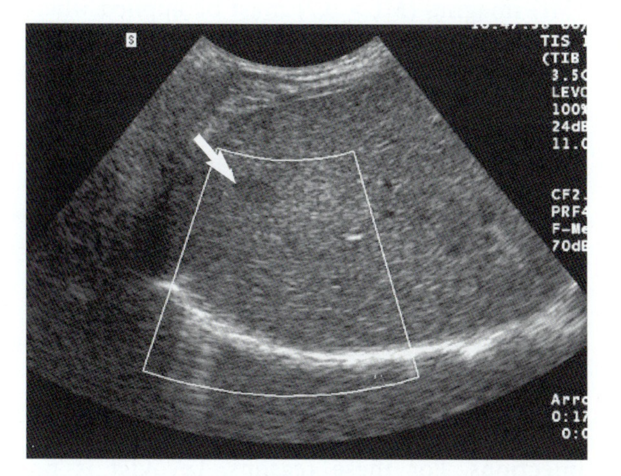

Fig. 5. Small hypoechoic FNH (*arrow*) indiscernible from metastasis

Focal fatty change presents as a hyperechoic area within the normal parenchyma and *focal fatty sparing* is a normal, relatively hypoechoic area in an otherwise hyperechoic fatty liver. Both lesion types are common in patients on chemotherapy. The size of the lesions may vary from less than a centimetre, to large areas covering several liver segments. Large areas of focal fatty change or sparing are readily diagnosed based on their characteristic 'geographical' or triangular shape without mass effect, while smaller lesions are often round or oval and are easily mistaken for metastases. A helpful differential diagnostic feature is their preponderance to occur at typical anatomical sites such as in segment IV at the insertion of the falciform ligament or in segment V near the main portal vein or the gallbladder fossa. On Doppler imaging, focal fatty change and sparing shows no abnormal vascularity and normal hepatic vessels crossing the lesion without displacement may be seen.

Multiple (fungal) *abscesses* sometimes occur in patients on chemotherapy (especially children) and they represent an important differential diagnosis of multiple lesions in patients on chemotherapy. Abscesses often do not have a typical cystic appearance, since their liquid portion contains corpuscular echogenic material. Their appearance can be identical to that of metastases, including the presence of a hypoechoic halo in fungal disease. Clinical signs and symptoms of infection may point towards the presence of an abscess.

Fatty Infiltration of the Liver and Metastases

Diffuse fatty infiltration of the liver, which often occurs during chemotherapy, can have substantial impact on US of focal liver lesions. On the one hand, it increases the reflectivity of the hepatic parenchyma and thus aids detection of lesions that would be isoechoic in a normal liver, and of hypoechoic lesions, since liver-to-lesion contrast is increased – one could call fatty infiltration a 'natural contrast agent'. On the other hand, severe fatty infiltration increases attenuation of sound by the liver and thus reduces penetration, which can obscure lesions in deeper liver areas. Further problems can occur when a small benign isoechoic lesion such as FNH or haemangioma, which remained undetected before chemotherapy, becomes visible as a 'new' hypoechoic lesion on follow-up. Such lesions are commonly misinterpreted as metastases (Fig. 4b).

Current Role and Limitations of Conventional US in Clinical Practice

As discussed above, there are no pathognomonic features of metastases on B-mode or colour Doppler and the differentiation of a single metastasis from other lesions is usually not possible. Such lesions are usually investigated further through the use of US contrast agents, other imaging modalities or sometimes biopsy. In a patient with a known primary malignancy, any focal liver lesion seen on unenhanced US must be regarded as suspicious of metastasis until proven otherwise. However, many lesions (25-50% of lesions ≤ 2 cm [3, 4]) will eventually prove to be benign, once contrast-enhanced US, other imaging tests or biopsy are used further to characterise the lesion.

The accuracy of unenhanced US for the assessment of hepatic metastases is lower than that of CEUS, CT and MRI. In series with true gold standard (intra-operative US or resection), its sensitivity ranges between 50% and 76% [8-12] (Table 2), which is considerably lower than that of CT and especially MRI. Problems of US for the detection of metastases are that the subdiaphragmatic areas of segments IVa and VIII are sometimes difficult to access and that there is poor liver-to-lesion contrast of almost isoechoic metastases, especially when small. For lesions smaller than 1 cm, the false negative rate is as high as 80% [9]. The false positive rate of US is in the order of 5-10% on a by patient basis and considerably higher on a lesion-by-lesion basis. For these reasons, CEUS, CT or MRI will be added to conventional US in most cancer patients for definitive liver staging, unless multiple metastases are clearly shown.

The role of US for follow-up of patients with hepatic metastases during chemotherapy is controversial. Its operator-dependant nature, and problems with reproducible image documentation limit its ability to clearly show small changes over time. In most cancer centres, CT or MRI are therefore preferred for follow-up imaging.

Contrast-Enhanced Ultrasound

Contrast Agents and Imaging Techniques

Two contrast agents are currently licensed for liver imaging in Europe: Levovist (Schering, Germany) and SonoVue (Bracco, Italy). The imaging technique varies according to the contrast agent chosen. Contrast-specific imaging modes exploiting non-linear bubble behaviour must be used with both agents to achieve clinically useful signal enhancement. Such imaging modes are now available on most medium and high end US systems.

Levovist, which was the first agent to be commercially available, has liver-specific properties during its late phase; this is advantageous for detection of metastases. High mechanical index (MI) imaging (MI > 0.7) must be applied when using Levovist. It provides signal enhancement due to strong non-linear signals from disrupting microbubbles. The disadvantage of this technique is the highly transient nature of the signals, which persist only for a few frames after insonation of an individual area, until the bubbles in the imaging plane are destroyed. To exploit the enhancement for clinical use, special scanning techniques such as rapid sweeping through the liver to image intact bubbles with each new frame or intermittent imaging have to be employed. Such scanning techniques are somewhat cumbersome and multiple sweeps through the liver are only possible with repeated injections. For these reasons, Levovist is no longer used on a large scale despite some very good results for detection and characterisation of focal liver lesions.

SonoVue, a more recent agent, provides strong and persistent signal enhancement due to its strong harmonic resonance at low (≤ 0.2) and very low (< 0.1) MI, where minimal or no bubble destruction occurs. This allows for continuous real-time imaging of a lesion during its vascular phase, as well as comprehensive surveying of the

Table 2. Sensitivity of conventional and contrast-enhanced US in detection of hepatic metastases; studies with true gold standard (IOUS ± resection) only

Author year	Contrast agent	No. patients	Sensitivity baseline	Sensitivity post-contrast
Clarke 1989 [8]	Only unenhanced	54	76%	-
Wernecke 1991 [9]	Only unenhanced	75	53%	-
Ohlson 1993 [10]	Only unenhanced	71	50%	-
Albrecht 2000 [11]	Levovist	35	70%	82%
Konopke 2005 [12]	SonoVue	56	53%	86%

liver in multiple planes during the delayed phase. Low MI imaging with SonoVue is now preferred in most instances, although it has weaker liver-specific properties than Levovist.

Several experimental agents such as Sonazoid (NC100100; Amersham Medical, UK) or BR14 (Bracco, Italy) combine the advantages of good enhancement at low MI with strong liver-specific properties. Early clinical studies have demonstrated the potential of such agents for detection of metastases. Unfortuna-tely, for commercial reasons, manufacturers are currently hesitant to continue the clinical development of such agents.

With real-time low MI imaging, the dynamic enhancement pattern and the vascular morphology of a lesion is assessed during the arterial (starting 10-20 seconds, and ending 25-53 seconds after injection) and portal-venous (starting 30-45 seconds and ending 120 seconds after injection) phases [13]. The delayed phase (> 2 minutes after injection) is particularly useful for detection of metastases as they show as non-enhancing defects. Characterisation is also improved by the late phase as the great majority of benign lesions show contrast up-take in this phase (see below).

Features of Metastases on Contrast-Enhanced Ultrasound

Metastases show characteristic dynamic features in all three phases after contrast injection (Figs. 6-8). All metastases have a predominantly arterial blood supply as opposed to a portal-venous one, but the degree of arterial perfusion is variable. Their appearance during the arterial phase of contrast-enhancement depends on the extent of arterial perfusion. Hypovascular metastases with relatively low arterial supply are common and typically occur in patients with adenocarcinoma or squamous cell carcinoma from gastrointestinal and other primaries. These lesions typically show rim enhancement of varying extents in the arterial phase. Hypervascular metastases are less common overall, they occur in patients with renal cell, thyroid or neuroendocrine carcinomas as well as with malignant melanoma and sarcoma and in about 25% of patients with breast cancer. During the arterial phase, hypervascular metastatic deposits show as homogeneously and strongly enhancing hyper-reflective and lesions, sometimes with non-enhancing necrotic areas. At the beginning of the portal-venous phase, the (rim) enhancement fades and the entire lesion becomes increasingly hyporeflective. In the delayed phase, both hypo- and hypervascular metastases almost invariably show as dark enhancement defects while the enhancement persists in normal liver parenchyma [7], independent of the contrast agent and imaging technique used. During the delayed phase metastases are often very well-defined, often with sharp, "punched out" borders (Figs. 7-10). Both portal-venous and delayed phase imaging markedly increase the contrast between the enhancing normal liver and the non-enhancing metastases and thus improve detection (Figs. 9, 10), see below for details.

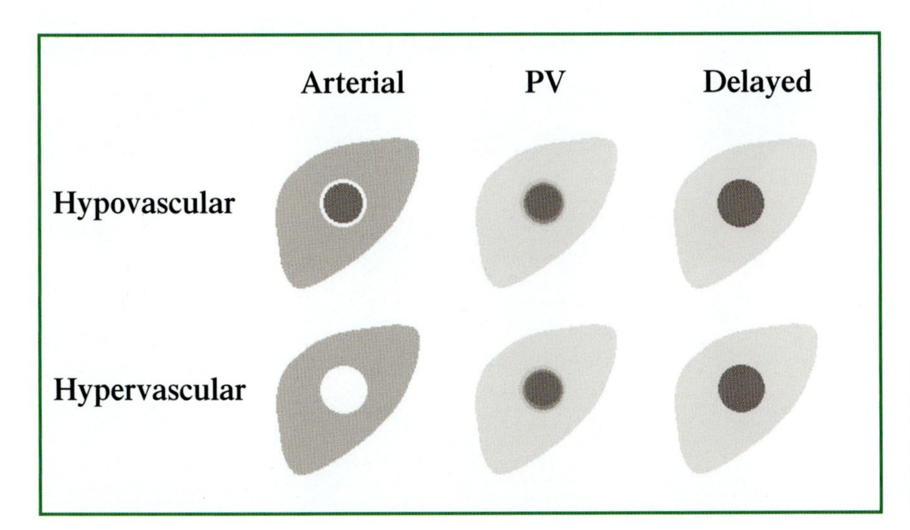

Fig. 6. Schematic display of the dynamic enhancement of hypo- and hypervascular metastases post-contrast injection during the arterial, portal-venous (PV) and delayed phase

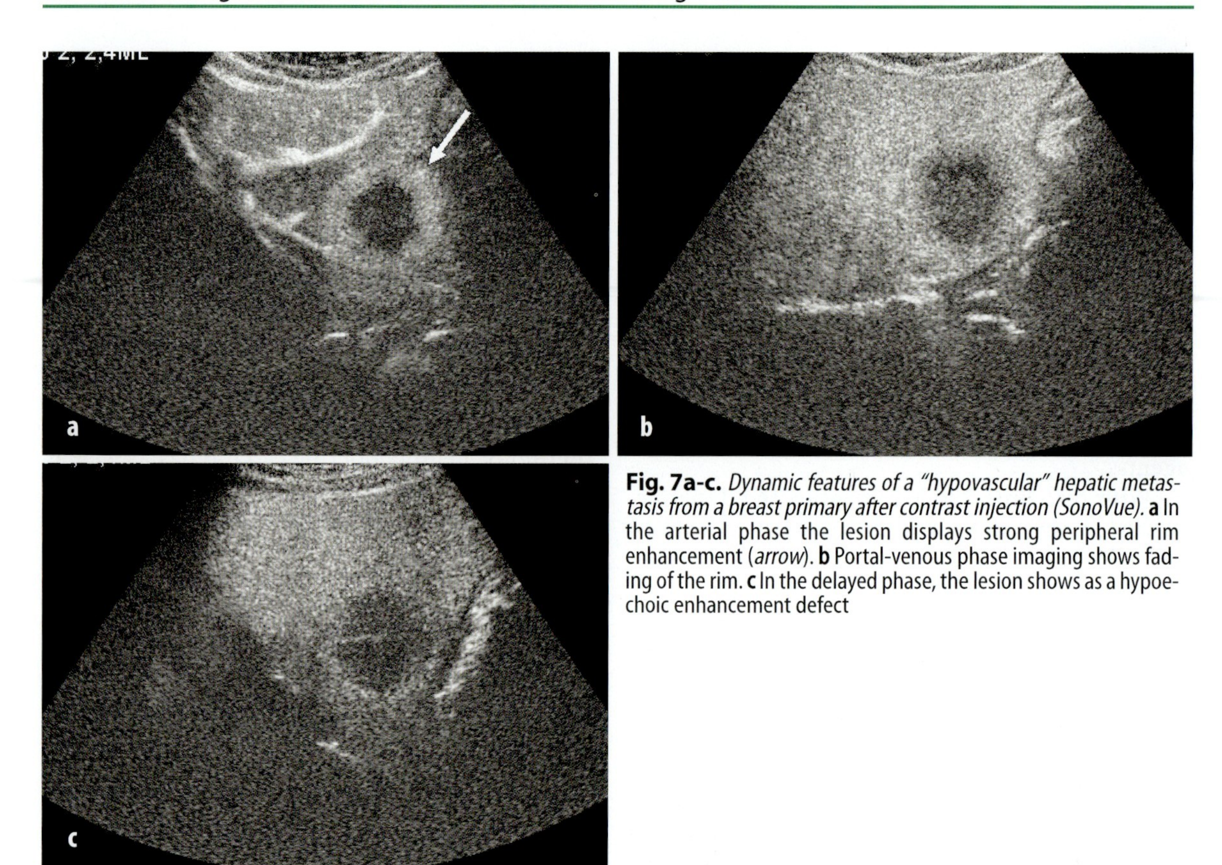

Fig. 7a-c. *Dynamic features of a "hypovascular" hepatic metastasis from a breast primary after contrast injection (SonoVue).* **a** In the arterial phase the lesion displays strong peripheral rim enhancement (*arrow*). **b** Portal-venous phase imaging shows fading of the rim. **c** In the delayed phase, the lesion shows as a hypoechoic enhancement defect

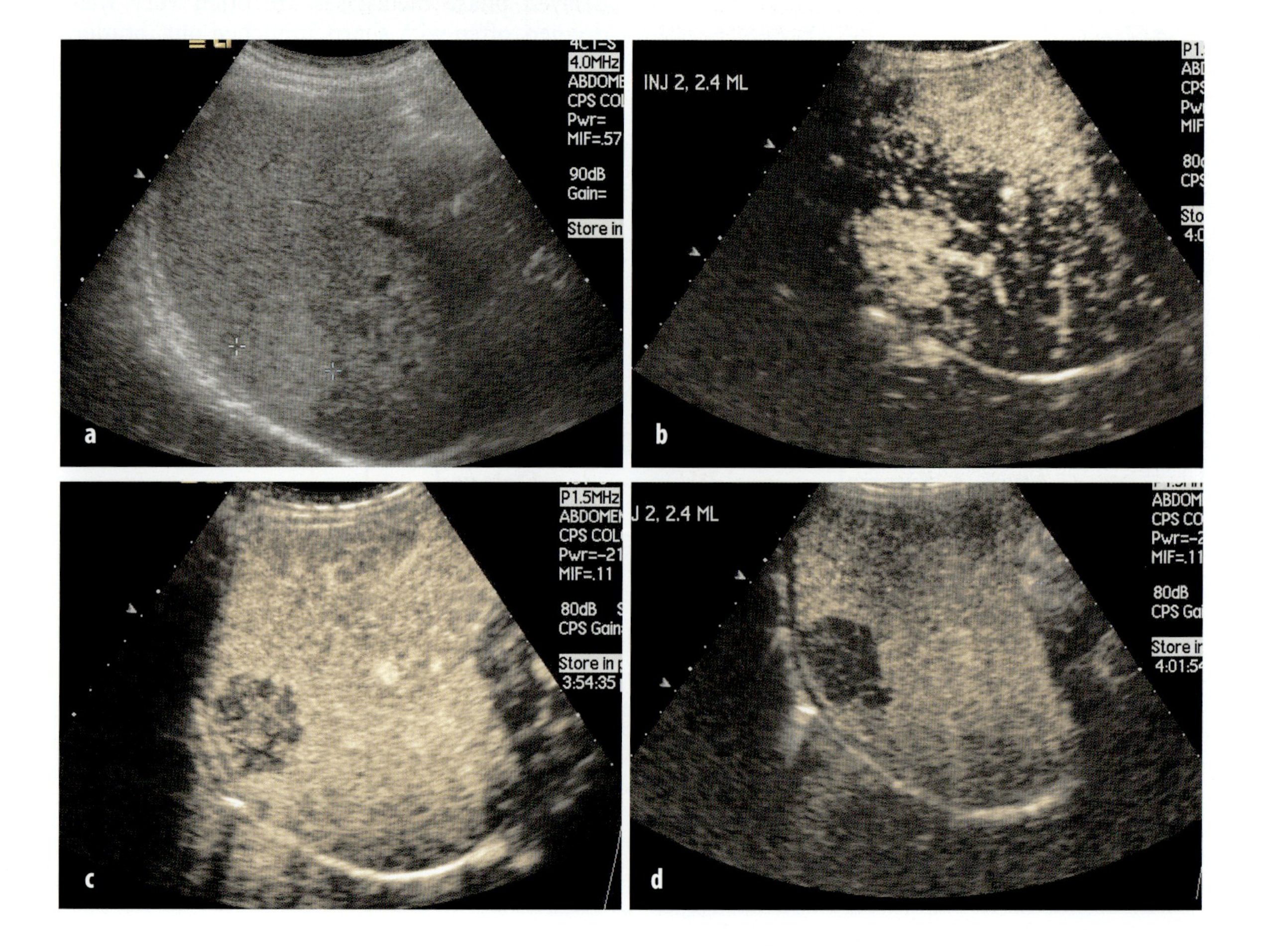

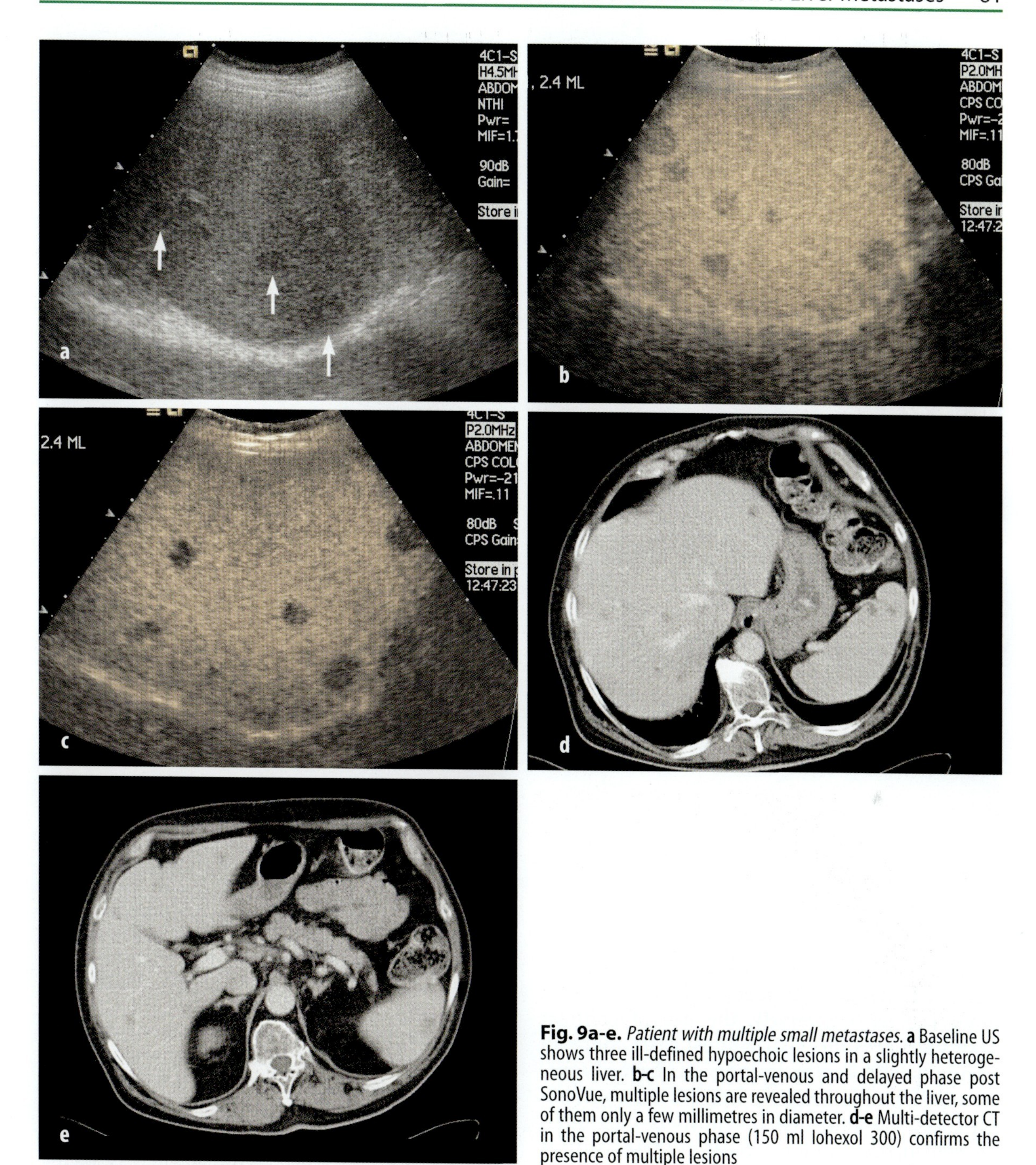

Fig. 9a-e. *Patient with multiple small metastases.* **a** Baseline US shows three ill-defined hypoechoic lesions in a slightly heterogeneous liver. **b-c** In the portal-venous and delayed phase post SonoVue, multiple lesions are revealed throughout the liver, some of them only a few millimetres in diameter. **d-e** Multi-detector CT in the portal-venous phase (150 ml Iohexol 300) confirms the presence of multiple lesions

← **Fig. 8a-d.** *Dynamic features of a "hypervascular" metastasis from a bronchogenic carcinoma after contrast injection (SonoVue).* **a** Conventional greyscale image shows a hyperechoic lesion. **b** During the arterial phase 18 seconds post injection, the lesion enhances homogenously while there is little contrast up-take by the liver parenchyma. **c** Portal-venous phase image (46 seconds post-injection) shows enhancement of normal liver and partial contrast wash-out from the lesion. **d** Delayed phase image (3:07 minutes post-injection) with persistent enhancement of the normal liver and complete contrast wash-out from the metastasis

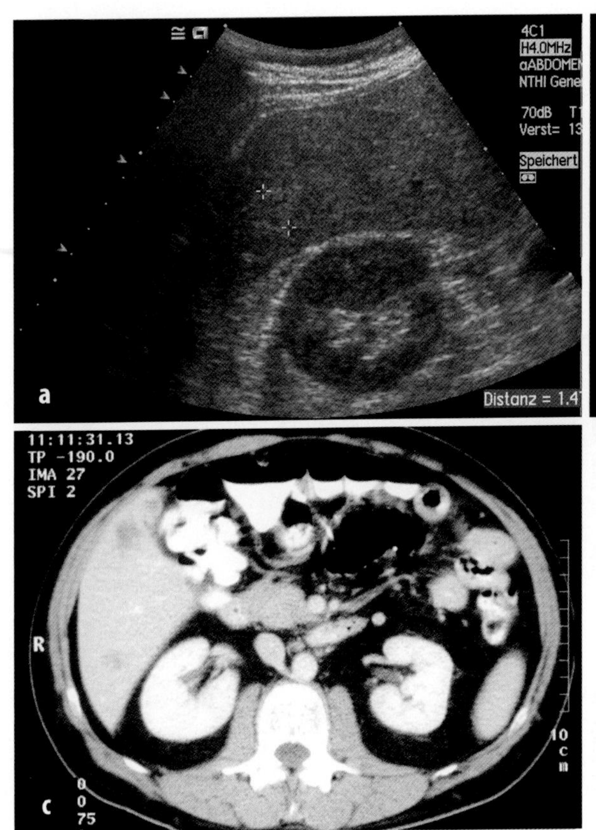

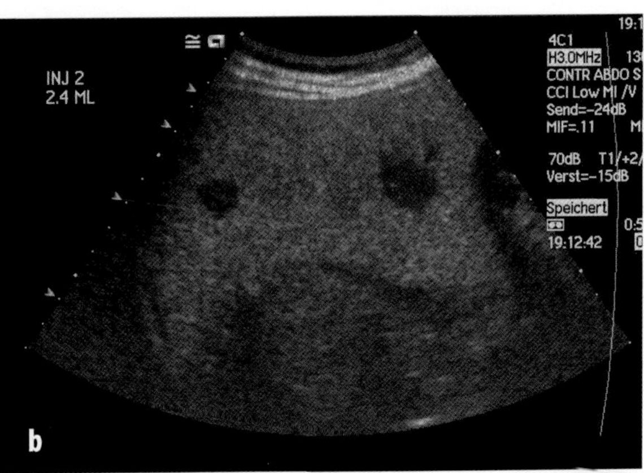

Fig. 10a-c. *Patient with colorectal carcinoma.* **a** Baseline US shows a nearly isoechoic lesion in Segment VI, measuring 1.5 cm. **b** In the delayed phase post SonoVue (2.5 minutes) the metastasis appears as a typical enhancement defect and is more easily visible. A second metastasis of 2 cm is now detected in segment V. **c** Spiral CT examination in portal-venous phase (150 ml Iohexol 300) confirms the presence of the two metastasis

Differential Diagnosis on Contrast-Enhanced US

As discussed above, unenhanced US is usually not able to reliably differentiate metastases from other lesions. Conversely, the use of contrast agents achieves this goal in most cases, since all common solid benign liver lesions have characteristic dynamic imaging features on contrast-enhanced US and their diagnosis is thus often unproblematic [7, 14-16]. Most of these features are analogous to those on dynamic CT and MRI.

Haemangiomas show a characteristic peripheral nodular arterial phase enhancement followed by gradual centripetal filling during the later phases (Fig. 11). The filling may be partial or complete. The speed of filling is size dependent: while small haemangiomas often fill within less than a minute, large lesions may take 5 minutes or more. The portal-venous and delayed enhancement of haemangiomas has been referred to as "lake-like". Many large haemangiomas will not fill completely and approximately 5-10% of smaller haemangiomas will show only minor peripheral filling (Fig. 12). This can lead to misinterpreted identification as metastases. In such instances it is important to carefully assess the arterial phase for peripheral nodular enhancement (haemangioma) versus rim enhancement (metastasis), although these can be confused in small lesions.

FNH appear as lesions with homogeneous enhancement in the arterial phase. In about 50% of FNH this is preceded by a typical spoke-wheel arterial pattern with centrifugal filling early in the arterial phase through a dominant feeding artery, lasting for a few seconds (Fig. 13). In the subsequent phases, the lesions show a similar degree of enhancement to the normal liver, due to the fact that they consist of a liver-like tissue. A non-enhancing central scar is frequently seen in larger FNH during the delayed phase (Fig. 13c). Delayed phase imaging is particularly useful for FNH, as they invariably show as isoechoic or hyperechoic lesions, often with a non-enhancing central scar that was previously invisible. They are thus easily differentiated from metastases. Small FNH especially may become completely occult in the delayed phase due to their liver-like contrast behaviour.

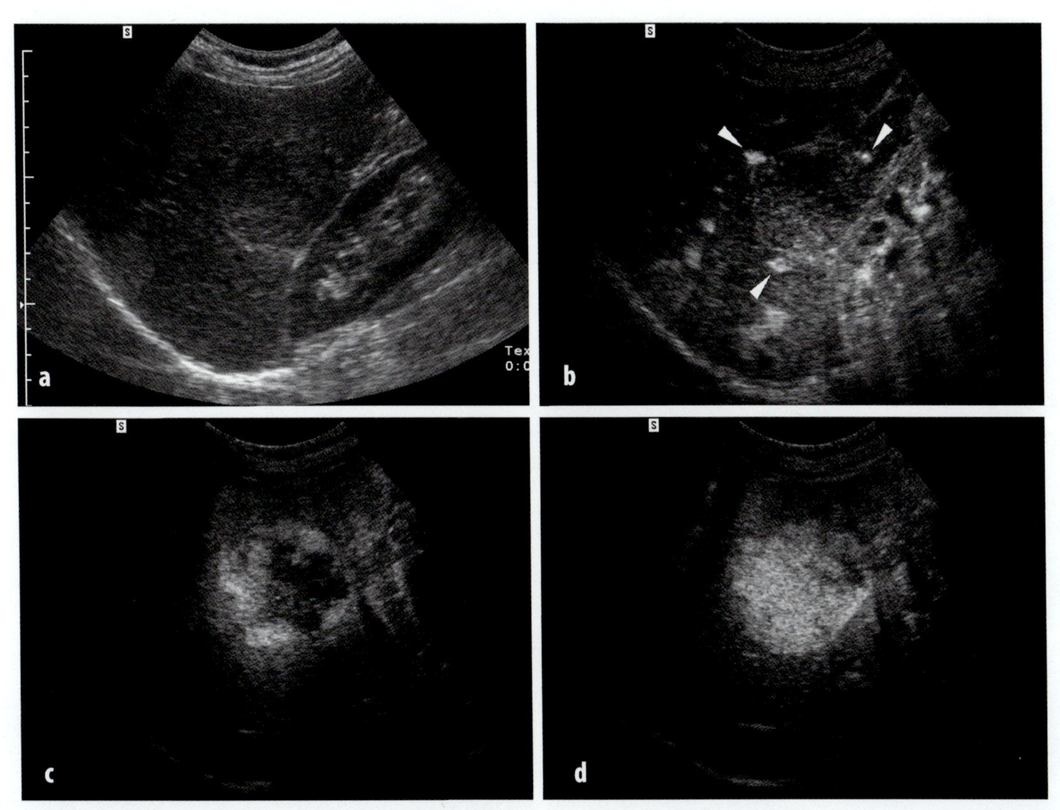

Fig. 11a-d. *Typical dynamic enhancement of a haemangioma using Sonazoid.* **a** Atypical baseline appearances: isoechoic lesion suspicious of metastases in a patient with colon carcinoma. **b** Arterial phase with peripheral nodular enhancement (*arrowheads*). **c** Partial centripedal fill-in in the portal-venous phase (45 seconds post injection). **d** Complete filling of the haemangioma in the delayed phase (3:30 minutes post-injection)

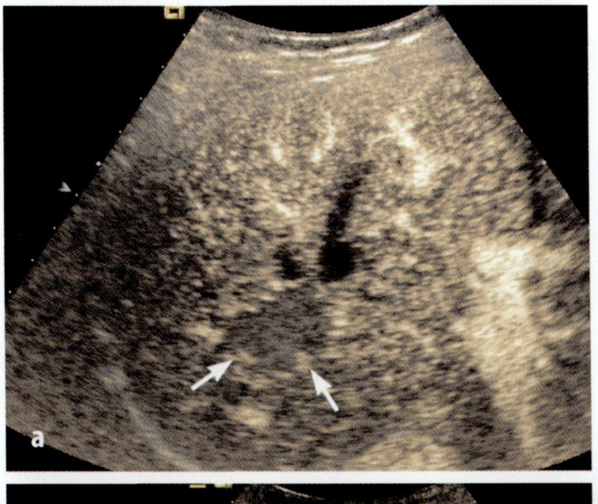

Fig. 12a-c. *Haemangioma with atypical partial filling after injection of SonoVue.* **a** Typical peripheral nodular enhancement (*arrows*) in the arterial phase. **b** Partial centripedal fill-in during the portal-venous phase. **c** No further filling of the haemangioma in the delayed phase. The centre of the lesion remains without contrast-enhancement throughout the entire examination. This can easily lead to confusion with metastases. The important differential diagnostic criterion is the arterial peripheral nodular enhancement typical of the haemangioma (versus rim enhancement, which is commonly seen in metastases)

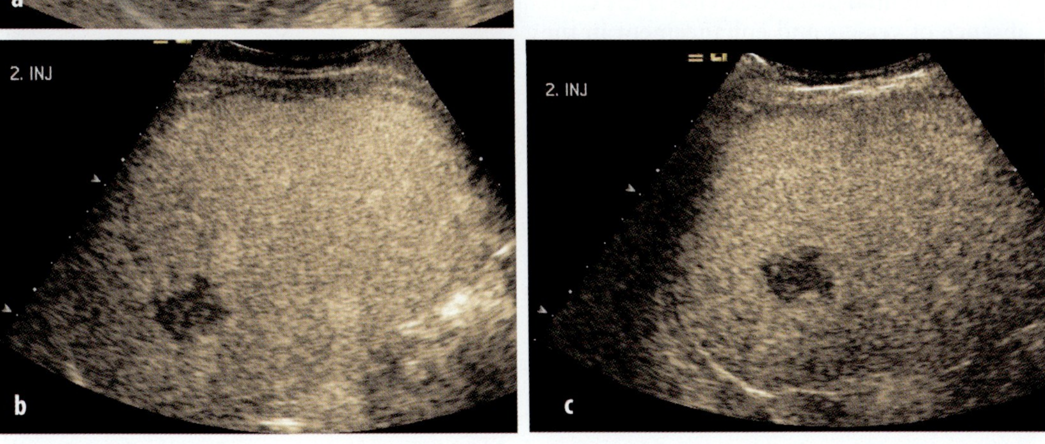

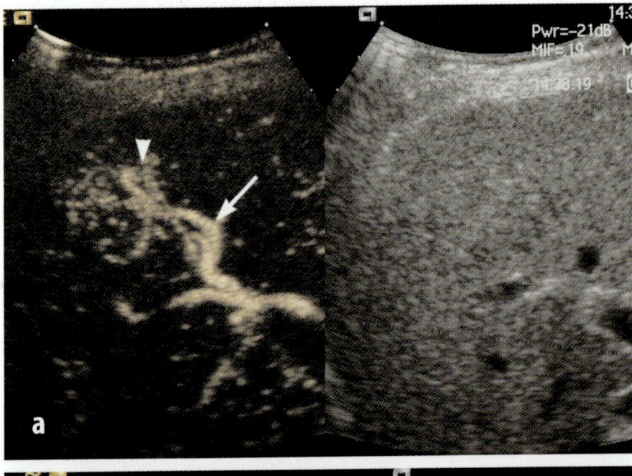

Fig. 13a-c. *Focal nodular hyperplasia post SonoVue.* **a** Large feeding artery (*arrow*) and spoke-wheel vascular pattern in the lesion (*arrowheads*) during the early arterial phase (14 seconds post injection). **b** Two seconds later the lesion is completely filled with contrast and appears hyperenhancing to normal liver. **c** In the portal-venous/delayed phase (2 minutes post injection) the lesion is isoenhancing to normal liver with the exception of a small hypoenhancing central scar (*arrowhead*)

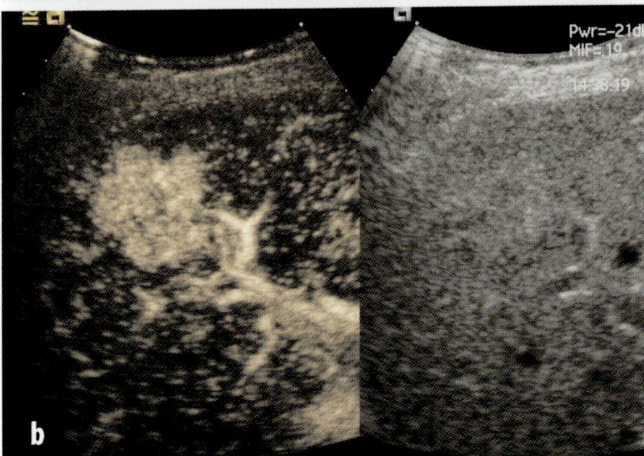

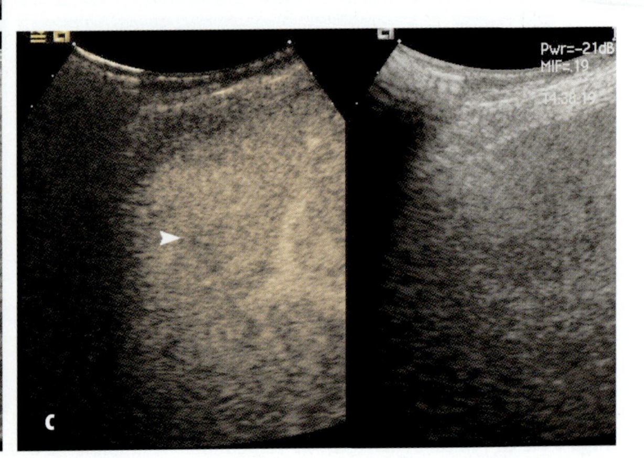

Focal fatty change and focal fatty sparing show the same contrast behaviour as normal liver parenchyma in all phases, since they contain no abnormal vessels and essentially consist of normal parenchyma. Normal vessels that cross the lesions without displacement are much more commonly seen than on conventional Doppler imaging, since much smaller vessels can be imaged. Again, these lesions usually disappear after contrast injection (Fig. 14).

Liver *abscesses* can be confused with metastases on CEUS since they also show rim enhancement in the arterial phase and produce enhancement defects in the subsequent phases. An important differential diagnostic clue is the complete absence of vessels and enhancement in the central liquid portion of an abscess, while even hypovascular metastases will display some weak but visible central enhancement due to small vessels, provided they are not necrotic.

Detection of Hepatic Metastases with CEUS

As with other imaging modalities, the use of contrast agents substantially improves the ability of US to detect liver metastases. As described above, metastases are seen as non-enhancing defects in an otherwise homogeneously enhancing liver in the portal-venous, and particularly in the delayed phase, after contrast injection. The impact on detection is most marked for small lesions below 1 cm in diameter (Fig. 9) and for lesions that are isoechoic on baseline US. On the other hand, small metastases are less readily detected than larger lesions even with the use of contrast agents and may still be missed.

The use of contrast agents improves the sensitivity of US in detection of individual lesions by about 20% in comparison to baseline, independent of the type of contrast agent used [11, 12, 17-20]. To the authors knowledge, only two studies with a real gold standard (intra-operative US ± resection) have been published [11, 12]: they showed a sensitivity of 82-86%, which is comparable to contrast-enhanced CT and MRI with non-specific Gadolinium chelates [21-24]. One of these studies compared CEUS and spiral CT and found that the detection rate of CEUS was almost identical to that of dual phase spiral CT (82% versus 80%) [11].

Specificity in diagnosing metastatic liver disease is also improved with USCA by up to 28% [18], since benign lesions show late phase enhancement similar to normal liver – independent of their arterial behaviour – and they

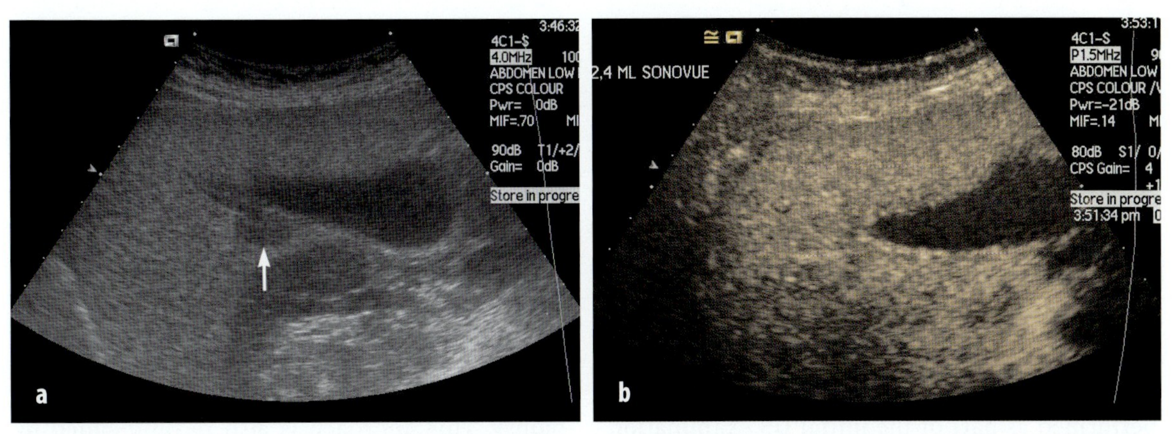

Fig. 14a, b. *Focal fatty sparing near the gallbladder in a patient with pharyngeal carcinoma.* **a** Unenhanced US shows a round hypoechoic lesion suggestive of a metastasis (*arrow*). **b** Homogeneous enhancement of the lesion in the delayed phase post SonoVue. The lesion is iso-enhancing to normal liver and becomes invisible

are thus usually not confused with metastases. Furthermore, equivocal findings such as focal areas of heterogeneous parenchyma on baseline US, which raise the possibility of metastases, can be assessed further with contrast agents. If homogeneous enhancement is seen, metastases can be ruled out.

Limitations of CEUS

Some of the limitations of baseline US also apply to CEUS. If sonographic visualisation of some parts of the liver is poor due to obesity or otherwise unfavourable anatomy, this will not improve with the use of contrast agents. This is particularly true for subcapsular regions near the dome of the diaphragm.

Penetration of contrast-specific imaging modes is usually limited to 12-15 cm. This may not be insufficient for full visualisation of the deep parts of the liver in larger patients, even if low frequencies are used. Scanning the patient on the left side is very helpful in order to overcome this limitation, as the liver moves forward towards the transducer at the anterior abdominal wall in this position. Fatty change of the liver aggravates the problem of limited penetration and in severe fatty infiltration, large parts of the liver may not be assessable by CEUS. Other imaging modalities should be used in such patients.

Current Role of CEUS in Clinical Practice

Contrast agents have greatly enhanced the role of US for liver imaging in oncology patients. There are two main indications for the use of contrast agents in this patient group: detection of metastases and characterisation of uncertain lesions.

Detection

According to the guidelines of the European Federation of Societies for Ultrasound in Medicine and Biology (EFSUMB) for the use of contrast agents in US [13], contrast agents should be used in 'all liver ultrasound scans to rule out metastases, unless conventional ultrasound shows clear evidence of these lesions'. This recommendation reflects the substantial improvement in sensitivity and the fact that the sensitivity of unenhanced US is too low to rule out metastases. Conventional US without contrast agents now has to be regarded as inadequate for ruling out metastases. The use of contrast agents is also recommended by the EFSUMB guidelines 'in selected cases, when clinically relevant for treatment planning, to assess the number and location of liver metastases as a complement to CT and/or MRI', since CEUS may show lesions that were missed by other imaging modalities. This obviously has important implications for planning of liver resection or local ablation. It is important to remember that CEUS is complementary to CT and/or MRI in such patients, and that it cannot replace the other modalities in the pre-operative or pre-interventional work-up, since CT and MRI give more comprehensive information about the liver and all other abdominal organs, including lymph nodes and peritoneum. The maximum information should be sought in these patients by combining several modalities. CT and/or MRI can, however, be replaced by CEUS for liver staging in patients with extra-abdominal tumours such as breast carcinoma, who usually do not require comprehensive abdominal imaging beyond the liver.

Characterisation

As discussed above, CEUS is ideally suited to characterise liver tumours in cancer patients, in whom 50-75% of lesions ≤ 2 cm represent metastases, while the remainder is benign. CEUS should be the first-line modality for the evaluation of lesions seen on baseline US. It should be performed as part of the initial US examination and, in most cases, it will provide a definitive lesion diagnosis. This approach avoids further imaging such as MRI or CT in many patients, especially when dealing with a benign lesion. It spares the patient from psychological stress while waiting for another examination. It is also cost-effective and makes the best use of the resources of a health care system, since the added cost of USCA is lower than that of an additional CT and especially of an MRI examination. CEUS can also be very useful in patients with a lesion that cannot be characterised on CT or even MRI. Not infrequently, such lesions can be characterised on CEUS, sparing the patient a biopsy. This approach is also recommended by the EFSUMB guidelines.

Key Points

- Conventional US without contrast agents is limited in its ability to detect metastases and to differentiate metastases from benign lesions.
- USCA substantially improves the ability of US to visualise metastases and thus increases the sensitivity of US for the detection of metastases, to a level that is comparable to spiral CT.
- CEUS provides reliable differentiation between metastases and benign lesions in most cases.
- USCA should be used in all oncology patients undergoing sonographic liver staging, unless metastases are clearly demonstrated by unenhanced US.

References

1. Edmunson H, Craig J (1987) Neoplasms of the liver. In: Schiff L (ed) Diseases of the liver. 8th ed, Lippincott, Philadelphia, p 1109
2. Karhunen PJ (1986) Benign hepatic tumours and tumour like conditions in men. J Clin Pathol 39:183-188
3. Jones EC, Chezmar JL, Nelson RC, Bernardino ME (1992) The frequency and significance of small (less than or equal to 15 mm) hepatic lesions detected by CT. AJR Am J Roentgenol 158:535-539
4. Kreft B, Pauleit D, Bachmann R, Conrad R, Kramer A, Schild HH. Häufigkeit und Bedeutung von kleinen fokalen Leberläsionen (2001) Rofo Fortschr Geb Rontgenstr Neuen Bildgeb Verfahr 173:424-429
5. Ishak KG, Rabin L (1975) Benign tumors of the liver. Med Clin North Am 59:995-1013
6. Wanless IR, Albrecht S, Bilbao J et al (1989) Multiple focal nodular hyperplasia of the liver associated with vascular malformations of various organs and neoplasia of the brain: a new syndrome. Mod Pathol 2:456-462
7. Hohmann J, Skrok J, Puls R, Albrecht T (2003) Characterization of focal liver lesions with contrast-enhanced low MI real time ultrasound and SonoVue. Rofo Fortschr Geb Rontgenstr Neuen Bildgeb Verfahr 175:835-843
8. Clarke MP, Kane RA, Steele G Jr et al (1989) Prospective comparison of preoperative imaging and intraoperative ultrasonography in the detection of liver tumors. Surgery 106:849-855
9. Wernecke K, Rummeny E, Bongartz G et al (1991) Detection of hepatic masses in patients with carcinoma: comparative sensitivities of sonography, CT, and MR imaging. AJR Am J Roentgenol 157:731-739
10. Ohlsson B, Tranberg KG, Lundstedt C et al (1993) Detection of hepatic metastases in colorectal cancer: a prospective study of laboratory and imaging methods. Eur J Surg 159:275-281
11. Albrecht T, Hoffmann C, Schmitz S et al (2000) Detection of liver metastases: comparison of contrast-enhanced phase inversion ultrasound and dual phase spiral CT with intraoperative sonographic correlation. Radiology 207:459
12. Konopke R, Kersting S, Saeger HD, Bunk A (2005) Detection of liver lesions by contrast-enhanced ultrasound - comparison to intraoperative findings. Ultraschall Med 26:107-113
13. Albrecht T, Blomley M, Bolondi L et al (2004) Guidelines for the use of contrast agents in ultrasound. Ultraschall Med 25:249-256

14. Dietrich CF, Ignee A, Trojan J et al (2004) Improved characterisation of histologically proven liver tumours by contrast-enhanced ultrasonography during the portal-venous and specific late phase of SHU 508A. 53:401-405
15. Strobel D, Raeker S, Martus P et al (2003) Phase inversion harmonic imaging versus contrast-enhanced power Doppler sonography for the characterization of focal liver lesions. Int J Colorectal Dis 18:63-72
16. Quaia E, Calliada F, Bertolotto M et al (2004) Characterization of focal liver lesions with contrast-specific US modes and a sulfur hexafluoride-filled microbubble contrast agent: diagnostic performance and confidence. Radiology 232:420-430
17. Albrecht T, Hoffmann CW, Schmitz SA et al (2001) Phase-inversion sonography during the liver-specific late phase of contrast-enhancement: improved detection of liver metastases. AJR Am J Roentgenol 176:1191-1198
18. Albrecht T, Blomley MJ, Burns PN et al (2003) Improved detection of hepatic metastases with pulse-inversion US during the liver-specific phase of SHU 508A: multicenter study. Radiology 227:361-370
19. Oldenburg A, Hohmann J, Foert E et al (2005) Detection of hepatic metastases with low MI real time contrast-enhanced sonography and SonoVue. Ultraschall Med 26:277-284
20. Bernatik T, Becker D, Neureiter D et al (2003) Detection of liver metastases–comparison of contrast–enhanced ultrasound using first versus second generation contrast agents. Ultraschall Med 24:175-179
21. Blakeborough A, Ward J, Wilson D et al (1997) Hepatic lesion detection at MR imaging: a comparative study with four sequences. Radiology 203:759-765
22. Soyer P, Levesque M, Caudron C et al (1993) MRI of liver metastases from colorectal cancer vs. CT during arterial portography. J Comput Assist Tomogr 17:67-74
23. Valls C, Andia E, Sanchez A et al (2001) Hepatic metastases from colorectal cancer: preoperative detection and assessment of resectability with helical CT. Radiology 218:55-60
24. Ward J, Naik KS, Guthrie JA et al (1999) Hepatic lesion detection: comparison of MR imaging after the administration of superparamagnetic iron oxide with dual-phase CT by using alternative-free response receiver operating characteristic analysis. Radiology 210:459-466

II.4

Guidance of Percutaneous Tumor Ablation Procedures

Luigi Solbiati, Massimo Tonolini and Tiziana Ierace

Introduction

Diagnostic imaging plays a key role in all steps of radiofrequency (RF) tumor ablation. It is used in the following ways:

1) detection of lesions and selection of patients for treatment;
2) targeting of lesions and guidance of the procedure;
3) immediate assessment of treatment results;
4) long-term follow-up.

Conventional, unenhanced ultrasound (US) is widely employed for screening liver disease, but variable sensitivity and well-known drawbacks limit its role in the staging of liver tumors. Furthermore, sonography represents the most commonly used imaging modality for the guidance of percutaneous ablative treatments owing to its availability, rapidity and ease of use. Differentiation of induced necrosis from a viable tumor is not possible with baseline and color Doppler sonography and therefore the immediate and long-term assessment of the therapeutic result is usually accomplished by contrast-enhanced helical computer tomography (CT) and magnetic resonance (MR).

In our experience, the use of contrast-enhanced ultrasound (CEUS) represents a significant improvement over conventional US for each of above-mentioned steps and has proven useful in achieving optimal patient management and treatment results [1].

Detection of Lesions and Selection of Patients

A wide range of treatment options is currently available for both primary and metastatic liver tumors. Therefore, timely detection and accurate quantification of neoplastic involvement at the time of diagnosis or during the course of the disease allows optimal patient management and treatment selection and may ultimately result in prolonged survival and possibly cure.

Adequate local tumor control is feasible with percutaneous RF ablation, provided that correct indications are respected. In most institutions patients with chronic hepatitis or cirrhosis without functional liver decompensation, portal thrombosis or extrahepatic tumor spread may undergo RF of one to four/five dysplastic lesions and/or hepatocellular carcinoma foci each not exceeding 4-4.5 cm. Hepatomas larger than 5 cm are usually treated by means of combined therapies (trans-arterial chemoembolization, ethanol injection, radiofrequency) [2-4]. Effective ablation of liver metastases requires the creation of a 0.5-1 cm 'safety margin' of ablated peritumoral liver tissue in order to destroy microscopical infiltrating tumor and therefore limit the incidence of local recurrence. In patients with previous radical treatment for colorectal, breast or other primary tumors, RF treatment is feasible when up to five liver metastases are present, each one not exceeding 3.0-3.5 cm in size [5-10].

Cross-sectional imaging modalities such as multiphasic contrast-enhanced helical CT and dynamic gadolinium-enhanced MR represent the mainstay for the staging of hepatic and extra-hepatic neoplastic involvement, whereas the use of hepatobiliary and reticuloendothelial-specific MR contrast agents may be helpful to maximize lesion detection in selected patients [11, 12].

The 'gold standard' for the detection of focal liver lesions is undoubtedly represented by intraoperative ultrasound (IOUS). Unenhanced B-mode US is cheap, fast, widely available and therefore commonly used for the screening of focal lesions in patients with chronic liver disease or with a history of cancer. Liver metastases display an extremely varied sonographic appearance, even within the same patient, as well as during the course of therapy [13].

The sensitivity of US is significantly affected by the operator's experience and available equipment, poor acoustic window due patient's body habitus and bowel gas distention, enlargement and inhomogeneity of the liver parenchyma due to steatosis, fibrosis, chronic liver disease and post-chemotherapeutic changes.

The rate of detection of hepatic metastases with unenhanced US is lower than that of CT and MR: reported sensivity ranges from 63% and 85%. The sensitivity of US is particularly poor for smaller focal lesions (less than 1 cm). Moreover, only limited characterization of focal liver lesions is possible with baseline US [13].

Contrast-enhanced ultrasound (CEUS) has proven to be a valuable tool to overcome the limitations of conventional US and to increase the detection of focal lesions for accurate disease staging [1, 13].

Contrast-specific US software systems (e.g., Pulse Inversion, Phase Inversion, Contrast-Tuned Imaging, Coherent Contrast Imaging, Contrast Pulse Sequencing) recently developed by the major US companies and all based upon the principle of wideband harmonic sonography, displaying microbubble enhancement in gray scale with optimal contrast and spatial resolution, allowed the evaluation of the microcirculation, thus prompting the evolution of CEUS from vascular imaging to tissue perfusion imaging [14].

Many authors employed CEUS examination in the late liver-specific phase 2-5 minutes after the administration of an air-based first generation contrast agent such as Levovist. Malignant tumors appear as hypoechoic defects in the brightly enhanced liver parenchyma, achieving both an increase in lesion conspicuity - particularly for infracentimetric lesions - and better characterization of lesions as malignant. Improvement in sensitivity for the detection of individual metastases was reported from 63-71% to 87-91%. Still, the examination has limited value in the deepest portions of the liver and in patients with an unsatisfactory sonographic window [15-18].

Second generation microbubble contrast agents such as SonoVue (sulphur hexafluoride) have higher harmonic emission capabilities and prolonged longevity. Their use, coupled with very low acoustic power (mechanical index (MI) values 0.1-0.2) that limits microbubble destruction, allows a continuous-mode CEUS examination. Signals from stationary tissues are cancelled and only harmonic frequencies generated by microbubbles are visualized. This imaging modality enables the display of both macro- and microcirculation: the enhancement is displayed in real-time over the arterial, early/full portal and delayed phases. The motion or color blooming artifacts characteristic of color and power Doppler sonography are not present. Although SonoVue has no liver-specific accumulation, significant enhancement persists in the liver parenchyma 4-5 minutes after the injection [1].

In our experience, continuous-mode CEUS can significantly improve the accuracy of US for the detection, characterization and staging of liver tumors, reaching very high sensitivity for the detection of both hyper- and hypo-vascular liver malignancies. In particular, in cancer patients, there is an increased conspicuity of small hypovascular metastases, with detection of satellite and additional previously invisible lesions, thus leading to a modification in the therapeutic approach, with exclusion of treatment in 25% of patients.

Given these capabilities of CEUS, to date in our institution, before performing ablative therapies, adequate diagnostic work-up includes laboratory tests and tumor markers along with conventional and contrast-enhanced US and at least one cross-sectional imaging modality (CT and/or MRI) are performed no more than 1 week prior to the therapeutic session.

Targeting of Lesions and Guidance of RF Ablation Treatment

Considerating its advantages, including nearly universal availability, portability, ease of use and low cost, US represents the modality of choice for the guidance of percutaneous interventional procedures. Quick and convenient real-time visualization of electrode positioning is a characteristic feature of sonography, whereas the same procedure may be cumbersome in CT and MR environments.

At our institution, pre-treatment CEUS examination is repeated as the initial step of the RF ablation session during the induction of anesthesia, in order to reproduce mapping of lesions as shown on CT/MRI examinations. Images and/or movie clips are again digitally stored to be compared with immediate post-ablation study.

Continuous-mode CEUS allows real-time targeting of lesions, that means precise needle insertion performed during the specific phase of maximum lesion conspicuity - in the arterial phase for highly vascularized lesions such as hepatocellular carcinoma and hypervascular metastases, and in the portal or equilibrium phases for hypovascular lesions such as colorectal and breast cancer metastases.

Real-time guidance of needle positioning during CEUS does not significantly prolong the total duration of the RF ablation session. In our opinion, this approach is mandatory for:

- small HCCs detected by CT/MR but not visible with unenhanced US against an inhomogeneous cirrhotic liver parenchyma: these lesions may be only reached during the transient arterial phase of CEUS in which they appear as hyperenhancing foci [19];
- small, usually infracentimetric hypovascular metastases, barely or not perceptible with unenhanced US but clearly evident as focal hypoenhancing nodules in the portal or late phase of CEUS;
- areas of residual untreated or locally recurrent tumor, both primary and metastatic: unenhanced US almost always cannot differentiate between coagulation necrosis and viable tumor, but the difference is usually straightforward during CEUS, in which viable tumor displays its native, characteristic enhancement pattern and coagulation necrosis is avascular.

Assessment of Treatment Results

Local treatment of neoplastic liver lesions with the application of radiofrequency ablation induces the formation of coagulation necrosis. Obtaining adequate necrosis and therefore effective tumor eradication may be limited by inhomogeneity of heat deposition and by the cooling effect of blood flow [20].

During the treatment, a progressively increasing hyperechogenic 'cloud' corresponding to gas microbubble formation and tissue vaporization appears around the distal probe and may persist for some minutes. B-mode sonographic findings observed during and after RF energy application (mostly the diameter of the hyperechoic region) represent only a rough estimate of the extent of induced coagulation necrosis and therefore are not useful to reliably assess treatment completeness [20, 21]. Similarly, color-flow and power Doppler US are unreliable to evaluate the adequacy of treatment of hepatocellular carcinomas treated with RF ablation. Furthermore, additional repositioning of electrodes may be hindered by the hyperechoic focus.

Assessment of the size of the induced coagulation necrosis and therefore of the completeness of the tumor ablation is usually accomplished for both hepatoma and for metastatic lesions by means of contrast-enhanced helical CT or MRI. Being practically unfeasible when ablations are performed in the interventional room, biphasic CT (or less frequently dynamic MRI) are performed on the first day or within one week of the RF ablation session and compared with baseline examinations to differentiate between treated regions and residual viable tumor requiring additional treatment [20]. Findings with both modalities can predict the extent of coagulation area to within 2-3 mm, as radiologic-pathologic correlation demonstrated in experimental and clinical studies [22].

Imaging features on immediate post-treatment CT/MR examinations, along with patterns of complete and partial necrosis, are discussed elsewhere in this book.

Most reported series demonstrate a high rate of apparently complete tumor necrosis on initial post-ablation evaluation, but local recurrences occur frequently and probably result from a lack of radicality [19, 23]. The achievement of incomplete tumor necrosis determines the need for additional treatment sessions with associated patient discomfort and increased costs.

Furthermore, delayed retreatment is often technically difficult owing to the unreliable discrimination of active tumor from coagulation necrosis with unenhanced sonography against an inhomogeneous liver parenchyma, due to chronic liver disease, steatosis and the presence of previously treated areas. Effective targeting of residual tumor foci is often impossible and retreatment has a higher failure rate [19, 24].

Therefore, imaging strategies that enable rapid assessment of the extent of tissue destruction induced by thermal ablation are desirable. Since the ablative treatment leads to the disruption of tumor vascularity, the demonstration of disappearance of any previously visualized vascular enhancement inside and at the periphery of the tumor by means of contrast-enhanced imaging methods is the hallmark of complete treatment of a focal liver tumor [25].

Since the introduction of first-generation ultrasound contrast agents, the use of microbubbles has allowed better depiction of microcirculation and parenchymal blood flow compared with conventional color and power Doppler. Initial experiences with enhanced color and power Doppler imaging addressed the evaluation of response of hepatocellular carcinoma to interventional treatments, including RF ablation. Better differentiation between perfused and non-perfused tissue and accurate detection of persistent viable HCC after ablation, compared with conventional color and power Doppler was demonstrated [26, 27]. Similarly, our group demonstrated that enhanced color/power Doppler sonography could detect residual tumor immediately after RF ablation of liver metastases, enabling repeated treatment sessions in some cases [28].

More recently, CEUS has been employed to reveal residual enhancement after ablation and has demonstrated optimal agreement and comparable accuracy in respect to helical CT, adopted as the 'gold standard' after different treatment modalities (percutaneous ethanol injection (PEI), transcatheter arterial chemoembolization (TACE), RF) for hepatocellular carcinoma [29, 30]. Meloni et al. [31] calculated an increase in sensitivity from 9.3% with contrast-enhanced power Doppler to 23.3% with pulse inversion CEUS for the detection of residual HCC after RF ablation.

In our protocol, immediate post-ablation evaluation using continuous-mode CEUS is performed 5 to 10 minutes after the assumed completion of the RF session, with the patient still under general anesthesia, employing a second generation contrast agent (SonoVue, Bracco, Milan, Italy) (Figs. 1-3). Comparison of immediate post-ablation images with stored pre-ablation scans is necessary. As visible on contrast-enhanced CT and MRI, a thin and uniform enhancing rim corresponding to reactive hyperemia may surround the periphery of the necrotic area.

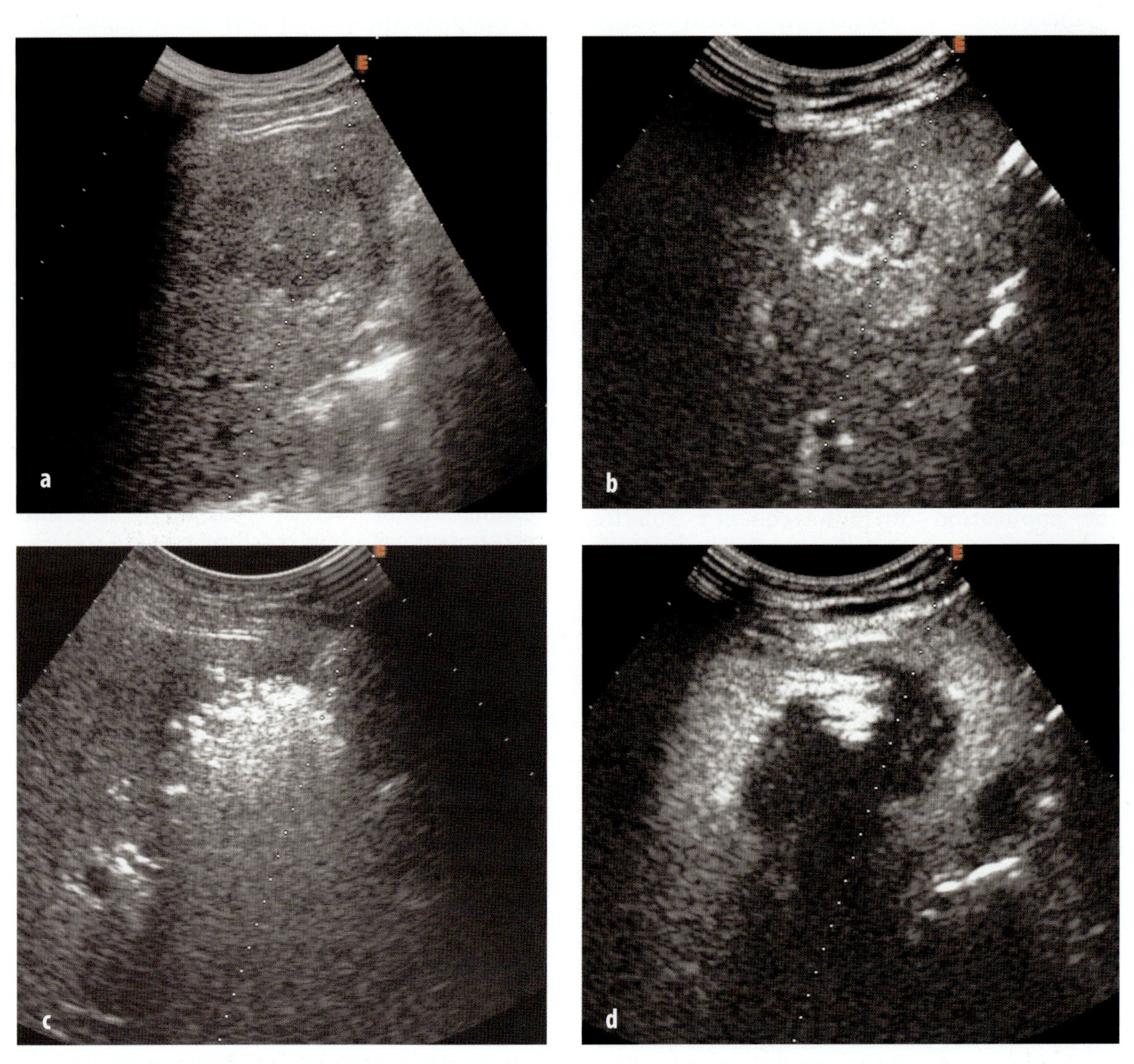

Fig. 1a-d. An hepatocellular carcinoma of 3.2 cm in size detected with B-mode US in segment VI in a patient with HCV-related cirrhosis (**a**). CEUS in arterial phase (**b**) shows poor and inhomogeneous enhancement of the lesion with ill-defined margins. At the end of the RF ablation treatment with single insertion of a cool-tip electrode, the tumor appears markedly hyperechoic due to the presence of gas produced by the ablation process (**c**). Five minutes after withdrawing the RF electrode, CEUS was repeated (**d**) and an oval, non-enhancing area, much larger than the treated HCC (meaning complete necrosis) was seen. The small hyperechoic area (formed by non-moving echoes) visible in the anterior portion of the necrotic lesion is due to residual post-ablation gas

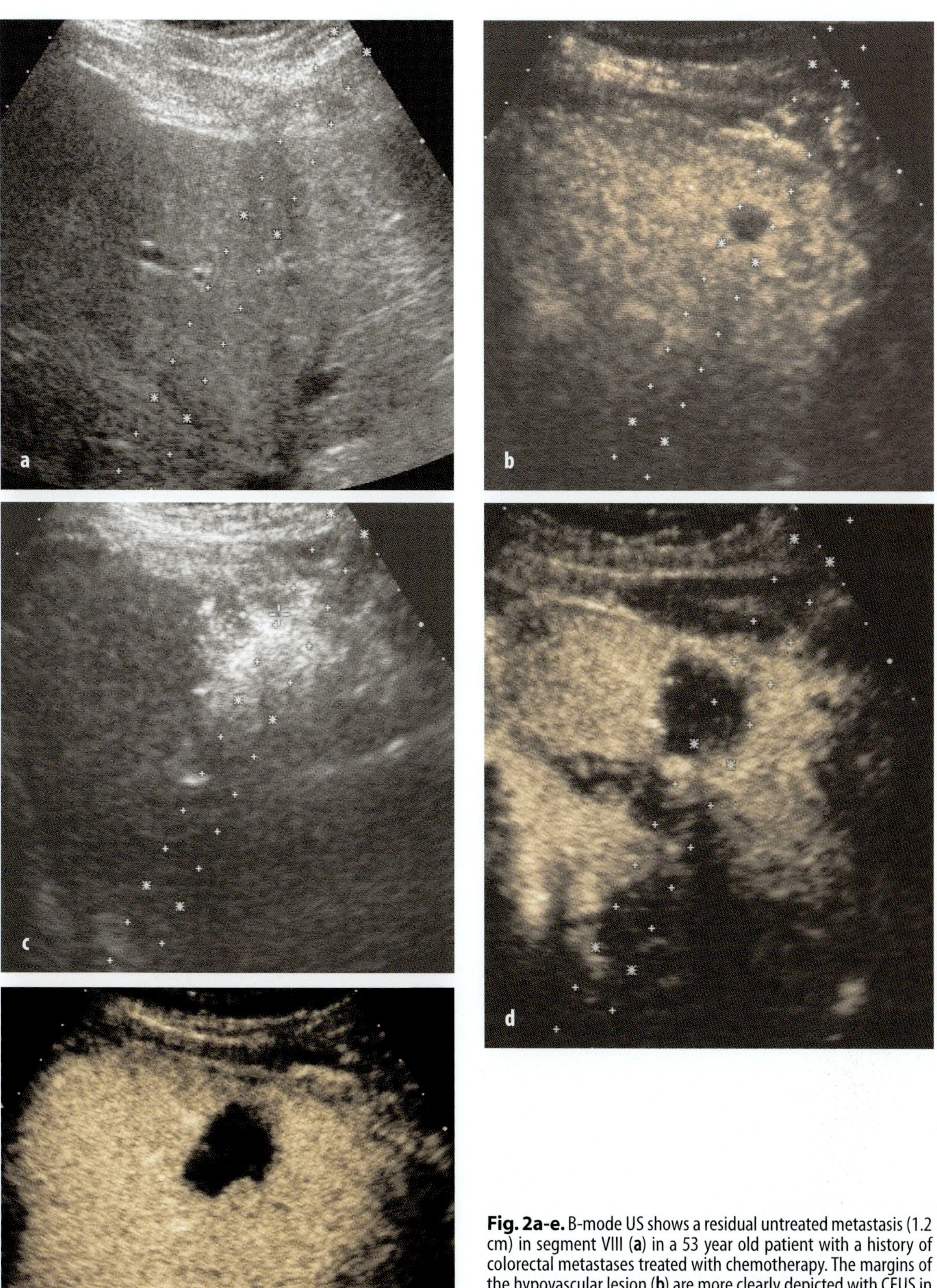

Fig. 2a-e. B-mode US shows a residual untreated metastasis (1.2 cm) in segment VIII (**a**) in a 53 year old patient with a history of colorectal metastases treated with chemotherapy. The margins of the hypovascular lesion (**b**) are more clearly depicted with CEUS in portal phase. RF ablation was performed with single insertion of cool-tip electrode. B-mode US shows a large hyperechoic area of gas formation (**c**). Six minutes after the end of the RF ablation, repeat CEUS in portal phase shows a non-enhancing area of coagulative necrosis larger in size than the metastatic lesion (**d**). In a three month follow-up study performed with CEUS, the necrotic area showed initial shrinkage but no residual enhancement or local recurrence (**e**)

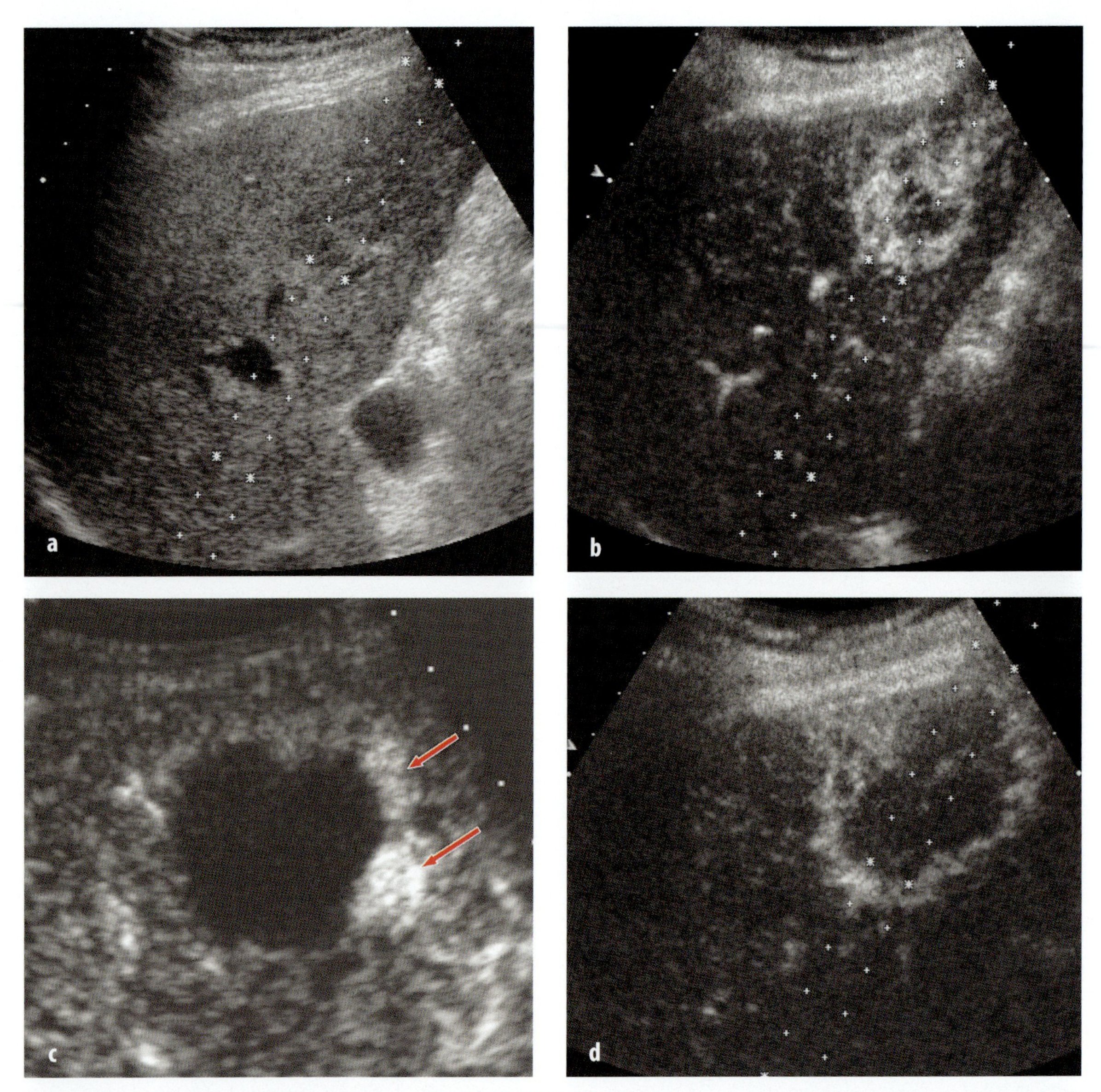

Fig. 3a-d. *A 4.3 cm hepatocellular carcinoma in segment IV in HCV-related cirrhosis.* Pre-treatment studies performed with B-mode US (**a**) and CEUS in arterial phase (**b**). A few minutes after the end of RF ablation with two insertions of cool-tip electrode, two small residual foci of enhancement (arrows) in arterial phase are shown by repeat CEUS (**c**). CEUS-guided re-treatment of the two foci were then performed during the same session and repeat CEUS shows complete necrosis of the tumor (**d**)

Residual viable tumor, usually located at the periphery of a lesion, maintains the enhancement behavior characteristic of native lesions as depicted on pre-treatment studies. Partial necrosis of HCC may be diagnosed when a portion of the original lesion still has hypervascular enhancement in the arterial phase. Residual untreated hypovascular metastases sometimes appear indistinguishable from necrosis in the portal and equilibrium phases: with CEUS, evaluation of the early phase is important, since viable tumor shows weak but perceptible enhancement [25].

If even questionable residual tumor foci with enhancement or vascular supply are depicted, we perform immediate CEUS-guided targeted retreatment and the treatment session ends only when complete avascularity is demonstrated (Fig. 3c). In our experience this approach greatly simplifies patient management and reduces costs by decreasing both the number of RF procedures and follow-up examinations.

At our institution, in the study period 2000-2002, no residual tumor was detected with CEUS in 176/199 liver malignancies treated: of these, CT depicted residual foci only in four cases (specificity 97.7%) which all had very small tumors (0.8-1.7 cm). In the remaining 23/199 tumors, single or multiple (1.0-2.2 cm) residual viable tumor portions were visible and immediately submitted to additional RF application in the same session until no further residual enhancement was detectable: in only two cases a 1.2-1.9 cm residual tumor was depicted by CT.

The routine adoption of CEUS (as the only technical improvement) achieved the final result of a decrease of partial necrosis from 16.1% to 5.1% in 429 hepatocellular and metastatic treated lesions.

Long-term Follow-up

Contrast-enhanced helical CT and, in some institutions, dynamic gadolinium-enhanced MRI are the mainstay for imaging follow-up of treated patients and the detection of local, remote intrahepatic and extrahepatic disease relapse [32-35]. Recently, the use of functional imaging with FDG has proven superior to cross-sectional studies [36].

At our institution, correlation of serum tumor markers with biphasic helical CT obtained every 3-4 months is employed in the long-term follow-up of patients treated for both primary and metastatic liver malignancies. Continuous-mode CEUS has proven to be of value to confirm or exclude doubtful or suspicious local recurrences or metachronous new lesions detected by cross-sectional imaging and to assess the possibility of their CEUS-guided retreatment.

Key Points

- Thanks to its nearly universal availability, portability, ease of use and low cost, ultrasound represents the modality of choice for the guidance of percutaneous interventional procedures.
- Continuous-mode CEUS allows real-time precise targeting of lesions during the specific phase of maximum lesion conspicuity: in the arterial phase for HCCs and hypervascular metastases and in the portal or equilibrium phases for hypovascular metastases.
- CEUS performed immediately at the end of the ablative session can reveal residual intralesional enhancement due to viable tumor tissue with accuracy comparable to that of helical CT, currently considered the 'gold standard' imaging modality for the assessment of tumor response to ablation.

References

1. Solbiati L, Tonolini M, Cova L, Goldberg SN (2001) The role of contrast-enhanced ultrasound in the detection of focal liver lesions. Eur Radiol 11: E15-E26
2. Livraghi T, Goldberg SN, Lazzaroni S et al (1999) Small hepatocellular carcinoma: treatment with radiofrequency ablation versus ethanol injection. Radiology 210:655-661
3. Livraghi T, Goldberg SN, Lazzaroni S et al (2000) Hepatocellular carcinoma: radiofrequency ablation of medium and large lesions. Radiology 214:761-768
4. Buscarini L, Buscarini E, Di Stasi M et al (2001) Percutaneous radiofrequency ablation of small hepatocellular carcinoma: long-term results. Eur Radiol 11:914-992
5. Solbiati L, Ierace T, Goldberg SN et al (1997): Percutaneous US-guided radio-frequency tissue ablation of liver metastases: Treatment and follow-up in 16 patients. Radiology 202:195-203
6. Solbiati L, Goldberg SN, Ierace T et al (1997) Hepatic metastases: percutaneous radio-frequency ablation with cooled-tip electrodes. Radiology 205:367-373
7. Solbiati L, Livraghi T, Goldberg SN et al (2001) Percutaneous radio-frequency ablation of hepatic metastases from colorectal cancer: long-term results in 117 patients. Radiology 221:159-166
8. Livraghi T, Goldberg SN, Solbiati L et al (2001) Percutaneous radio-frequency ablation of liver metastases from breast cancer: initial experience in 24 patients. Radiology 220:145-149
9. De Baere T, Elias D, Dromain C et al (2000) Radiofrequency ablation of 100 hepatic metastases with a mean follow-up of more than 1 year. AJR Am J Roentgenol 175:1619-1625
10. Solbiati L, Ierace T, Tonolini M et al (2001) Radiofrequency thermal ablation of hepatic metastases. Eur J Ultrasound 13:149-158
11. Sica GT, Ji H, Ros PR (2000) CT and MR imaging of hepatic metastases. AJR Am J Roentgenol 174:691-698
12. Valls C, Andia E, Sanchez A et al (2001) Hepatic metastases from colorectal cancer: preoperative detection and assessment of resectability with helical CT. Radiology 218:55-60
13. Harvey CJ, Albrecht T (2001) Ultrasound of focal liver lesions. Eur Radiol 11:1578-1593

14. Lencioni R, Cioni D, Bartolozzi C (2002) Tissue harmonic and contrast-specific imaging: back to gray scale in ultrasound. Eur Radiol 12:151-165
15. Harvey CJ, Blomley MJK, Eckersley RJ et al (2000) Hepatic malignancies: improved detection with pulse-inversion US in the late phase of enhancement with SHU 508A – early experience. Radiology 216:903-908
16. Albrecht T, Hoffmann CW, Schmitz SA et al (2001) Phase-Inversion sonography during the liver specific late phase of contrast-enhancement: improved detection of liver metastases. AJR Am J Roentgenol 176:1191-1198
17. Quaia E, Bertolotto M, Forgacs B et al (2003) Detection of liver metastases by pulse inversion harmonic imaging during Levovist late phase: comparison with conventional ultrasound and helical CT in 160 patients. Eur Radiol 13:475-483
18. Albrecht T, Blomley MJK, Burns PN et al (2003) Improved detection of hepatic metastases with pulse-inversion US during the liver-specific phase of SHU 508A: Multicenter study. Radiology 227:361-370
19. Numata K, Isozaki T, Ozawa Y et al (2003) Percutaneous ablation therapy guided by contrast-enhanced sonography for patients with hepatocellular carcinoma. AJR Am J Roentgenol 180:143-149
20. Goldberg SN, Gazelle GS, Mueller PR (2000) Thermal ablation therapy for focal malignancy. A unified approach to underlying principles, techniques, and diagnostic imaging guidance. AJR Am J Roentgenol 174:323-331
21. Leyendecker JR, Dodd GD, Halff GA et al (2002) Sonographically observed echogenic response during intraoperative radiofrequency ablation of cirrhotic livers: pathologic correlation. AJR Am J Roentgenol 178:1147-1151
22. Goldberg SN, Gazelle GS, Compton CC (2000) Treatment of intrahepatic malignancy with radiofrequency ablation: radiologic-pathologic correlation. Cancer 88:2452-2463
23. Chopra S, Dodd GD 3rd, Chintapalli KN (2001) Tumor recurrence after radiofrequency thermal ablation of hepatic tumors: spectrum of findings on dual-phase contrast-enhanced CT. AJR Am J Roentgenol 177:381-387
24. De Baere T, Elias D, Dromain C (2000) Radiofrequency ablation of 100 hepatic metastases with a mean follow-up of more than 1 year. AJR Am J Roentgenol 175:1619-1625
25. Rhim H, Goldberg SN, Dodd Gd 3rd (2001) Essential techniques for successful radiofrequency thermal ablation of malignant hepatic tumors. Radiographics 21:S17-31
26. Choi D, Lim HK, Kim SH et al (2001) Hepatocellular carcinoma treated with percutaneous radio-frequency ablation: usefulness of power Doppler US with a microbubble contrast agent in evaluation therapeutic response-preliminary study. Radiology 221:447-454
27. Cioni D, Lencioni R, Rossi S (2001) Radiofrequency thermal ablation of hepatocellular carcinoma: using contrast-enhanced harmonic power Doppler sonography to assess treatment outcome. AJR Am J Roentgenol 177:783-788
28. Solbiati L, Goldberg SN, Ierace T (1999) Radio-frequency ablation of hepatic metastases: postprocedural assessment with a US microbubble contrast agent – early experience. Radiology 211:643-649
29. Ding H, Kudo M, Onda H et al (2001) Evaluation of posttreatment response of hepatocellular carcinoma with contrast-enhanced coded phase-inversion harmonic US. Comparison with dynamic CT. Radiology 221:712-730
30. Numata K, Tanaka K, Kiba T et al (2001) Using contrast-enhanced sonography to assess the effectiveness of transcatheter arterial embolization for hepatocellular carcinoma. AJR Am J Roentgenol 176:1199-1205
31. Meloni MF, Goldberg SN, Livraghi T et al (2001) Hepatocellular carcinoma treated with radiofrequency ablation. Comparison of pulse inversion contrast-enhanced harmonic sonography, contrast-enhanced power Doppler sonography and helical CT. AJR Am J Roentgenol 177:375-380
32. Choi H, Loyer EM, DuBrow RA et al (2001) Radiofrequency ablation of liver tumors: assessment of therapeutic response and complications. Radiographics 21:S41-S54
33. Catalano O, Lobianco R, Esposito M et al (2001) Hepatocellular carcinoma recurrence after percutaneous ablation therapy: helical CT patterns. Abdom Imaging 26:375-383
34. Dromain C, De Baere T, Elias D et al (2002) Hepatic tumors treated with percutaneous radio-frequency ablation: CT and MR imaging follow-up. Radiology 223: 255-262
35. Sironi S, Livraghi T, Meloni F et al (1999)Small hepatocellular carcinoma treated with percutaneous RF ablation: MR imaging follow-up. AJR 173: 1225-1229
36. Anderson GS, Brinkmann F, Soulen MC et al (2003) FDG position emission tomography in the surveillance of hepatic tumors treated with radiofrequency ablation. Clin Nucl Med 28:192-197

II.5

Follow-up of Oncology Patients Undergoing Chemotherapy

Nathalie Lassau, Jérome Leclère and Pierre Péronneau

Introduction

The phenomenon of neoangiogenesis, defined as the formation of new vessels from existing vessels, is a key stage in the development of malignant tumours. Tumours smaller than 2 mm absorb nutrients through passive diffusion. Above this size, the existing vascular network is no longer sufficient and cancer cells secrete angiogenic substances to induce the creation of new vessels that will irrigate the tumour. The invasive potential of a tumour is thus strongly linked to its vascularisation [1-3].

New treatments based on antiangiogenic substances are the object of promising research for cancer treatment and have been developed in order to destroy new vessels. In view of the large number of new target drugs and treatment modalities that are under development, there is a great need for early reliable imaging indicators of tumour responses. Many of these developments have been linked to the evaluation of anti-angiogenic drugs [4].

Overall survival rate is the best objective parameter of efficacy of the treatments, but this parameter is obtained too late, as the effect on the tumour must be determined as soon as possible in order to institute another treatment if necessary. Tumour response, or objective response, is based on changes in the number and size of measurable primary or secondary tumour 'targets' [5]. These parameters are obtained more rapidly than survival data, but their reliability is highly dependent on the quality of comparative clinical and especially radiological measurements of tumour targets. The guidelines defining the method of measurement of solid tumours and response criteria are no longer adapted to technical progress in imaging. A process is currently underway to update these guidelines and a new set of criteria has recently been proposed, taking into account advances in imaging [7]. These criteria are still based on measurement of the size of the target lesion. The use of this single criterion to evaluate the response to treatment needs to be discussed in the light of the new technologies able to provide information on tumour composition, metabolism or neovascularisation, modifications which reflect the response to treatment before a reduction of the tumour volume can be detected [7].

With the recent evolution of technologies, Doppler Ultrasonography (DUS) has been developed. DUS allows both morphological studies of tumours and an accurate analysis of tumour vascularity [8]. The use of contrast media has strongly increased the detectability of intratumour vessels. Quantification of intratumoural vascularity allows a more objective analysis and a better reproducibility than the qualitative evaluation of the Doppler signal from tumour vessels.

These improvements in DUS accuracy are due not only to the technological evolution of the devices, but also to the use of ultrasound contrast agents, with advances including:

- the use of digital devices allowing signal processing and improving image quality by increasing the signal-to-noise ratio;
- the development of high-frequency probes clearly increasing axial and lateral resolutions;
- the use of contrast agents considerably strengthening the Doppler signal coming from the microvessels and improving functional imaging;
- the set up of perfusion software connected to working stations opening the way to an objective quantification of the Doppler signal enhancement, allowing kinetic studies with a collection of numerical parameters.

Several years ago, research using animals showed that DUS can visualise tumour angiogenesis *in vivo*, by detecting tumour vessels of 100μm in diameter in real-time [9]. Since 1999, we have carried out research in animals [10] and humans [11] that has shown that an early decrease or a disappearance of tumour vascularity evaluated by DUS reflected the efficiency of chemotherapy, before any decrease in tumour volume was seen. A study concerning patients with metastases from melanoma and receiving an innovative treatment consisting of an isolated limb perfusion of antiangiogenic drugs, demonstrated that an early disappearance of lesion vascularisation, detected by DUS, was predictive of a complete response even before the modification of the lesion's volume. On the contrary, an increase in tumour vascularity reflected tumour progression [12]. The use of contrast agents optimises this detection, allowing the visualisation of vessels of 40 μm in diameter [13].

Recent Doppler ultrasound techniques, especially contrast-enhanced harmonic imaging, combined with perfusion software can be used to study microvascularisation of superficial tumours as well as deep ones, in order to evaluate the efficacy of therapeutic novelties aiming to block tumour angiogenesis (e.g., Thalidomide, Neovastat, Sugen, tumour necrosis factor alpha [TNFα]) [14].

The president of the European Organisation for Research and Treatment of Cancer (EORTC), Alexander Eggermont [15], discussing the quest for early predictors and surrogate markers for response, explained that contrast-enhanced Doppler ultrasound (CEDUS) represents a relatively simple, practical and cheap procedure. One of our studies demonstrated that a CEDUS exam performed as early as one day after the start-up of an isolated limb-TNF perfusion for locally advanced sarcomas is of good predictive accuracy [16].

Baseline Ultrasound

The role of US examination during the follow-up of a patient treated by chemotherapy for liver metastases is to evaluate the number of tumours, tumour size and tumour location in the different segments of the liver. The greatest, or three diameters of tumour target, are measured using electronic calipers and the values are compared with those of the anterior examination in order to determine if there is an objective response, i.e., a stable or a progressive disease. Tumour response evaluation using sonography is not recommended in the case of clinical trials, where CT scanning is the gold standard. Sonography can be used only in case of protocols using drugs of known efficacy. Currently, colour or power Doppler has no recognised role in these evaluations, although some studies have used it. These techniques are used only to detect malignant neovasculature. Power Doppler is generally used because the flow direction is not important for this application. Power Doppler US has the advantages of low noise, relative angular independence, and increased dynamic signal range, which make it more sensitive and specific than conventional colour Doppler. For each study, the US examinations must be standardised in particular for the wall filter, the colour gain, the pulse frequency and the persistence. The focusing depth must be of less than 12 cm. A slow movement of the transducer is important to achieve the highest sensitivity without artefact. The adjustment is different for each type of sonograph and must be recorded in a specific program.

Two methodologies have been applied to evaluate anti-angiogenic treaments in liver tumours.

The first of these methodologies involves a visual scoring system to quantify the neovascularisation that has been used and applied to liver tumours, as well as other tumours. This method was used to evaluate the anti-angiogenic effect of thalidomide in hepatic metastasis from renal cell carcinoma. The hepatic tumour target must be scanned by continuously displacing the probe (3.5-4.4 MHz) across successive transverse and longitudinal sections. These sonographic scans must be recorded on digital videotapes and reviewed by one or two radiologists to quantify the number of vessels. In general, the number is computed as the mean value from the longitudinal and transverse scans to an already validated method [17]. A second methodology has been used in a prospective study testing thalidomide for the treatment of advanced hepatocellular carcinoma [18]. The evaluation of angiogenesis for follow-up imaging was carried out on only one lesion per patient. The tumour is carefully scanned in all directions, and the radiologist selects and stores the image of the tumour section with maximal colour signals for later analysis. After that, the radiologist marked the contour of the tumour margin with the cursor. Quantification of the vascular colour signal in the region of interest (ROI) is carried out by software using the DICOM video image. The vascularity index is calculated by dividing the number of coloured pixels by the number of total pixels in the area. This technique is similar to the digitised analysis of microvessel density studied by immunohistochemistry.

Results showed that colour or power Doppler were capable of selecting good responders earlier than the Response Evaluation Criteria In Solid Tumors (RECIST) and World Health Organization (WHO) morphological criteria. Nevertheless, there are several limitations, relating to:

- the tumour patterns: the depth of the tumour, for example (segment II), diffuse tumour infiltration, tumours treated by transarterial chemoembolisation.
- the protocol: the reproductibility of the evaluation of neovascularisation - it is very important for each study to impose a single setting in order to minimise variability between patients and examinations.

Contrast Ultrasound Features

The objective of our first study in hepatic metastasis was to propose CEDUS as an early predictor of tumour response or primary resistance to Imatinib in GIST patients treated with Imatinib (STI 571, Glivec, Gleevec, Novartis Pharmaceuticals), according to the French BFR14 trial.

Gastrointestinal stromal tumors (GIST) arise from the interstitial cells of Cajal of the GI tract [19]. Both localised and advanced recurrent GISTs are associated with a dismal prognosis and major resistance to conventional chemotherapy [20, 21].

Imatinib is a newly-developed tyrosine kinase inhibitor recently tested in clinical trials on patients with unresectable GISTs [22-25].

This molecularly targeted treatment [26] induces strong changes in the tumour structure, such as decreased tumour vascularity, hemorrhage or necrosis, consistent with a therapeutic response with or without a change in tumor volume [27]. Classic WHO or RECIST morphological criteria based on tumour size measurements often fail to accurately appraise tumour response to Imatinib. Morphological and functional imaging modalities such as contrast-enhanced magnetic resonance imaging (MRI), computed tomography (CT) or positron emission tomography (PET) should preferably be combined to assess tumor response. Both morphological and perfusion data are provided by DUS with contrast agent injection [28].

Thirty patients, with metastatic or recurrent malignant GISTs were prospectively included in this study. A total of 59 lesions were studied with CEDUS the day before starting oral therapy. 40 were hepatic metastases and 19 were recurrent intraperitoneal tumours. All patients were given a single daily dose of 400 mg of Glivec orally.

A Doppler US was performed one day before starting treatment, and at day 1, day 7, day 14, 2 months, 3 months, 6 months, 9 months, and 1 year. The mean follow-up period was 145 days ± 23 SD. US imaging was performed by two radiologists using an Aplio sonograph (Toshiba, Japan), with a 4.4 MHz C37 convex array or a 12 MHz linear transducer equipped with Dynamic Flow (DF) perfusion software which, thanks to wide-band Doppler technology, provided imaging of flow with excellent spatial resolution, a rapid imaging rate and suppression of the blooming effect. Contrary to conventional colour Doppler based on a long emission of narrow-bandwidth pulses, the DF uses a short emission of broad-bandwidth pulses. In this way, the spatial resolution of the detected signal is comparable to B-mode imaging.

As this technique is very sensitive to small movements, it is difficult to separate information related to slow flow of microvascularisation and that connected with movements of close tissues. A specific algorithm (Doppler Signal Processing) is used in order to answer this need. The efficacy of this method will be particularly useful for the study of tissue perfusion combined with use of contrast agents. The result is a natural combination of display of tissues and flow, contributing to the suppression of the blooming phenomenon.

CEDUS examinations were performed in four steps:

1. The morphological study was performed in B-mode. It allowed identification of the target lesion and selection of the best acoustic window for its assessment. The largest diameter of each lesion was measured with calipers and the tumour volume was measured using the three perpendicular diameters.
2. Injection of sonographic contrast agent.

Before June 2003, we used Levovist (58 exams), administered via an intravenous bolus injection (10 ml at a concentration of 400 mg/ml). Levovist (SHU 508 A, Schering, Germany) is a suspension of micrometer-sized microparticles of galactose and microscopic gaseous bubbles combined with a very weak concentration of palmitic acid prepared by shaking 4 g of microparticles in sterilised water. This yields a suspension of 10 ml at a concentration of 400 mg/ml that must be administered via an intravenous bolus injection.

Since June 2003, we have used Sonovue (Bracco, Italy) administered as an intravenous bolus injection (127 exams) (4.8 ml at a concentration of 8 μl/ml). It consists of microbubbles (from 100 to 500 million/ml with a diameter 2-8 μm) constituted of a shell of phospholipids containing sulphur hexafluoride. One of the characteristics of this gas is its weak solubility in water and therefore low diffusion in the blood. This contrast agent has been conceived to withstand blood pressure in order to obtain a longer half-life. The active part of the product is represented by the interface between the gas and the liquid phase of the dispersion. This interface reflects the ultrasound more strongly than blood, thus largely enhancing the blood echogenicity.

The reconstruction system (a vial with sodium chloride added) is very simple to use. The reconstructed suspension is stable for 6 hours and it is injected as a bolus of 4.8 ml into a peripheral vein. Adverse effects are not serious; they are transient and regress spontaneously.

To study the anti-angiogenic effect of treatment, the totality of solution (Levovist or Sonovue) must be injected in bolus in order to obtain the maximal of intensity reflecting the perfusion of tumour.

When there were multiple tumours in the same patient, target lesions were selected so that several lesions could be evaluated on the same US slice. Patients whose target lesions could not be evaluated on a single slice had a second injection with the same amount of contrast agent but long enough after the first injection (10-15 minutes) to allow the effects of the first injection to disappear.

3. Dynamic study. The use of contrast agent to study hepatic tumours permits access to both microvascularisation and perfusion tissue. These functional studies could be obtained with a contrast agent in destructive mode or in non-destructive mode, using the non-linear characteristics of second-generation contrast agents. The Doppler parameters remained constant between studies of the same patient and between examinations of different patients. First, we used DF in destructive mode with Levovist. When contrast agents are destroyed by ultrasound they transmit a signal that is very energetic and ripe with harmonics, thus the signal is detected when the microbubbles are destroyed by a high mechanical index (MI) (MI > 0.7) with conventional ultrasonography imaging (B-mode or colour and power Doppler). This technology in destructive mode was initially used to evaluate the anti-angiogenic effect of STI-571 in hepatic metastasis of GISTs. This technology is still used by some groups to evaluate vascularisation in HCC [29].

We next used a non-destructive mode with pulse subtraction, and then the Vascular Recognition Imaging (VRI) program.

Concerning the pulse subtraction mode, microbubbles, moving or static, are detected from a sequence of two ultrasound emissions of identical amplitude, but of opposite phases. Moreover, the MI is very weak (0.1-0.2), in order to avoid destroying the contrast agent. Once received, the two signals of opposite signs are added up. The fundamental component is automatically eliminated. This means that the signals sent back by the tissues are not visualised on the screen. The non-linearity of the signal originating from the microbubbles, due to the fact that their expansion is more important than their compression under acoustic pressure, makes it possible to visualise only the contrast agents.

This selective visualisation of contrast agent enables the kinetics of the contrast uptake, the density, and the presence or absence of microbubbles in the analysed area to be appreciated in real-time.

This mode of perfusion detection is more sensitive than the destructive mode. The major inconvenience is that the examination is initiated without first visualising the tumour, generating difficulties when studying the curve of contrast uptake over time, which permits quantification of several criteria, in respect to the morphological patterns.

We are now using new VRI software. VRI couples harmonic imaging with pulse subtraction and DF after injection of Sonovue. This sonographic method is original because B-mode imaging of tissue and of different coloured microbubbles can be visualised simultaneously but independently, thanks to 'Advanced Dynamic Flow' (ADF).

Two emission processes were used at a low MI (0.05-0.2) in order to avoid destroying contrast agent microbubbles, and were combined as follows: (1) emission/reception with a fundamental frequency for imaging tissue in grey-scale and (2) an emission/reception sequence involving the harmonic response of bubbles (ADF) for differentiated detection of moving and static microbubbles. This technique allows: (1) conservation of anatomical marks before and during an examination with contrast agent; (2) differential analysis of microvessels with information on flow direction (red/blue) and perfusion (green); (3) individualised or simultaneous imaging depiction of data related to tissue or microbubbles. The originality of this imaging method comes from the simultaneous, but independent visualisation of the tissue imaging in fundamental B-mode and the contrast agent imaging in different colours.

This new and very sophisticated tool helps to detect ultrasound contrast agents using current applications and it will take part in widening the spectrum in the future.

Total gain was the only parameter that the operator could modify. This gain was regulated

according to the depth of the target lesion. This parameter had no impact on the data used for quantification. The operator selected the slice passing through the largest tumor diameter and then the probe remained fixed in this plane for the dynamic study of contrast uptake. After injection of contrast agent, signal enhancement of intratumor neovessels was evaluated visually in real-time and the dynamic sequence was recorded on a digital tape.
4. Doppler US images were reviewed by two radiologists. The percentage of the tumour surface taking up contrast agent was visually evaluated based on the consensus of two readers, on the selected single-2D image when contrast uptake was maximal. Digitised quantification of contrast uptake was performed on the same selected single-2D US scan. After selecting this image, the lesion was outlined in order to determine a ROI. Photoshop software was used to quantify the percentage of pixels exhibiting signal enhancement by the contrast agent, using the following equation: contrast-enhanced pixels/total number of pixels in the ROI. At each examination, this percentage of contrast uptake was compared with the value observed the day before treatment started.

In all cases, Doppler US examinations were technically feasible without any complications.

A total of 185 CEDUS examinations were performed. Initial tumour contrast uptake evaluated with CEDUS before treatment was predictive of the future response: 71% (mean percentage of contrast uptake) in tumours in the group of good responders versus 41% (mean percentage of contrast uptake) in the group of poor/non-responders. Abundantly vascularised tumors (> 70%) had a better response to Imatinib than poorly vascularised tumours. A strong correlation ($p < 10^{-4}$) was found between the decrease in tumour contrast uptake at day 7, day 14 and 2 months after the beginning of treatment, and tumour response (Figs. 1-3). At day 14, the mean percentage of tumour contrast uptake decreased from 71% to 31% in tumors with a good response. This mean percentage remained at 43% in lesions exhibiting a poor response at 2 months.

In this study, CEDUS allowed early and accurate evaluation of the efficacy of Glivec. Decreased contrast uptake, assessed by CEDUS 7 and 14 days after the beginning of treatment was correlated with a good response at 2 months. The objectives of our ongoing studies are to correlate the percentage of the early decrease in contrast uptake on CEDUS with progression-free survival and to determine whether a further rise in contrast uptake after an initial response is predictive of future resistance to Glivec. Currently, we are extending this study to evaluate the detection of active residual GIST cells in selected necrotic masses. Biopsies of tissue exhibiting new neovascularisation could be performed to characterise secondary resistance to Glivec in order to propose other treatment options (such as surgical resection, radio-frequency ablation or different drugs) to refractory patients [30].

In another study, we evaluated Dynamic Contrast-Enhanced Doppler Ultrasound (DCE-US) with perfusion software (VRI) and contrast agent injection as a predictor of tumour response, progression-free survival (PFS) and overall survival (OS) in thirty patients with a metastatic renal cell carcinoma (RCC) who were already enrolled in a double-blind randomised study [31].

Patients were given an anti-angiogenic treatment (BAY-9006). Sorafenib is an efficient anti-tumour treatment that has demonstrated significant inhibition of neovascularisation in xenograft models of human cancers [32, 33]. Several authors have demonstrated the efficacy of this new drug in refractory solid tumours in phase I and II studies [34].

Since 2004, several teams have proposed novel trial designs and endpoints to evaluate new agents in RCC. For example, Rini et al. [35] proposed time to progression as a novel endpoint. In our study, 10 patients had liver metastases. Examinations were performed at baseline, and after 3 and 6 weeks on sorafenib or a placebo, in patients with tumour targets that were accessible to DCE-US.

A total of 85 DCE-US examinations were performed. The dynamic study was performed after injection of 4.8 ml of Sonovue at a concentration of 8 μl/ml (intravenous bolus injection). Signal enhancement of intratumour neovessels was evaluated visually in real-time and the dynamic sequence was recorded on a digital tape. We chose one to two lesions per patient. Qualitative and quantitative evaluations were performed:

Qualitative analysis: the percentage of contrast uptake throughout the lesion was evaluated by the radiologist conducting the examination and validated by two radiologists.

Quantitative analysis: quantification of mean contrast uptake by digital analysis of images was performed in the following manner: (1) the tumour was outlined using Adobe Photoshop, which automatically discriminates colours, distinguishing two zones in two different tonalities; (2) the image was analysed with the Matrox Inspector software, which quantifies image pixels, allowing discrimination of the tonalities and evaluation of the percentage of perfused tissue.

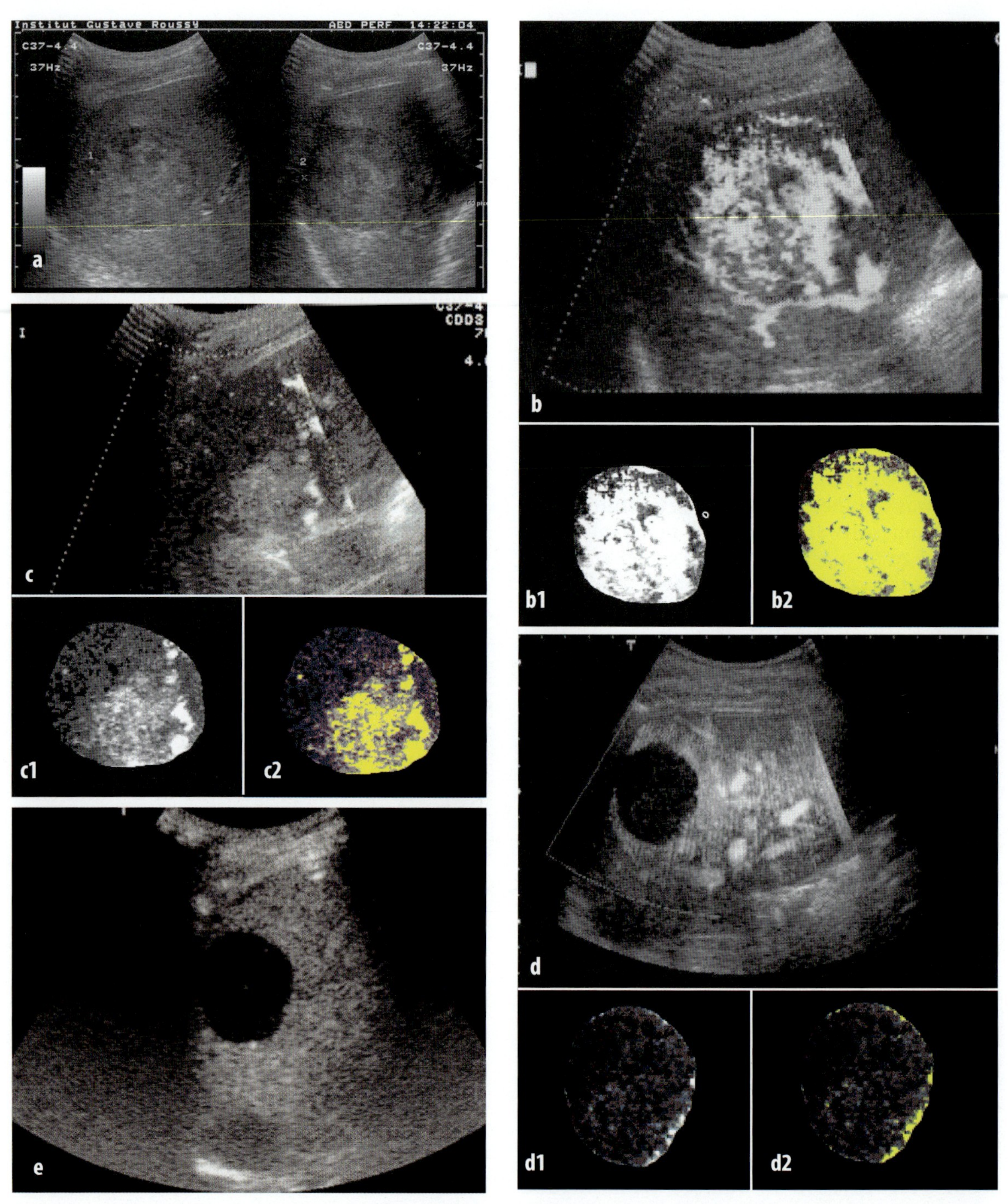

Fig. 1a-i. *A hepatic metastasis (segment VI-VII) from a GIST in a 69 year old man.* **a** US imaging at day -1 shows that the tumor measured 53 x 51 x 49 mm. **b** DUPSCA at day -1 shows parenchymal vascularisation with contrast uptake throughout the tumour estimated at 80%, with contrast uptake quantified by Photoshop. **c** At day 1 the percentage of contrast uptake is about 30%, with contrast uptake quantified by Photoshop. **d** At 2 months the percentage of contrast uptake is 0%, with contrast uptake quantified by Photoshop. **e** At 12 months the percentage is still 0% at DUPSCA. **f** At 15 months DUPSCA shows an initial tumour recurrence. **g** At 18 months DUPSCA shows an increase of contrast uptake of about 80% without size modification. **h** At 24 months, DUPSCA shows a contrast uptake of 100%, with a strong tumoral progression. **i** At 27 months DUPSCA shows 10% contrast uptake after modification of therapy

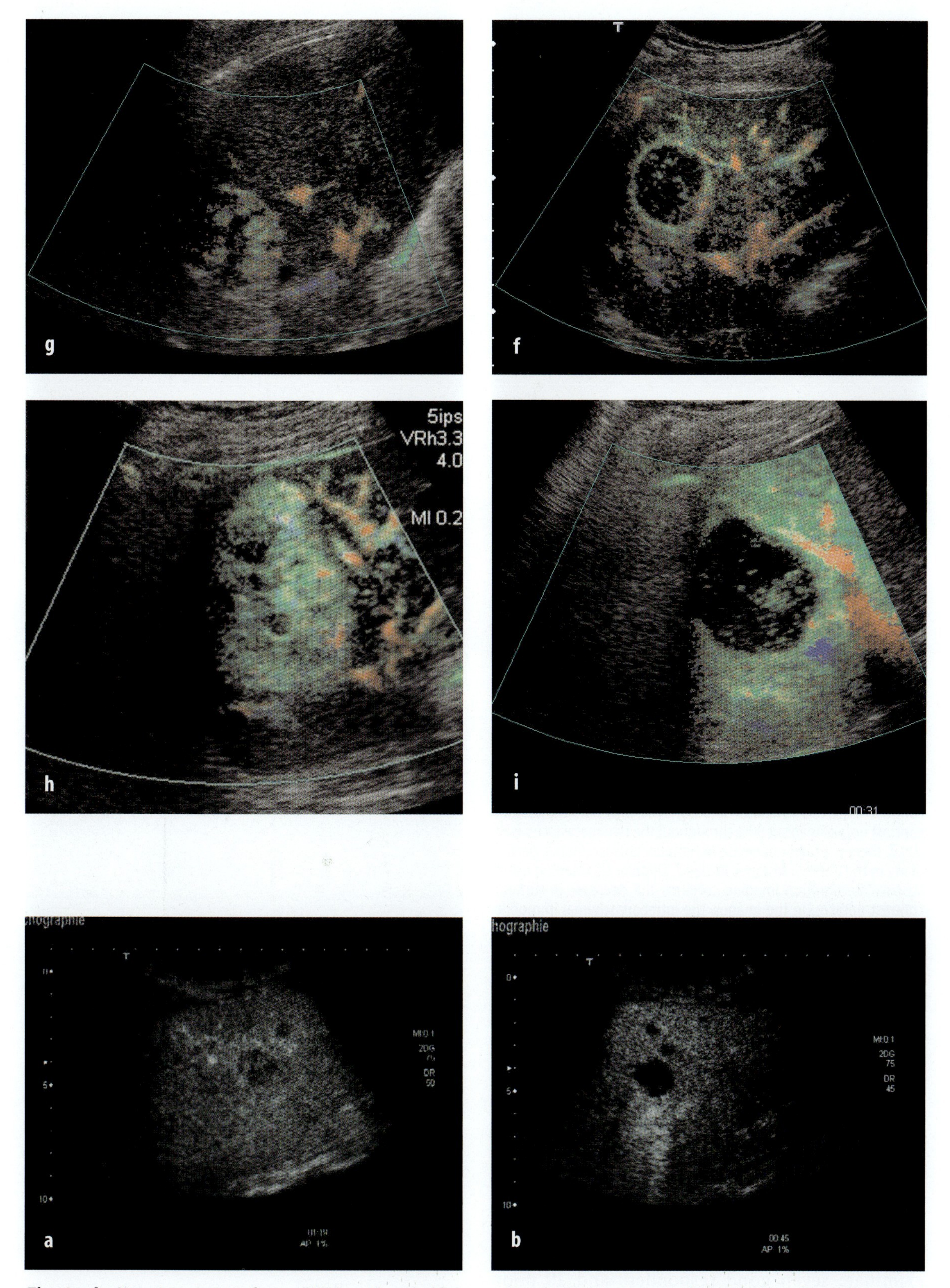

Fig. 2a, b. *Hepatic metastasis from a GIST in a 39 year old woman.* Doppler US imaging using 'Contrast Tissue Discriminator' and Sonovue injection. **a** The day before treatment, contrast uptake is estimated at more than 90% throughout the tumour. **b** At day 14, there is no tumour contrast uptake, indicating treatment efficiency

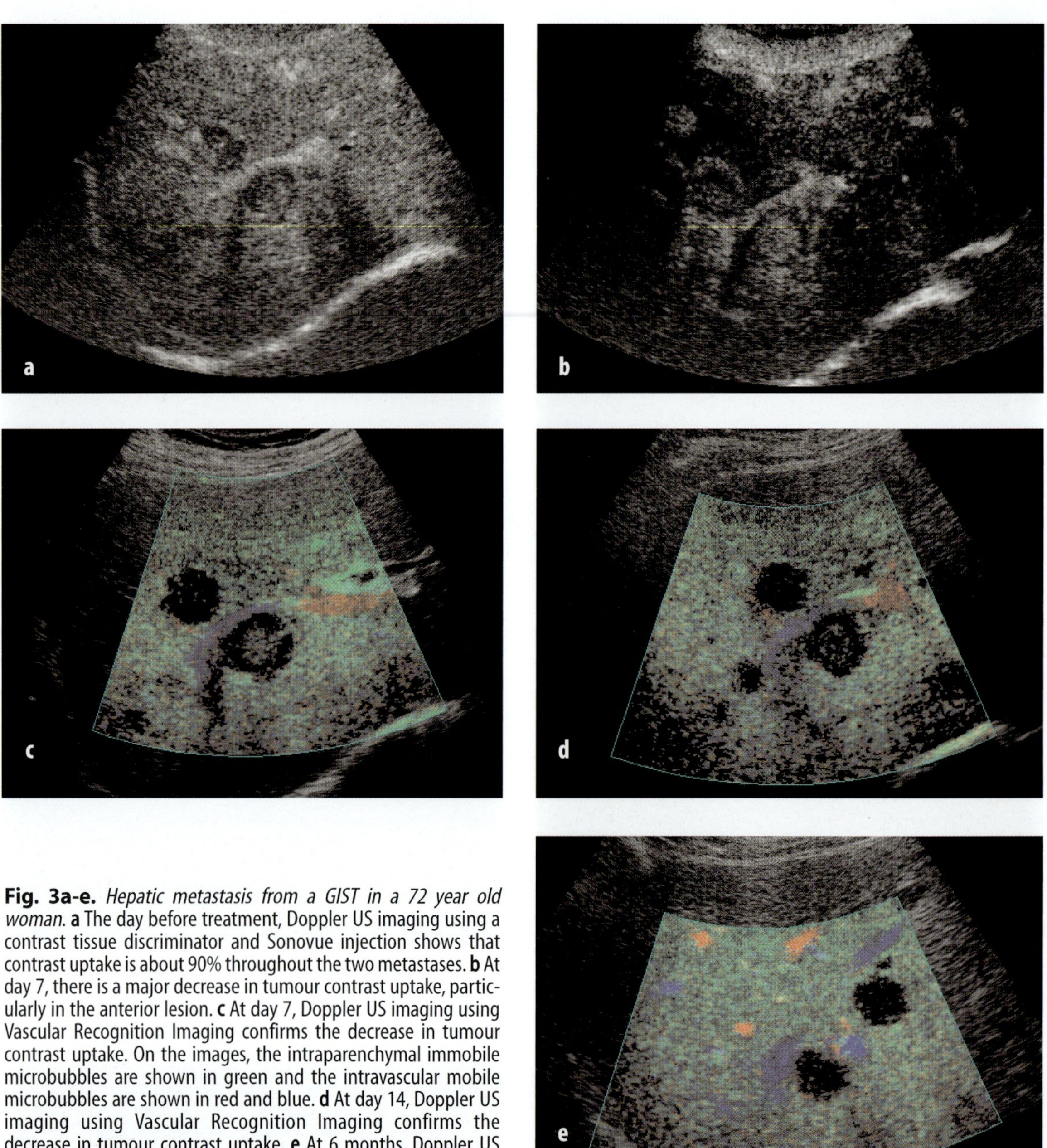

Fig. 3a-e. *Hepatic metastasis from a GIST in a 72 year old woman.* **a** The day before treatment, Doppler US imaging using a contrast tissue discriminator and Sonovue injection shows that contrast uptake is about 90% throughout the two metastases. **b** At day 7, there is a major decrease in tumour contrast uptake, particularly in the anterior lesion. **c** At day 7, Doppler US imaging using Vascular Recognition Imaging confirms the decrease in tumour contrast uptake. On the images, the intraparenchymal immobile microbubbles are shown in green and the intravascular mobile microbubbles are shown in red and blue. **d** At day 14, Doppler US imaging using Vascular Recognition Imaging confirms the decrease in tumour contrast uptake. **e** At 6 months, Doppler US imaging using Vascular Recognition Imaging confirms the total tumour necrosis without contrast uptake

The combination of a decrease in contrast uptake exceeding 10%, and stability or a decrease in tumour volume allowed us to discriminate seven good responders and 20 poor responders at 3 weeks (Fig. 4). There was a statistically significant difference in PFS ($p = 0.002$) and OS ($p = 0.01$) between good and poor responders. In ten patients treated with sorafenib, DCE-US also appears to predict PFS.

Role of Contrast Ultrasound in Clinical Practice

Despite significant advances in medical imaging in the recent past, quantification parameters need to be developed to objectively assess the efficacy of these new treatments. Anti-angiogenic treatments target tumour vessels and rapidly induce

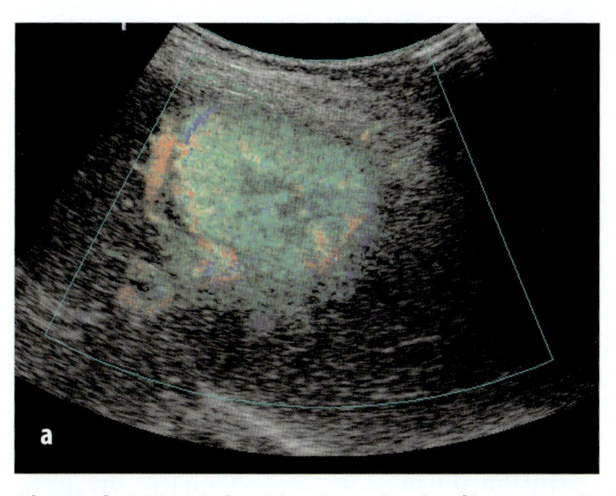

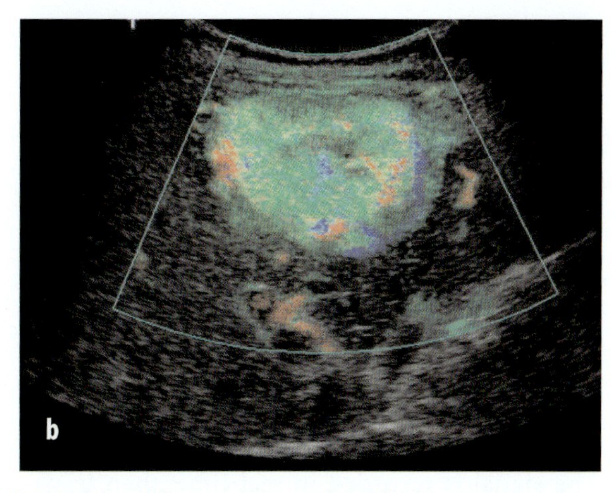

Fig. 4a, b. DCE-US before (**a**) and 3 weeks after (**b**) treatment by BAY-9006 (phase III) in a poor responder with a liver metastasis from an RCC

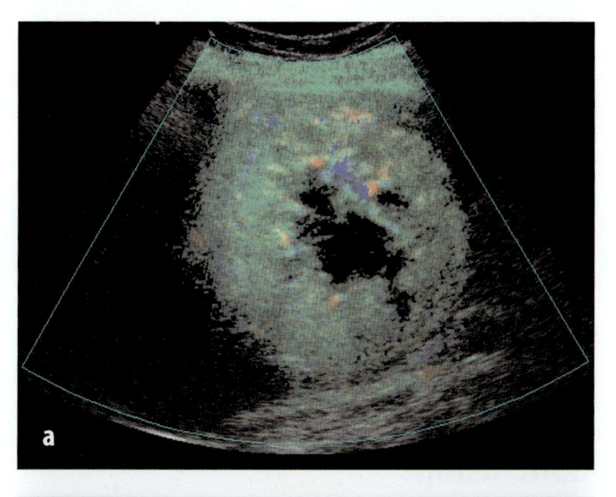

Fig. 5a-c. *Hepatic metastasis from liver metastasis from an RCC in a 62 year old woman.* DCE-US before (**a**) and after 2 (**b**) and 4 weeks (**c**) of treatment with BAY-9006 with interferon (trial phase I) in a good responder with a liver metastasis from an RCC. The contrast uptake was estimated at 80, 60 and 40% respectively

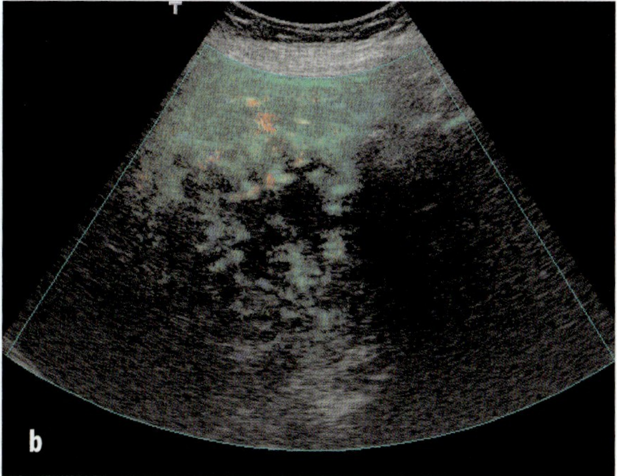

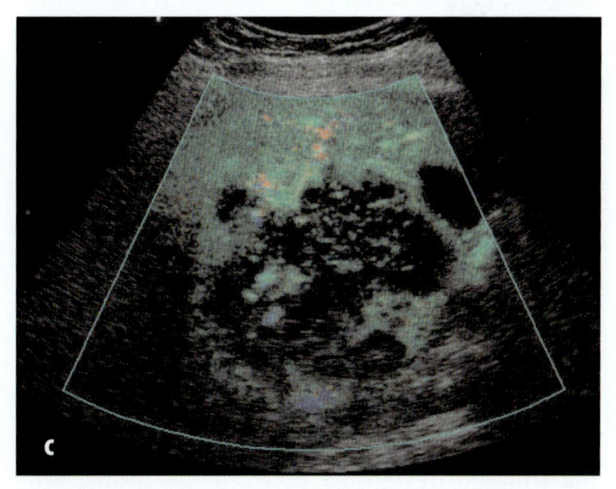

functional changes, such as a decrease in tumour perfusion or a decrease in blood flow before the tumour volume even decreases. At the time, oncologists add functional imaging as DCE-MRI, CT-scan or CT-Pet in phase I, II or III trials, using anti-angiogenic treatments. Currently, DCE-US is used in several trials at our institution with different therapeutics such as Avastin in chronic hepatitis C (CHC), Bay-9006 and interferon in RCC (Fig. 5), Bay-9006 DTIC in melanoma, AVE 8062 in phase I or AB1010 in GIST. All these functional changes should be quantified as early as possible with quantitative parameters obtained using a non-invasive method.

Concerning the methodological aspect of the number of targets evaluated, Mazumdar et al. [36] used a mathematical model, showing that it is preferable to choose fewer targets, as this lowers the risk of errors. Thus, in our studies only one or two targets were selected to perform this quantification.

New ultrasonic detection modes and new modeling methods are appearing for the quantification and evaluation of microvascularisation and perfusion. These new modes are using latest generation contrast agents as perfusion tracers, which backscatter an ultrasonic signal when they are subjected to an acoustic pressure field. The signal is recorded in real-time, then transferred to a software program that computes the contrast kinetics in the area of interest, i.e., the tumour for the field of cancer research. Quantitative parameters, in other words, parameters that take into account all injection parameters (e.g., injected volume, length and dynamics of the injection), can then be extracted from the kinetic data as research has shown that such data can be linked to hemodynamic parameters.

To date, clinical examinations use only semi-quantitative parameters (e.g., maximum enhancement, time at which the maximal enhancement occurs, area under the curve, and mean transit time [MTT]) obtained from the kinetics of the onset of contrast.

In order to perform this quantification in our on-going studies, linear computations are needed and we work from raw data. The raw data are obtained by the equipment just before the compression to the DICOM display. We carry out an acquisition over at least 3 minutes, and store the data on a workstation. The specific software (CHI-Q, Toshiba) is able to track the lesion to overcome the problem of patient movement. Criteria such as maximum enhancement, time of obtaining maximal enhancement, the area under the curve, and MTT, are computed from the linear raw data in the workstation. Contrast uptake kinetic curves modeling is then carried out.

Data are analysed on a personal computer using Excel 9.0 software (Microsoft Corporation, USA) with the Solver algorithm (Microsoft Corporation, USA), which minimises the sum of the squared deviations between the model and the experimental data. The contrast uptake curves are modeled off-line by two equations: a sigmoid equation is first used between the start of contrast uptake (V_0) until the maximum (V_{max}) so-called 'wash-in' phase.

$$V^t = V_o + \frac{V_{max} - V_o}{1 + \left\{\frac{t}{Tc}\right\}^p}$$

Where V_0 is the initial value, V_{max} is the maximal value recorded , Tc is the half-rise time and p is correlated to the contrast uptake speed.

A second equation is used after this maximum contrast uptake and corresponds to a simple hyperbole during the 'wash-out' phase.

Both equations are preferred to commercial ones, which give only moderate approximations of perfusion curves.

To avoid calculation errors due to bolus injection time variations, each time parameter was normalised according to the latency time (T_L), below which no contrast is taken up.

Two parameters were used to quantify the perfusion during the wash-in phase: the peak intensity (PI), defined as the difference between V_{max} and V_0; and the time-to-peak intensity (T_{PI}), defined as the difference between T_{max} and T_L. PI and T_{PI} were calculated from linear values. The MTT is taken into account to quantify the contrast uptake during the wash-out phase, this corresponds to the duration during which the uptake is superior to $V_{max}/2$.

The design of DCE-US programs is adapted according to the specific action of molecules. In general, a baseline is always performed one day before treatment, early evaluations are carried out between the first and seventh day after the beginning of treatment and we always perform a DCE-US at the same time as the standard morphological imaging generally performed after two months.

Conclusion

Many new functional imaging techniques, with their strengths, weaknesses and costs, are expected to reach the clinic for early assessment of tumour response to new drugs in development. These allow an evaluation of the efficacy of innovative treatments in oncology, such as the anti-angiogenic and anti-vascular treatments that are in full expansion and are aimed at the destruction of tumour vascularisation.

In ultrasonography, the combination of perfusion software and contrast agents gives rise to a functional imaging method. The access to raw data and the development of software using the tracking of lesions permits a more precise and objective quantification of treatment efficiency to be performed.

Key Points

- The early and functional evaluation of new treatments in oncology is a main goal. At present, technical advances in Doppler ultrasonography allow the detection of neovascularisation for superficial and deep malignant tumours in order to evaluate the efficiency of new treatments such as anti-angiogenic molecules.
- Contrast agent injection improves the efficiency of this technique and developments in perfusion software optimise this detection. Slow flows in tumour microvessels can be detected.
- Treatment response can be predicted early, based on changes in vascularisation before volume modification.

References

1. Folkman J (1971) Tumour angiogenesis: therapeutic implications. N Engl J Med 285:1182-1186
2. Folkman J (1995) Angiogenesis in cancer, vascular, rheumatoid and other disease. Nat Med 1:27
3. Miller JC, Pien HH, Sahani D, Sorensen AG, Thrall JH (2005) Imaging angiogenesis: applications and potential for drug development. J Natl Cancer Inst 97:172-187
4. Rehman S, Jayson G (2005) Molecular Imaging of antiangiogenic agents. The Oncologist 10:92-103
5. World Health Organisation Offset Publication, editor (1979) WHO Handbook for Reporting Results of Cancer Treatment Geneva (Switzerland)
6. Therasse P, Arbuck SG, Eisenhauer EA et al (2000) New guidelines to evaluate the response to treatment in solid tumours. European Organization for Research and Treatment of Cancer, National Cancer Institute of the United States, National Cancer Institute of Canada. J Natl Cancer Inst 92(3):205-216
7. Schwartz L (2004) Conventional and novel techniques for therapeutic response assessment. Radiological Society North America (RSNA). 90th Scientific Assembly and Annual Meeting, Chicago. Proc Radiology 115
8. Cosgrove D (2003) Angiogenesis imaging. Ultrasound. the British Journal of Radiology 76:S43-S49
9. Lassau N, Paturel-Asselin C, Guinebretière JM et al (1999) New haemodynamic approach to angiogenesis: colour and pulsed Doppler ultrasonography. Invest Radiol 34:194-198
10. Asselin C, Lassau N, Guinebretière JM et al (1999) The in vivo murineinterleukin-12 transfer by the Semliki Forest Virus induces B16 tumour regression through inhibition of tumour blood vessel formation monitored by Doppler ultrasonography. Gene Therapy 4:606-615
11. Escudier B, Lassau N, Couanet D et al (2002) Phase II trial of thalidomide in renal-cell carcinoma. Ann Oncol 13(7):1029-1035
12. Hochedez P, Lassau N, Bonvalot S et al (2003) Treatment of local recurrent melanomas by isolated limb perfusion: value of Doppler ultrasonography. J Radiol 84(5):597-603
13. Lassau N, Koscielny S, Opolon P et al (2001) Evaluation of contrast-enhanced colour Doppler ultrasound for the quantification of angiogenenis in vivo. Invest Radiol 36:50-55
14. Lassau N, Lamuraglia M, Leclere J, Rouffiac V (2004) Functional and early evaluation of treatments in oncology: interest of ultrasonographic contrast agents. J Radiol 85(5):704-712
15. Eggermont AM (2005) Evolving imaging technology: contrast-enhanced Doppler ultrasound is early and rapid predictor of tumour response. Ann Oncol 16(7):995-996
16. Lassau N, Lamuraglia M, Vanel D et al (2005) Doppler US with perfusion software and contrast medium injection in the early evaluation of isolated limb perfusion of limb sarcomas: prospective study of 49 cases. Ann Oncol 16(7):1054-1060
17. Lassau N, Chawi I, Rouffiac V et al (2004) Interest of colour Doppler ultrasonography to evaluate a new anti-angiogenic treatment with thalidomide in metastatic renal cell carcinoma. Bull Cancer 91(7-8):629-635
18. Hsu C, Chen CN, Chen LT et al (2005) Effect of thalidomide in hepatocellular carcinoma: assessment with power doppler US and analysis of circulating angiogenic factors. Radiology 235(2):509-516
19. Connolly EM, Gaffney E, Reynolds JV (2003) Gastrointestinal stromal tumours. Br J Surg 90:1178-1186
20. Berman J, O'Leary TJ (2001) Gastrointestinal stromal tumor workshop. Hum Pathol 32:578-582
21. Emory TS, Sobin LH, Lukes L et al (1999) Prognosis of gastrointestinal smooth-muscle (stromal) tumors: dependence on anatomic site. Am J Surg Pathol 23:82-87
22. Joensuu H, Roberts PJ, Sarlomo-Rikala M et al (2001) Effect of the tyrosine kinase inhibitor STI571 in a patient with a metastatic gastrointestinal stromal tumor. N Engl J Med 344:1052
23. van Oosterom AT, Judson I, Verweij J et al (2001) Safety and efficacy of imatinib (STI571) in metastatic gastrointestinal stromal tumours: a phase I study. Lancet 358:1421-1423

24. van Oosterom AT, Judson IR, Verweij J et al (2002) Update of phase I study of imatinib (STI571) in advanced soft tissue sarcomas and gastrointestinal stromal tumors: a report of the EORTC Soft Tissue and Bone Sarcoma Group. Eur J Cancer 38[Suppl 5]:S83-S87
25. Verweij J, van Oosterom A, Blay JY et al (2003) Imatinib mesylate (STI-571 Glivec, Gleevec) is an active agent for gastrointestinal stromal tumours, but does not yield responses in other soft-tissue sarcomas that are unselected for a molecular target. Results from an EORTC Soft Tissue and Bone Sarcoma Group phase II study. Eur J Cancer 39:2006-2011
26. Savage DG, Antman KH (2002) Imatinib mesylate-a new oral targeted therapy. N Engl J Med 346:683-693
27. Chen MY, Bechtold RE, Savage PD (2002) Cystic changes in hepatic metastases from gastrointestinal stromal tumors (GISTs) treated with Gleevec (imatinib mesylate). AJR Am J Roentgenol 179:1059-1062
28. Lassau N, Lamuraglia M, Chami L et al (2005) Gastro-intestinal stromal tumours treated with Imatinib: Monitoring response with contrast-enhanced ultrasound. AJR (in press)
29. Hotta N, Tagaya T, Maeno T et al (2005) Advanced dynamic flow imaging with contrast-enhanced ultrasonography for the evaluation of tumour vascularity in liver tumours. Clin Imaging 29: 34-41
30. Shankar S, vanSonnenberg E, Desai J et al (2005) Gastri-intestinal stromal tumour: new nodule-within-a -mass pattern of recurrence after partial response to imatinib mesylate. Radiology 235(3):892-898
31. Lassau N, Lamuraglia M, Chami L et al (2005) Doppler-ultrasonography with perfusion software and contrast agent injection as an early evaluation tool of metastatic renal cancers treated with the Raf-Kinase and VEGFR inhibitor: a prospective study. J Clinic Onco 3[Suppl 16]:209. ASCO Annual Meeting Proceedings
32 Wilhelm S, Chien DS (2002) BAY 43-9006: preclinical data. Curr Pharm Des 8(25):2255-2257
33. Wilhelm SM, Carter C, Tang L et al (2004) BAY 43-9006 exhibits broad spectrum oral antitumour activity and targets the RAF/MEK/ERK pathway and receptor tyrosine kinases involved in tumour progression and angiogenesis. Cancer Res 64(19):7099-7109
34. Sridhar SS, Hedley D, Siu LL (2005) Raf kinase as a target for anticancer therapeutics. Mol Cancer Ther 4(4):677-685
35. Rini BI, Weinberg V, Shaw V et al (2004) Time to disease progression to evaluate a novel protein kinase C inhibitor, UCN-01, in renal cell carcinoma. Cancer 101(1):90-95
36. Mazumdar M, Smith A, Debroy P, Schwartz L (2005) A theorical approach to choosing the minimum number of multiple tumors required for assessing treatment response. J Clin Epidemiol 58:150-153

II.6

Quantification of Microbubble Enhancement in Liver Imaging

Martin Krix and Stefan Delorme

Introduction

With contrast-enhanced ultrasound (CEUS), the perfusion of an examined region can be entirely detected, i.e. the blood flow per tissue unit, including the capillary blood flow. Since US interacts with the microbubbles directly, the bubbles are detected regardless of their motion. Theoretically, CEUS techniques are ultimately sensitive, able to detect each microbubble individually. Furthermore, perfusion can be visualized in real-time, using low-mechanical index (MI) US techniques.

Unlike other contrast agents used in radiology, US contrast agents are confined to the intravascular space. Thus, complex and sometimes inaccurate pharmacokinetic models to describe the contrast agent distribution in tissue are not necessary in order to quantify perfusion using CEUS.

In summary, CEUS is a promising and competitive tool for the detection of tissue perfusion. In the following text, CEUS methods and techniques are explained. These techniques are used to quantify microbubble enhancement, particularly in the liver.

Contrast US Features of Quantitative Methods

Technical Requirements

To quantitatively describe CEUS examinations, the wash-in and wash-out of the contrast agent is followed in a dynamic fashion. Therefore, measures must be taken to ensure that the examined region does not move during the examination, otherwise any plot of contrast over time would not make sense. Usually, the transducer is kept in approximately in the same position and, if necessary, the patient is instructed to stop breathing or to breathe superficially. Furthermore, video sequences (either analogue or digital) of the dynamic process have to be recorded, and digital post-processing is required. Automatic software tools are commercially available and are recommended, since they permit the rapid and easy analysis of the obtained image series.

Low-MI US techniques allow the detection of microvascularity in real-time with a high spatial resolution. These techniques require the use of a second-generation US contrast agent. SonoVue (Bracco, Italy), which has microbubbles stabilized by phospholipids, contains sulphur hexafluoride and is an example of an US contrast agent which is optimised for low-MI imaging, and approved for liver examinations. Furthermore, US devices should operate a contrast-specific pulse- or phase-inversion technique. Novel contrast-specific US techniques (CPS, Siemens-Acuson; VRI, Toshiba) are preferable, since they allow for the additional separation of the contrast-enhanced signal from the background.

Perfusion Curves

Perfusion curves describe the US signal intensity over time after a contrast bolus injection in a region of interest. Several rather descriptive parameters are used to characterize such curves, like the maximum enhancement after contrast bolus injection, the time to peak enhancement, the slope to maximum, or the area under the entire perfusion curve (Fig. 1). These parameters are quantifiable and relatively easy to obtain, but they do not directly characterize perfusion itself, or, for example, local blood volume. They may nevertheless be considered as indirect perfusion

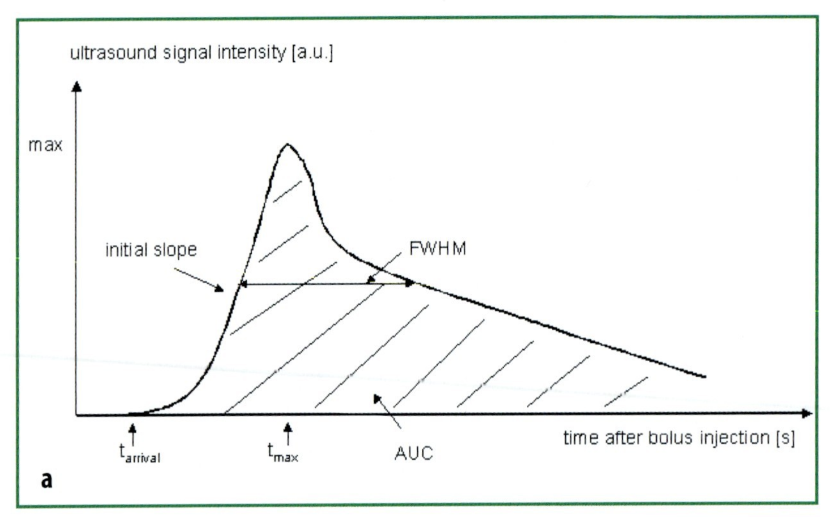

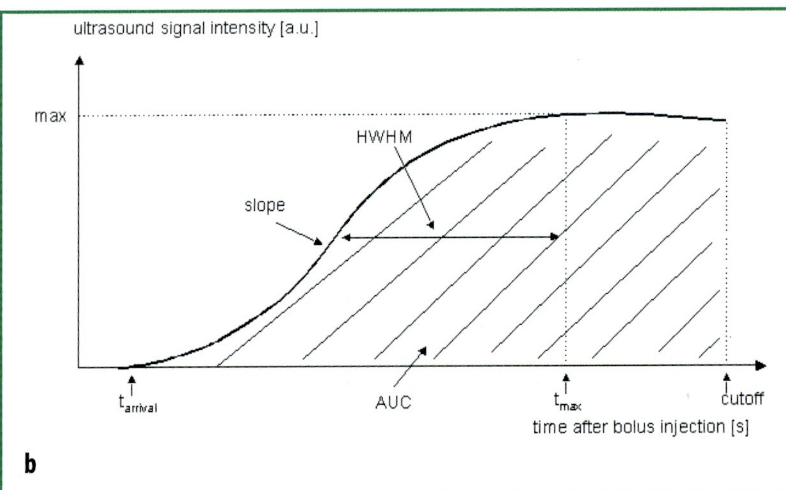

Fig. 1a, b. *Perfusion curves: ultrasound signal intensity over time after bolus injection.* **a** Arterially-perfused tissue shows typical behaviour, with an early increase to maximum followed by an exponential-like decrease. **b** In liver tissue the additional portal-venous supply causes a slow increase to a plateau at late phase. Several indirect perfusion parameters can be derived from the perfusion curve. max=maximum; AUC=area under the curve; FWHM=full width half maximum; HWHM=half width half maximum; t_{max}=time to maximum; $t_{arrival}$=time of contrast arrival; a.u.=arbitrary units

markers, and have been used in clinical examination of the brain, kidney or prostate using contrast-enhanced ultrasound [1-3].

Particular Aspects in the Liver

Perfusion curves can be derived using a normal injection protocol of the US contrast agent (e.g., bolus injection of 2.4 ml SonoVue). In tissues that are predominantly arterially supplied (as are most organs or malignant tumors), the perfusion curve has a typical shape with a rapid increase of contrast-enhancement and an exponential-like decrease after reaching a maximum (Fig. 1a). Liver metastases show similar dynamics, and perfusion curves derived from contrast-enhanced liver examinations show that CEUS is much better able to reflect the arterial perfusion of liver metastases than contrast-enhanced computed tomography [4]. Fortunately, the dynamics of contrast-enhancement in benign liver lesions are considerably different, helping to better characterization liver lesions.

The perfusion curves in healthy liver tissue differ completely to those in other organs, due to the portal-venous blood supply. The enhancement shows a slow increase, which reaches a plateau at the portal-venous phase, followed by a very slow decrease (Fig. 1b). For a comprehensive analysis of the complex blood supply of the liver, a separation between the arterial and portal-venous flow is required. This, however, is not possible using simple perfusion curves.

Classic Tracer Kinetics Modelling

Mathematical models are widely used and allow the calculation of perfusion by analyzing the contrast signal intensity in the examined region of interest (ROI) and comparing it with the input function derived from the arterial enhancement in the feeding vessels [5]. Such methods work very well in anatomical regions, where an input function can be derived (e.g., brain perfusion using dynamic MRI).

US has the disadvantage that it is in principle a two-dimensional examination method. Thus, it is difficult to perform an extraction of an input function and a measurement of the tissue enhancement simultaneously.

Particular Aspects in the Liver

It is even more difficult to obtain an input function in the liver due to the liver's double blood supply. Nevertheless, methods to modulate the arterial input of contrast agent and thereby differentiating the hepatic flow have been proposed. A possible approach is to suddenly interrupt the contrast agent flow (negative bolus) by destroying the microbubbles in the feeding vessels with additional high-energy US pulses for a certain time during a continuous infusion [6]. The intention of these studies was to assist in the diagnosis of metastatic liver disease and cirrhosis, where changes in the liver transit time of the blood supply have been reported.

Replenishment Kinetics

Replenishment kinetics uses the potential of US to destroy contrast agents if the output power is high enough. After such destructive US pulses (using a high-MI US 'flash'), it can be assumed that the examined slice is void of microbubbles, and that these will again progress into the slice from the outside, where they are still present. The analysis of such replenishment kinetics (US signal intensity over time after destruction) can provide several direct perfusion parameters. It has been shown that the initial increase of the refilling curve indicates the mean blood flow velocity (~m/s) in the ROI, and the plateau of signal intensity that will be reached after the complete replenishment is a parameter proportional to the local blood volume (~ml). According to a model of Wei, a parameter proportional to the perfusion (l/s·mg) can then be calculated via the product of blood velocity and blood volume [7]. This method has been used successfully and accurately for the measurement of tissue perfusion in several organs. An important application is the assessment of myocardial microcirculation in echocardiography [8].

The established model of Wei assumes a constant velocity of refilling and neglects the fact that contrast agent will re-enter the slice through vessels of varying callipers and directions (Fig. 2a). His model was chosen for mainly practical reasons, essentially because of its simplicity, but is far from being a consistent description of the refilling process (Fig. 2b, d). Therefore, other models have been proposed that attempt a more valid analysis of replenishment kinetics [9, 10]. One example is a multivessel model (Fig. 2c,e), which was previously developed to calculate tumor perfusion [11]. In addition, this multivessel model can be used together with a single bolus injection instead of the usually required continuous infusion of contrast agent used when analyzing replenishment kinetics.

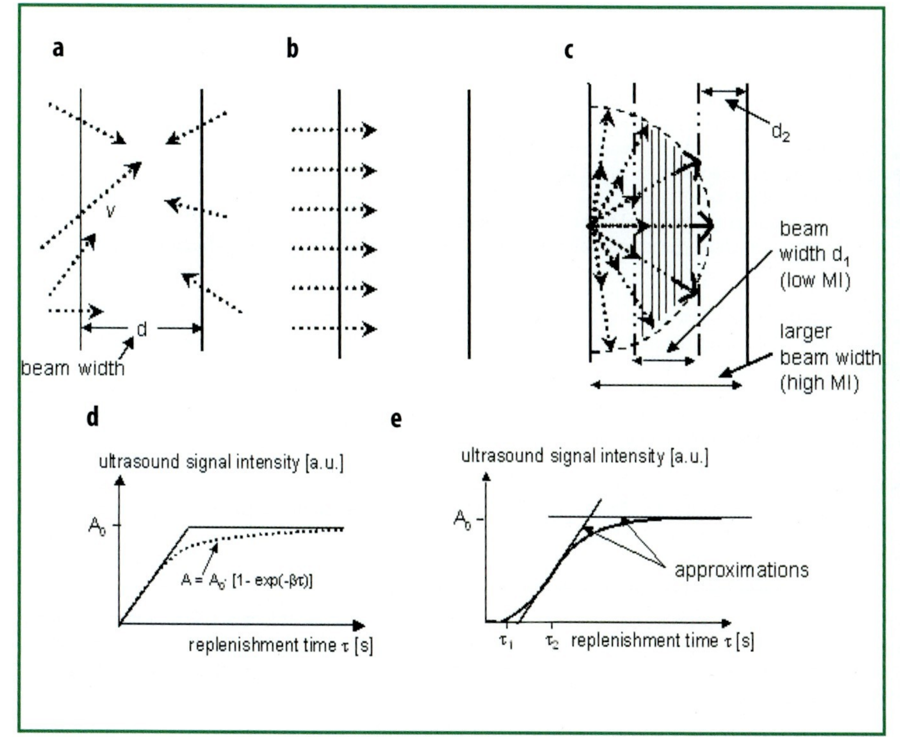

Fig. 2a-e. *Models to describe replenishment kinetics.* **a** The arrows describe the individual blood flow velocities found in a region of interest determined by the ultrasound beam width, which destroys the microbubbles. An established model assumes an exponential increase of ultrasound signal intensity asymptotically reaching a plateau A_0 after local destruction of the microbubbles (**d**). Its mathematical model neglects the physiological variations in the flow rate and its direction depending on the alignment of the blood vessels inside the region of interest (**b** compared to **a**). The multivessel model (**c**) is taken into account, which results in a more extensive mathematical description (see Fig. 3), even when the complex refilling process with 'flash'/low-MI imaging (two different US beam widths have to be considered) is additionally included. t_1, t_2=start of different phases of replenishment

Particular Aspects in the Liver

Quantification of tissue perfusion using CEUS of the liver is a challenge. One difficulty is that the arterial and the portal-venous blood supply need to be assessed separately. This is hardly possible whenever replenishment kinetics are obtained during a continuous infusion of contrast agent. Furthermore, the contrast agent might pool in the liver parenchyma, which biases perfusion measurements. One possible method to separate the arterial and the portal-venous phase of liver perfusion and to minimize pooling effects is to use a bolus injection. It has been shown, using a modified multivessel model (Fig. 3), that quantification of liver perfusion is possible with replenishment kinetics after a single bolus injection of US contrast agent [12] (Fig. 4). For this, the additional time dependence of the systemic contrast agent concentration after bolus injection has to be taken into account by measuring the perfusion curve before and after the refilling, and interpolating the contrast agent concentration, which would be expected during the replenishment. Using repetitive destructive pulses, the arterial and portal-venous perfusion of the normal liver can be assessed separately and compared with that of liver lesions. However, since different normalization parameters have to be used, a direct comparison of the blood volumes calculated for the arterial and portal-venous phase is not possible using this method (Fig. 3).

Transit Time Measurement

Besides perfusion imaging, which allows a direct assessment of the liver tissue, analysis of the flow dynamics measured in the larger hepatic vessels is an alternative approach in functional liver imaging. The hepatic transit time can be measured with CEUS of the liver, if the difference between the contrast agent dynamics of the arterial and the hepatic venous system is analyzed. Some approaches have used more global transit times, which are easier to calculate, such as the contrast arrival time in the hepatic veins after bolus injection. It has been shown that this CEUS method provides important information about the hemodynamic changes in

Quantification of liver perfusion using flash/low-MI imaging after contrast bolus injection

Influencing variables

Flash/low-MI imaging

Bubbles outside the region where replenishment is detected (low-MI technique), can also be destroyed due to tissue movement and due to the different beam widths of the low-MI and flash-imaging.

-> initial phase of replenishment:

$A_1 = 0$ for $\tau < \tau_1$ τ, time after replenishment subsequently, a more complex replenishment behaviour follows

Multivessel model

Takes into account the fact that the contrast agent will re-enter the slice through vessels of varying calipers and directions.

-> two other different phases of replenishment have to be considered:

$A_2 = A_0 \cdot [2/(3d_1) v_{mean} \tau - d_2/d_1]$ for $\tau_1 < \tau < \tau_2$, $d_2 < d_1$ (beam widths, see figure 2)

The gradient of a linear approximation results in the mean blood velocity v_{mean}.

$A_3 = A_0 \cdot [1 - \Sigma_1 g (d_1^2 - d_1 d_2)/(v_1 \tau)^2]$ for $\tau < \tau_2$

The maximum plateau A_0 is a parameter proportional to the blood volume.

v_{mean}, mean blood flowvelocity, g_1, weighting factor of each blood flowvelocity v_1 inside the region of interest.

Contrast bolus injection

The additional time dependence of the systemic contrast agent concentration after bolus injection has to be taken into account by measuring the perfusion curve before and after the refilling, and interpolating the contrast agent concentration, which would be expected during the replenishment.

Normalized values have to be used for the blood volume, which are different for the arterial and portal-venous phase. Therefore, a direct intra-individual comparison of arterial and venous blood volume parameters is not possible.

Arterial and portal-venous blood supply

The destructive pulses (flash) have to be used repeatedly. To obtain normalized values at the arterial phase, the arterial perfusion curve without using a flash has to be measured additionally (second bolus injection).

Fig. 3. Overview of the influencing variables in the quantification of liver perfusion using replenishment kinetics. The clinically verified, more complex replenishment kinetics using flash/low-MI imaging requires a different mathematical model. Furthermore, the additionally time dependence of the microbubble concentration has to be taken into account when using a bolus injection of microbubbles, in order to separate the arterial from the portal-venous blood supply

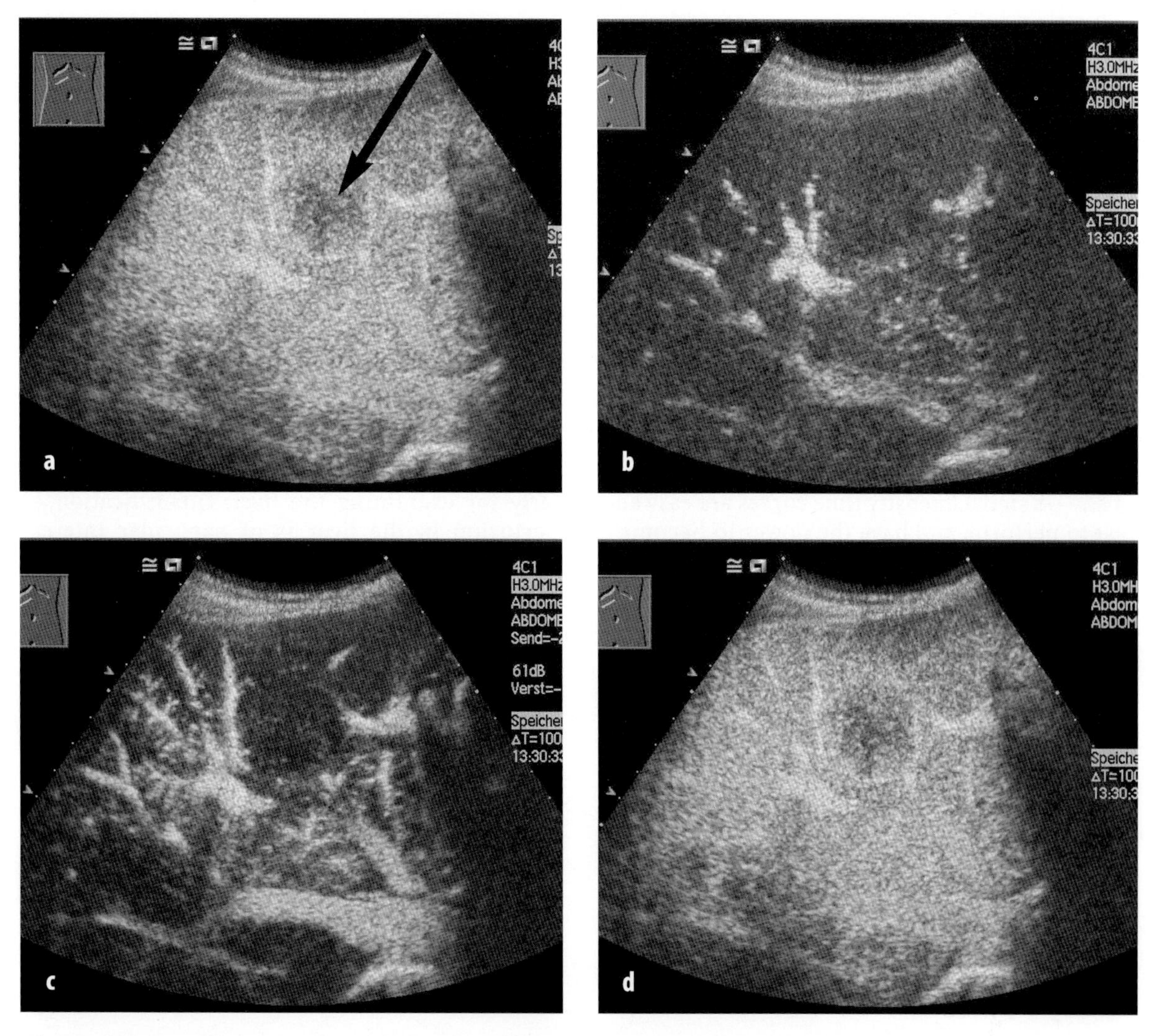

Fig. 4a-d. Contrast-enhanced US after injection of 2.4 ml SonoVue in low-MI imaging (**a**: 29 s after bolus injection). Microbubble replenishment can be visualized in real-time in normal liver tissue and liver metastases (*arrow*) using 'flash'/low-MI imaging. **b-d** 1 s, 2 s, and 7 s after microbubble destruction (late arterial phase) (reprint with permission [12a]

liver cirrhoses [13], and can predict disease severity non-invasively in patients with hepatitis [14]. Furthermore, it has been proposed as an indicator of hepatic spread in the liver in oncological patients, since a significant reduction of the hepatic transit time has been described in patients with hepatic metastases, compared to controls [14, 15]. Recently, hepatic transit time has been used as an indicator of the therapeutic response to radio-frequency ablation of liver tumors [17].

Limitations

An important precondition to quantify perfusion with CEUS is that the signal intensity of the chosen US parameter has to correlate with the concentration of the US contrast agent. High-frequency, raw data of the CEUS examinations are considered as gold standard. However, these data are commonly not available on most US devices. Therefore, the video signals of the US device are often used. Here, low-MI US often delivers greyscale equivalent values. However, these US signals have limitations, since the background signal from the non-enhanced tissue is relatively large and the US signals may not be linearly associated with the local concentration of the US contrast agent. More contrast-specific US techniques (such as CPS from Siemens-Acuson) may have advantages, since they permit the separate assessment of the background tissue and the contrast-enhanced signal. Furthermore, using these techniques in very low-MI imaging (<0.2 MI) may reduce possible microbubble destruction caused by the low-MI pulses and thus can further improve quantification of microvascularity.

General US limitations, such as the influence of depth or focus adjustment are self-explanatory, but may limit the general acceptance of CEUS in functional imaging compared to other non-invasive radiological modalities, in particular compared to MRI. In the liver, an US examination of the organ's whole circumference can be difficult to achieve, which may limit the use of CEUS in the assessment of liver perfusion.

A comprehensive analysis of liver perfusion using replenishment kinetics is still complex and time-consuming. Those applications will be reserved to dedicated study protocols in the near future. On the other hand, software-based analyses of any US signal intensity time curves are easy and fast to perform, and have the power to become a clinical tool also in liver examinations.

Role of Quantitative Perfusion Imaging using Contrast US in Clinical Practice

Perfusion is a recognized parameter of tissue viability and functionality. Its measurement can be useful in the detection and characterization of various pathological changes such as ischemia, inflammation, or neoplasia. Thus, perfusion imaging is an important part of the growing field of functional imaging, which may become indispensable for the characterization of many diseases.

Quantification is a prerequisite for many applications in functional imaging, in particular in perfusion imaging. Important indications are the evaluation of tumor or organ perfusion (e.g., brain, heart, or kidney), particularly during follow-up or therapy monitoring. For such examinations, valid and reproducible quantitative tools are required.

Particular Aspects in the Liver

CEUS is a sensitive and reliable method, particularly for examining the liver. Quantification of perfusion in the liver is of particular interest when examining the liver tissue itself (e.g., after transplantation) or malignant hepatic lesions (e.g., for differential diagnosis or monitoring). Since US is more advantageous for the examination of focal lesions, CEUS perfusion imaging can be useful particularly in follow-up examinations of liver lesions. Promising applications are the monitoring of local ablative therapies (e.g., radio-frequency ablation or radiation therapy [18]) or systemic treatment, especially if it has perfusion-related effects (e.g., anti-angiogenic drugs). Both aspects may be increasingly needed in the near future.

Key Points

- CEUS is a promising method for the sensitive detection of microvascularization in real-time, and the accurate quantification of tissue perfusion.
- In the near future, novel treatment strategies - like local ablative therapy of liver lesions or systemic antiangiogenic treatment - will increasingly require dedicated tools such as quantitative CEUS for perfusion monitoring.
- Analysis of the contrast agent dynamics after bolus injection in the ROI (perfusion curve) provides several indirect vascularization parameters. A direct quantification of perfusion is possible using the replenishment kinetics of the microbubbles.
- Additionally, measurement of the hepatic transit time might be a valuable tool for the diagnosis of liver disease.

References

1. Seidel G, Meyer-Wiethe K, Berdien G et al. (2004) Ultrasound perfusion imaging in acute middle cerebral artery infarction predicts outcome. Stroke 35:1107-1111
2. Levefre F, Correas JM, Briancon S et al.(2002) Contrast-enhanced sonography of the renal transplant using triggered pulse-inversion imaging: preliminary results. Ultrasound Med Biol 28:303-314
3. Strohmeyer D, Frauscher F, Klauser A et al. (2001) Contrast-enhanced transrectal color doppler ultrasonography (TRCDUS) for assessment of angiogenesis in prostate cancer. Anticancer Res 21(4B): 2907-2913

4. Krix M, Kiessling F, Essig M et al. (2004) Low mechanical index contrast-enhanced ultrasound better reflects high arterial perfusion of liver metastases than arterial phase computed tomography. Invest Radiol 39:216-222
5. Johnson G, Wetzel SG, Cha S et al. (2004) Measuring blood volume and vascular transfer constant from dynamic, T(2)*-weighted contrast-enhanced MRI. Magn Reson Med 51:961-8
6. Rhee R, Rubin J, Carson P, Fowlkes JB (2003) Modulated acoustic interruption of contrast agent flow for hepatic flow differentiation. Ultrasound Med Biol 29[Suppl 1: S109-S110
7. Wei K, Jayaweera AR, Firoozan S et al (1998) Quantification of myocardial blood flow with ultrasound-induced destruction of microbubbles administered as a constant venous infusion. Circulation 97:473-483
8. Lepper W, Belcik T, Wei K et al (2004). Myocardial Contrast Echocardiography. Circulation 109:3132-3135
9. Lucidarme O, Franchi-Abella S, Correas JM et al (2003) Blood flow quantification with contrast-enhanced US: "entrance in the section" phenomenon-phantom and rabbit study. Radiology 228:473-479
10. Pollard RE, Sadlowski AR, Bloch SH et al (2002) Contrast-assisted destruction-replenishment ultrasound for the assessment of tumor microvasculature in a rat model. Technol Cancer Res Treat 1:459-470
11. Krix M, Kiessling F, Farhan N et al (2003) A multivessel model describing replenishment kinetics of ultrasound contrast agent for quantification of tissue perfusion. Ultrasound Med Biol 29:1421-1430
12. Krix M, Plathow C, Kiessling F et al (2004) Quantification of perfusion of liver tissue and metastases using a multivessel model for replenishment kinetics of ultrasound contrast agents. Ultrasound Med Biol 30:1355-1363

12a. Krix M (2005) Quantification of enhancement in contrast ultrasound: a tool for monitoring of therapies in liver matastases. Eur Radiol Suppl 15[Suppl 5]:E104-E108

13. Albrecht T, Blomley ML, Cosgrove DO et al (1999). Non-invasive diagnosis of hepatic cirrhosis by transit-time analysis of an ultrasound contrast agent. Lancet 353:1579-1583
14. Lim AK, Taylor-Robinson SD, Patel N et al (2005) Hepatic vein transit times using a microbubble agent can predict disease severity non-invasively in patients with hepatitis C. Gut 54:128-133
15. Blomley MJ, Albrecht T, Cosgrove DO et al (1998) Liver vascular transit time analyzed with dynamic hepatic venography with bolus injections of an US contrast agent: early experience in seven patients with metastases. Radiology 209:862-866
16. Bernatik T, Becker D, Neureiter D et al (2004) Hepatic transit time of an echo enhancer: an indicator of metastatic spread to the liver. Eur J Gastroenterol Hepatol 16:313-317
17. Zhou X, Strobel D, Haensler J, Bernatik T (2005) Hepatic transit time: indicator of the therapeutic response to radiofrequency ablation of liver tumours. Br J Radiol 78:433-6
18. Krix M, Plathow C, Essig M et al (2005) Monitoring of liver metastases after stereotactic radiotherapy using low-MI contrast-enhanced ultrasound–initial results. Eur Radiol 15:677-684

II.7

Intra-Operative Contrast Ultrasound in Liver Surgery

Edward Leen, Susan Moug and Paul G. Horgan

Introduction

Intra-operative ultrasound (IOUS) is the gold standard for the detection of liver tumours, and dictates the surgical management of patients undergoing liver resection. The appropriate use of contrast agents will improve the performance of any imaging modality. The value of contrast agents in computed tomography (CT) and magnetic resonance (MR) for the detection of liver metastases is predictably unquestioned in current practice, such that it would even be considered unethical if they were not routinely applied. However, the application of contrast agents to percutaneous ultrasound (US) in general is relatively new and is now gradually gaining support in routine clinical practice. Its extension to IOUS is a natural pathway to improving the detection and characterisation of liver tumours, which may further impact on surgical decision making.

Background

Hepatocellular carcinomas (HCC) and colorectal cancer liver metastases (CLM) are the two most common malignancies of the liver, associated with a dismal outcome of zero survival at five years if left untreated. The worldwide incidence of hepatocellular carcinoma is increasing, most noticeably in North America and Europe, as a result of increasing numbers of patients with hepatitis C and chronic liver disease. In the western world, colorectal cancer accounts for 14% and 16% of cancer deaths in men and women, respectively, with approximately 25% of patients having liver involvement at the time of initial presentation and up to 50% developing hepatic metastases during the course of their disease [1, 2].

Patients with early stage HCC should be offered the surgical therapeutic options of transplantation or resection [3]. Transplantation offers a four-year overall survival rate of 75% and a four-year recurrence-free survival rate of 83%. However, few can benefit from transplantation given the shortage of living donors and the eligibility of patients according to the 'Milan criteria' for transplantation (i.e, decompensated cirrhosis, solitary tumour smaller than 5 cm and up to three lesions smaller than 3cm) [4]. Liver resection still offers a potential for cure for those patients with a solitary lesion and relatively well preserved liver function.

For patients with colorectal hepatic metastases, surgical resection is the treatment of choice, with 10-20% of patients being candidates for potentially curative resection. Resection should be considered if there is no unresectable extrahepatic disease, if all liver deposits can be resected with a free clearance margin of 1 cm and if there is adequate liver reserve. The five-year survival rates vary from 25-40% [5-6]. 75% of those who undergo liver resection will develop recurrence and of these, the liver is involved in 50%. 64-85% of all recurrences appear within the first two years [5]. Repeat liver resection in these patients still has a five-year survival of 30-40% with comparable post-operative mortality or morbidity to that of single hepatectomy [7-8]. Results of growth rate studies of hepatic metastases support the hypothesis that these metastases were present at the time of liver resection but remained 'occult', i.e., undetected by IOUS, CT and/or MRI scans [9].

Traditionally, contrast-enhanced CT and MR imaging have been used to stage colorectal hepatic metastatic disease. IOUS has been shown to yield significant new information not identified on pre-operative imaging, which determines resectability and/or changes the operative plan in up to 50% of patients; it is considered the gold standard and is thereby achieving universal usage [10-13]. However, of those patients who develop recurrence following apparently curative liver resection, the 50% hepatic recurrence rate underlines the limitation of IOUS itself; clearly small lesions are easily missed if they have acoustic characteristics similar to those of the adjacent hepatic parenchyma. It is recognised that patient outcome is highly dependent upon the ability to define the true extent of the metastatic disease; therefore the need for a more accurate imaging technique cannot be overemphasised, as it would enable more precise as well as more aggressive treatment of the liver metastases using adjunctive therapies.

More recently, there has been increasing interest in the use of contrast agents during extra-corporeal sonography of the liver to improve the detection of liver metastases. US contrast agents consist of microbubbles of air or gases of low solubility, stabilised by a lipid, surfactant or polymer shell. Analogous to CT or MR, it is the relative distribution of the contrast agents between normal tissue and the lesion that makes the lesion more visible and easier to characterise [14, 15]. IOUS with an echo-enhancer was first used in 1990 by a group of Japanese workers evaluating the effectiveness of carbon dioxide as a contrast agent in the detection of small HCCs using fundamental imaging mode [16]. In their preliminary report they showed that contrast-enhanced IOUS (CE-IOUS) detected additional lesions in two of nine patients whose lesions had not been identified on IOUS. The difficulty in using carbon dioxide, which is an unstable echo-enhancer with poor reproducibility is well known, it also had to be injected directly into the hepatic artery or the portal vein and is associated with significant artifacts. Recent advances in harmonic imaging combined with the development of contrast agents with liver specificity have markedly improved the sensitivity of extra-corporeal sonography for the detection of small metastases, which may be equal to or even superior to that of CT or MR in some cases [17]. The question is whether the use of contrast agents in combination with IOUS using non-linear harmonic imaging modes improves the detection of occult liver metastases, or has any impact on the surgical management of patients undergoing liver resection.

Contrast-Enhanced Intra-Operative US Technique

There are specific US equipment requirements that enable contrast-enhanced US imaging. Nonlinear harmonic imaging software capability is a prerequisite. At present there is only one equipment manufacturer (Philips, USA) that produces a dedicated high frequency finger probe (CT8-4) with pulse inversion harmonic (PIH) imaging capability designed specifically for liver imaging. The advantage of this curvilinear probe is that it has good penetration, wide field of view and enables scanning from the posterior aspect of the liver as well as over the dome of the right lobe. Nonetheless, the use of a percutaneous low frequency end-fire probe, combined with the use of percutaneous high frequency end-fire probes with non-linear imaging mode capability may be adequate to examine the whole liver, albeit with limitations.

At operation, all patients undergo thorough abdominal and pelvic exploration for extrahepatic disease, and the liver is subsequently mobilised off the diaphragm for improved sonographic visualisation of the liver. Bimanual palpation of the liver is then carried out followed by hepatic sonography using a high-frequency finger probe designed for liver scanning. The IOUS and CE-IOUS scans are performed co-operatively by an experienced surgeon and radiologist. Sonography is performed in a systematic fashion, inspecting the liver parenchyma for previously diagnosed as well as additional lesions and for any major vascular or biliary involvement.

Following the baseline fundamental (± colour Doppler mode) and PIH mode scans, a bolus intravenous injection of 3-4 mL of contrast agent, SonoVue (Sulphur hexafluoride gas stabilised by phospholipid-shell) (Bracco, Italy) is administered via the central venous line, followed by a 10 ml of normal saline flush, and repeat US scanning is performed in the PIH mode. SonoVue is a new second-generation microbubble contrast agent (mean size: 2.5 micron; 90% measuring less than 8 micron in diameter). The US gain, focal zone and output power (Mechanical index [MI]: 0.02-0.04) settings are standardised. Scanning of both lobes of the liver before and after contrast administration is performed in a standardised fashion in axial, sagittal and oblique sweeps to ascertain complete liver coverage. Following contrast administration, the normal liver enhances uniformly and the hepatic malignancies are easily identified, appearing as dark, contrast free, filling defects during the portal venous and delayed sinusoidal phases (Figs, 1, 2). The persistent enhancement of the normal liver parenchyma in the late sinusoidal phase lasts for up to three minutes.

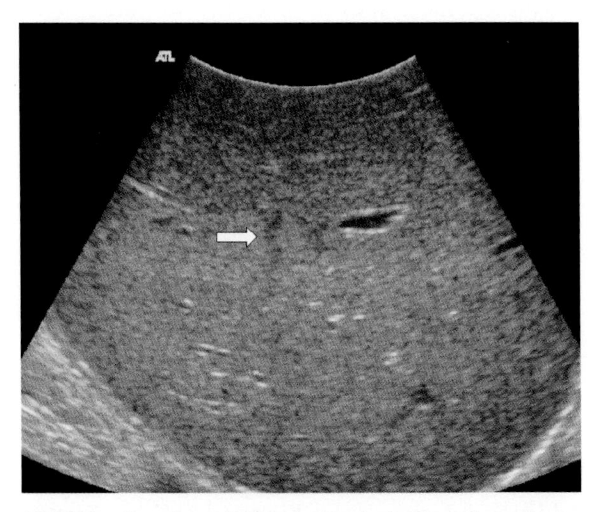

Fig 1. Baseline scan on fundamental mode showing sub-centimeter metastasis with surrounding halo

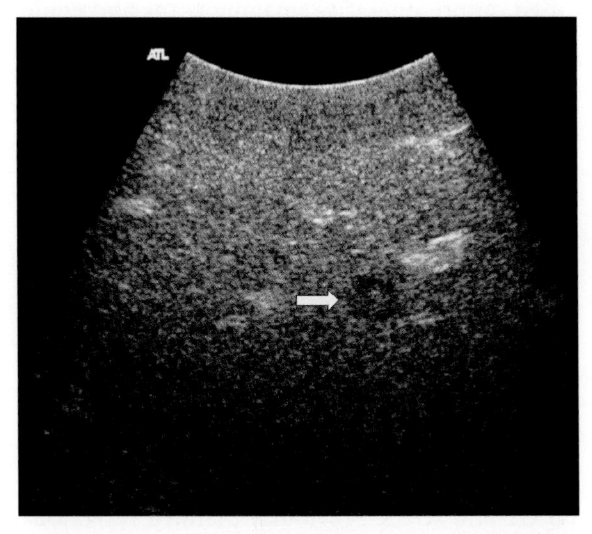

Fig. 2. Post-contrast scan on non-linear imaging mode showing improved delineation and contrast between the metastasis and normal liver in the late phase

Characterisation of Focal Liver Lesions with CE-IOUS

There is some speculation as to the mechanism underlying the prolonged enhancement of the liver parenchyma in the late phase; there is no evidence of phagocytosis of SonoVue by the reticuloendothelial cells, unlike agents such as Levovist (Schering, Germany) or Sonazoid (GE, Norway). The persistence of the agent within the normal liver may be due to the very slow flow within the sinusoids. Indeed, there is some experimental evidence in rats that microbubble agents containing perfluorocarbon gas enhance the normal liver by virtue of the slow flow within the sinusoids [18]. Malignant lesions, such as metastases and hepatocellular carcinomas, are devoid of sinusoids and are almost exclusively fed by abnormal arterial channels associated with complex shunts leading to rapid contrast wash-out; as a result there is a relative absence of contrast accumulation relative to normal liver in the late parenchymal phases. Indeed, all metastases and the vast majority of HCCs appear as filling defects on a background of bright liver parenchyma. Furthermore, the demonstration of hypervascularity in the arterial phase in small nodules is a diagnostic indicator of HCCs in patients with liver cirrhosis. Although focal nodular hyperplasias (FNH) have a rich arterial supply, there is relative accumulation of contrast in the late phases because they consist of normal functioning hepatic tissue similar to adjacent normal sinusoids with very slow wash-out - the majority of the FNHs are of higher or isoechogenicity in the late phase. The slow blood flow within the haemangiomas, which consist of vascular spaces lined with endothelial cells, is well known; persistent and/or progressive accumulation of contrast in the late phases occurs in over 95% of cases. Irrespective of the vascular enhancement pattern, if the lesion is hyperechoic based on the late phase alone, the probability of it being benign is over 95%.

CE-IOUS of Liver Metastases

More recently, we assessed the value of CE-IOUS in 60 consecutive patients undergoing liver resection of metastases [19]. The technique for IOUS and CE-IOUS is described above. The number of metastases identified on CT and/or

MR, IOUS and CE-IOUS were counted, sized and mapped according to Couinaud classification on a liver schematic chart for each modality and in real-time for all the sonographic examinations. Benign cysts were not included in the counts. The excised liver segments or lobes were sectioned at pathology to obtain a true pathologic gold standard of the lesions. Correlation with resection/biopsy histopathology findings was also performed. Changes in surgical management following CE-IOUS compared with that made after IOUS were documented (e.g., abandoned resection, more extensive resection, limited resection or combined resection with radiofrequency ablation).

A total of 107 lesions were identified on histopathology findings of biopsies and resected tissues and of these, 103 were confirmed metastases and four were haemangiomas. The number of correctly identified metastases on CT and/or MRI combined, IOUS and CE-IOUS were 79, 84 and 101, respectively. There was a statistically significant increase in the number of detected metastases on CE-IOUS compared with IOUS and also with combined CT/MRI (p = 0.029 and p= 0.047, respectively). No statistical difference was observed in the number of metastases detected between IOUS and combined CT/MRI (p= 0.53). For CT/MRI, IOUS and CE-IOUS, the sensitivity was 76.7%, 81.5%, and 96.3%, respectively; accuracy was 73.8%, 78.5% and 96.3%, respectively; the positive predictive value was 95.2%, 95.5% and 98.0%, respectively. The mean (± SD) size of the lesions identified on CT/MRI/IOUS combined and CE-IOUS were 2.73 (± 1.46) cm and 1.71 (± 1.57) cm, respectively. The median size of the additional lesions identified on CE-IOUS was 0.8 cm (Fig. 3). The smallest metastasis identified was 4 mm in diameter.

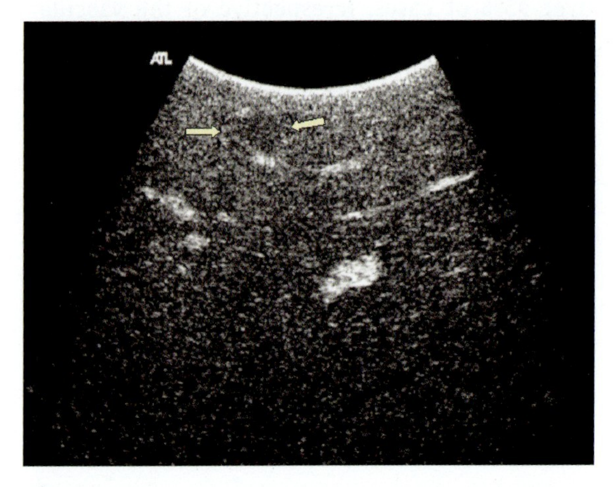

Fig. 3. Post-contrast scan on non-linear imaging mode showing additional sub-centimeter metastasis in the late phase not seen on IOUS, CT or MRI scans

Actual Change in Surgical Management as a Result of CE-IOUS

Of the 60 patients, CE-IOUS was not performed in three patients; two patients had peritoneal metastases at exploration and one patient had widespread metastases on a background of fatty liver on the basis of IOUS. Of the remaining 57 patients, there was no alteration in the surgical management in 40 patients. CE-IOUS detected no additional lesion in 37 of the 40 patients; in two cases there were additional lesions but they did not entail any extended resection or adjunctive surgical manoeuvres. In another patient, one of the lesions was wrongly diagnosed on IOUS and CT as metastasis and was accurately identified as a benign haemangioma on CE-IOUS.

In contrast, new information identified on CE-IOUS alone altered the surgical plan in the remaining 17 of 57 patients (29.8%). Additional hepatic metastases were detected in 11 cases (19.3%), which extended to a tri-segmentectomy in three cases, additional non-segmental wedge resection in two patients and radio-frequency ablations of the additional lesions in six cases, as an adjunct to the planned hepatic lobectomy. All additional lesions were biopsied and confirmed as metastasis prior to radio-frequency ablation; all biopsies and radio-frequency ablations were performed using CE-IOUS guidance. In two patients (3.5%) there were less lesions than identified on pre-operative imaging scans and could not be confidently excluded on IOUS alone, which resulted in an alteration to the original surgical plan from right hepatectomy to excision of three segments in one patient and removal of segment VII/VIII plus a metastatectomy in the other. CE-IOUS also confirmed presence of an arterio-venous malformation in one patient (1.8%) that was not identified on IOUS and was previously diagnosed as apparent solitary metastasis on CT.

In two patients (3.5%), IOUS also accurately diagnosed a solitary benign haemangioma, with characteristic peripheral nodular enhancement progressively filling-in over the vascular and late phases, that was wrongly identified as metastasis on CT and IOUS. Previously planned resections were therefore not carried out. In one case the tumour margin could be clearly visualised on CE-IOUS to be too close to the inferior vena cava for resection and it was ablated instead. New findings on CE-IOUS alone also altered IOUS/CT/MRI hepatic staging in 35.1% (20 of 57) of patients.

Clinical Perspective

In this study, the sensitivity of CE-IOUS for the detection of liver metastases is significantly higher than that of IOUS and that of CT/MR combined. CE-IOUS detected additional lesions not identified on IOUS or CT/MR in 13 patients (22.8%) and the smallest of the additional lesions measured 0.4 cm. A key question is whether the detection of these additional lesions really matters. One might argue that small lesions measuring less than 5 mm (if left undetected) might be eradicated by adjuvant chemotherapy. However, this remains uncertain; as yet adjuvant chemotherapy following liver resection is not routinely administered in most centres. Surprisingly, the median size of the additional lesions identified by CE-IOUS in this study is 8 mm, which is larger than the threshold size of lesions identified by conventional IOUS (5 mm), and thus they may potentially impact on the eventual patient outcome. The median clinical risk score of those 13 patients with additional lesions was 2 before CE-IOUS and did not significantly change after CE-IOUS (median Score 2) [20]. One would only anticipate a change in the clinical risk score for those patients with solitary lesion at CT/MRI/IOUS; in this study three of those 13 patients (23.1%) had solitary lesions before CE-IOUS. However, the numbers are far too small for any proper analysis. Clearly, follow-up studies of larger cohorts of patients are needed.

There is still some debate as to the value of IOUS during hepatic resection, with its impact on surgical management ranging from 7-44% [10-12]. As previous suggested, the impact variations between studies might be explained partly by the difference in the adequacy and extent of the pre-operative imaging studies; clearly, the higher the performance of CT/MR, the lower the impact of IOUS. Moreover, resectability/irresectability is no longer the sole surgical issue with the advent of extensive/adjunctive surgical/interventional maneuvers; the more aggressive the surgeon/interventional radiologist in proceeding with these maneuvers, the higher the impact of IOUS. Similar considerations may be applied to the impact of CE-IOUS on surgical plans; any additional information provided by CE-IOUS alone that would alter surgical management may depend on the adequacy of IOUS and also on the quality and the extent of the pre-operative imaging scans. Our surgical/interventional approach might be considered as 'aggressive' and the optimum protocol for imaging had been selected using top of the range equipment. Ultimately, the true value of CE-IOUS can only be judged by the outcome of these patients.

Nevertheless, the preliminary results of this study are compelling. In this study, additional findings based on CE-IOUS alone altered the surgical plan in 29.8% of patients. Lesional characterisation was also improved with CE-IOUS as a result of its ability to image contrast-enhancement in real-time. It could be argued that the four patients with benign lesions wrongly diagnosed on CT and IOUS would have been spared laparotomy if MRI had been performed pre-operatively; on the other hand the value of performing both MR and CT in all patients undergoing liver resection remains debatable. Whilst the arterio-venous malformation lesion missed on IOUS and CT would have been diagnosed on Doppler US mode, the latter is not routinely performed. Nonetheless, even if they were to be excluded, a change in surgical management in the remaining 13 patients would still be clinically significant. Moreover, CE-IOUS alone identified additional lesions in a total of 13 patients (22.8%) and exclusively guided biopsy and radio-frequency ablation of new lesions in 10.5% of cases.

CE-IOUS of Hepatocellular Carcinomas

The impact of CE-IOUS for the assessment of cirrhotic patients with HCCs undergoing liver resection was reported in a short note by an Italian group in 2004 [21]. In this preliminary report, of the 13 patients with HCCs studied, CE-IOUS improved on the accuracy of IOUS for HCCs; of the 11 additional lesions detected by IOUS as HCCs, eight and three lesions were confirmed to be benign and malignant, respectively. No benign lesions showed any enhancement during the arterial phase, whilst the three additional HCCs did. Four of the eight patients with benign lesions still had their liver resection. In effect, CE-IOUS changed the surgical management in four of the 11 patients (36.4%). CE-IOUS did not detect any additional lesions. It is worth highlighting that CE-IOUS was performed with an end-fire percutaneous probe not designed for intra-operative scanning of the liver with obvious limitations, as described above.

Limitations of CE-IOUS

There are some limitations to the CE-IOUS technique. PIH capability is a prerequisite and as yet is not widely available for the intra-operative US finger-probes. Although such new technology is relatively cheap, there would be the additional cost of the contrast agent and any upgrade of existing conventional equipment. IOUS probes with PIH capability are a tenth of the cost of a top-of-the-range US scanner, and the cost of the US contrast agent is about half that of an MRI liver-specific contrast agent (in the UK, SonoVue costs £40 [$72] per vial, which is made up to a volume of 5ml).

In order to minimise the disruption of the microbubbles to prolong enhancement and maintain uniformity, scanning is performed at a much lower US output power (MI range: 0.02-0.04), which renders the US screen display dark until the arrival of contrast. This can be compensated for, to some extent, by increasing the ultrasound gain; the spatial resolution is also lower compared with that of the fundamental mode. These require some degree of observer adaptation with the obvious learning curve, which may be up to 3 weeks. Furthermore, the duration of the contrast-enhancement is shorter, with a mean duration of 2-3 minutes compared with the 4-5 minutes of enhancement obtained from lower frequency probe scans; this may also be related to some of the interactions with the general anesthetics as well as the positive pressure ventilation, which may disrupt the microbubbles. After the liver parenchymal enhancement has completely vanished (usually 5 minutes from the injection time), the injection of the same dose of SonoVue can be safely repeated (total safe dose per patient is 10ml of SonoVue in 3 doses) to complete the examination. We can anticipate future software optimisation for improved sensitivity to SonoVue.

Key Points

- Contrast-enhanced intra-operative ultrasound is an essential tool for staging patients undergoing liver resection
- It is also vital in the guidance of adjunctive radio-frequency ablation of lesions that are occult on conventional intra-operative ultrasound.

References

1. O'Brien MJ (1988) Cancer of the colon and rectum: current concepts of etiology and pathogenesis. Br J Med Sci 157: 5-15
2. McArdle CS, Hole D, Hansell D et al (1990) A prospective study of colorectal cancer in the West of Scotland: a ten year follow-up. Br J Surg 77:206-208
3. Bruix J, Sherman M, Llovet JM et al (2001) Clinical management of hepatocellular carcinoma. Conclusions of the Barcelona-EASL Conference. J Hepatol 35:421-430
4. Mazzaferro V, Regalia E, Doci R et al (1996) Liver transplantation for the treatment of small hepatocellular carcinoma in patients with liver cirrhosis. N Eng J Med 334:693-699
5. Scheele J, Strang R, Altendorf-Hofmann A, Paul M (1995) Resection of colorectal liver metastases. World J Surg 19:59-71
6. Fong Y, Cohen AM,Fortner JG, Enker WE et al (1997) Liver resection for colorectal metastases. J Clin Oncol 15:938-46
7. Adam R, Bismuth H, Castaign D et al (1997) Repeat hepatectomy for colorectal liver metastases. Ann Surg 225:51-62
8. Fernandez-Trigo V, Shamsa V, Sugarbaker PH et al (1995) Repeat liver resections from colorectal liver metastases. Surgery 117:296-304
9. Finlay IG, Meek D, Brunton F, McArdle CS (1988) Growth rate of hepatic metastases in colorectal carcinoma. Br J Surg 75:641-644
10. Conlon R, Jacobs M, Dasgupta D, Lodge JPA (2003) The value of intraoperative ultrasound during hepatic resection compared with improved preoperative magnetic resonance imaging. Eur J Ultrasound 16:211-216
11. Jarnagin WR, Bach AM, Winston CB et al (2001) What is the yield of intraoperative ultrasonography during partial hepatectomy for malignant disease? J Am Coll Surg 192:577-82
12. Cervone A, Sardi A, Conaway GL (2000) Intraoperative ultrasound is essential in the management of metastatic colorectal liver lesions. Am Surg 66:611-5
13. Charnley RM, Morris DL, Dennison AR et al (1991) Detection of colorectal liver metastases using intraoperative ultrasonography. Br J Surg 78:45-48
14. Leen E, Horgan P (2003) Ultrasound contrast agents for hepatic imaging with nonlinear modes. Curr Probl Diagn Radiol 32:66-87
15. Wilson SR, Burns PN (2001) Liver mass evaluation with ultrasound: the impact of microbubble contrast agents and pulse inversion imaging. Semin Liver Dis 21:147-59
16. Takada T, Yasuda H, Uchiyama K et al (1990) Contrast-enhanced intraoperative ultrasound of small hepatocellular carcinomas. Surgery 107:528-32
17. Albrecht T, Blomley MJ, Burns PN et al (2003) Improved detection of hepatic metastases with pulse-inversion US during the liver-specific phase

of SHU 508A: multicenter study. Radiology 227:361-370
18. Kono Y, Steinbach GC, Peterson T et al (2002) Mechanism of parenchymal enhancement of the liver with a microbubble-based US contrast medium: an intravital microscopy study in rats. Radiology 224:253-257
19. Leen E, Ceccotti P, Glen P et al (2005) Potential value of CE-IOUS during partial hepatectomy for metastases: an essential investigation before resection. Ann Surg (in press)
20. Fong Y, Fortner J, Sun RL et al (1999) Clinical score from predicting recurrence after hepatic resection for metastatic colorectal cancer: analysis of 1001 consecutive cases. Ann Surg 230:309-321
21. Torzilli G, Del Fabbro D, Olivari N et al (2004) Contrast-enhanced ultrasonography during liver surgery. Br J Surg 91:1165-1167

II.8

European Guidelines in Liver Contrast Ultrasound

Riccardo Lencioni, Clotilde Della Pina, Dania Cioni, Laura Crocetti and Carlo Bartolozzi

Introduction

Detection and characterization of focal liver lesions is an important and challenging issue. Hepatocellular carcinoma (HCC) is the fifth most common cancer [1]. The liver is the organ most frequently involved by metastases. In addition, benign liver lesions, such as hemangioma and focal nodular hyperplasia (FNH), have a high prevalence in the general population. Several imaging modalities and diagnostic protocols have been used in attempts to optimize detection and characterization of focal liver lesions.

Ultrasound (US) is the most commonly used liver imaging modality. Unfortunately, US has limited sensitivity for the detection of small tumor nodules. Moreover, US findings are often non-specific, as there is enough variability and overlap in the appearance of benign and malignant liver lesions to make a definite distinction problematic. Computed tomography (CT) and magnetic resonance (MR) imaging are commonly used to clarify questionable US findings and to provide a more comprehensive assessment of the liver parenchyma.

Recently, the introduction of microbubble contrast agents and the development of contrast-specific techniques have opened up new prospects in liver US [2]. Contrast-specific techniques produce images based on non-linear acoustic effects of microbubbles and display enhancement in gray-scale, maximizing contrast and spatial resolution. The goal of improving the US assessment of focal lesions was initially pursued through scanning the liver with high mechanical index techniques. With these techniques, the signal is produced by the collapse of the microbubbles. The main limitations of this destructive method is that it produces a transient display of the contrast agent. Thus, it requires intermittent scanning, and a series of sweeps have to be performed in an attempt to cover the whole liver parenchyma. The advent of second-generation agents - that have higher harmonic emission capabilities - has been instrumental in improving the ease and the reproducibility of the examination [3]. In fact, a lower, non-destructive mechanical index can be used, thus enabling continuous real-time imaging. Over the past few years, several reports have shown that real-time contrast-enhanced US can substantially improve detection and characterization of focal liver lesions with respect to baseline studies [4].

With the publication of the guidelines for the use of contrast agents in liver US by the European Federation of Societies for Ultrasound in Medicine and Biology (EFSUMB), contrast-enhanced US has entered into clinical practice [4]. The guidelines define the indications and recommendations for the use of contrast agents in focal liver lesion detection, characterization, and post-treatment follow-up. In this paper, we discuss the impact of EFSUMB guidelines on diagnostic protocols currently adopted in liver imaging with regard to four clinical scenarios: (1) characterization of focal liver lesions of incidental detection; (2) diagnosis of HCC in patients with cirrhosis; (3) detection of hepatic metastases in oncology patients; and (4) guidance and assessment of the outcome of percutaneous tumor ablation procedures.

Characterization of Incidental Focal Liver Lesions

Characterization of focal lesions of incidental detection is one of the most common and sometimes troublesome issues in liver imaging.

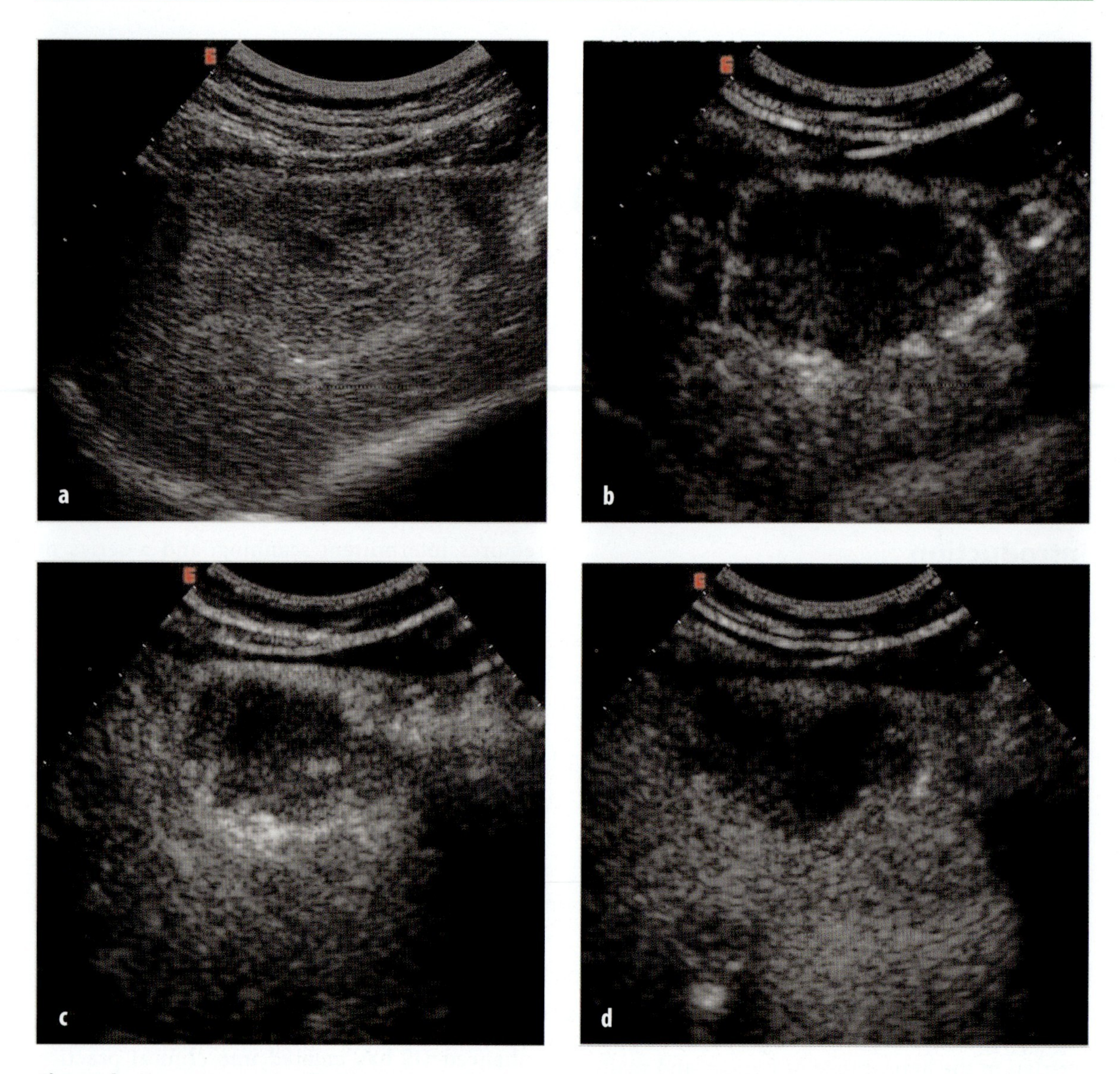

Fig. 1a-h. *Hemangioma.* At baseline US, the lesion has atypical features and appears as an iso-hypoechoic nodule (**a**). At contrast-enhanced US, the lesion shows peripheral nodular enhancement in the arterial phase (**b**) with centripetal filling in the portal-venous and delayed phases (**c**, **d**). The enhancement pattern resembles that observed at multidetector CT (**e**, baseline; **f**, arterial phase; **g**, portal-venous phase; **h**, delayed phase)

Unsuspected lesions, in fact, are frequently detected in patients who have neither chronic liver disease nor history of malignancy during an US examination of the abdomen. While a confident diagnosis is usually made on the basis of US findings in cases of simple cysts and hemangiomas with typical hyperechoic appearances, lesions with non-specific US features require further investigation [5]. The patient is typically referred for contrast-enhanced CT or contrast-enhanced MR imaging of the liver.

EFSUMB guidelines recommend the use of contrast agents to diagnose benign focal lesions not characterized at baseline study. This statement is based on the ability of contrast US to allow analysis of lesion vascularity. In fact, lesions that most frequently cause incidental findings – such as hemangioma and focal nodular hyperplasia – typically show contrast-enhanced US patterns that closely resemble those at contrast-enhanced CT or contrast-enhanced MR imaging. Most liver hemangiomas

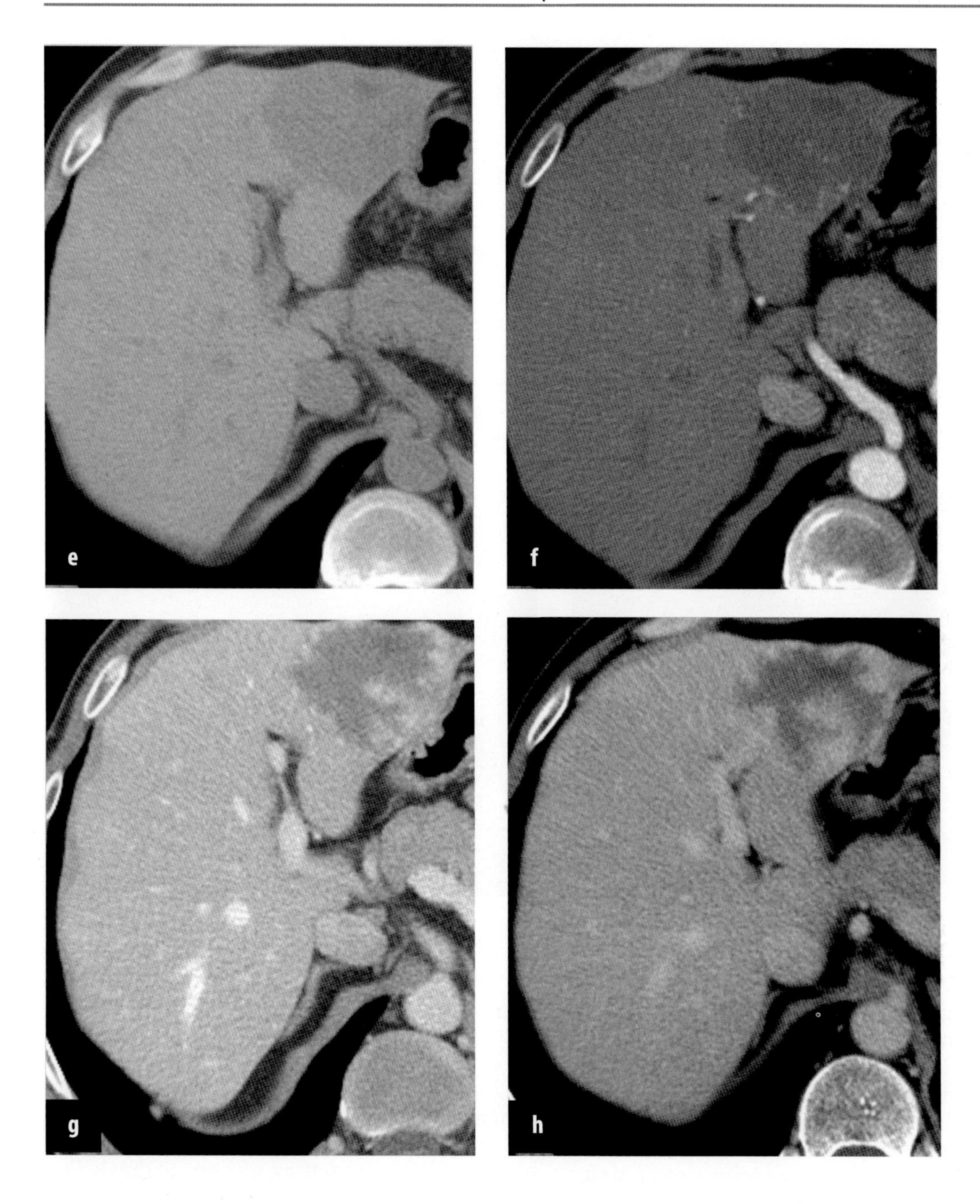

show peripheral nodular enhancement during the early phase, with progressive centripetal fill-in, leading to lesion hyperechogenicity in the late phase (Fig. 1). In two recent series, this characteristic features have been shown in 78-93% of hemangiomas [6, 7]. Focal nodular hyperplasia shows central vascular supply with centrifugal filling in the early arterial phase, followed by homogeneous enhancement in the late arterial phase. In the portal phase the lesion remains hyperechoic relative to normal liver tissue, and becomes isoechoic in the late phase (Fig. 2). This pattern has been observed in 85-100% of focal nodular hyperplasias [6, 8]. Therefore, it appears that in most liver lesions incidentally discovered at the baseline US study, detection of typical enhancement patterns after contrast injection may enable a quick and confident diagnosis, possibly avoiding the need for more complex and expensive investigations.

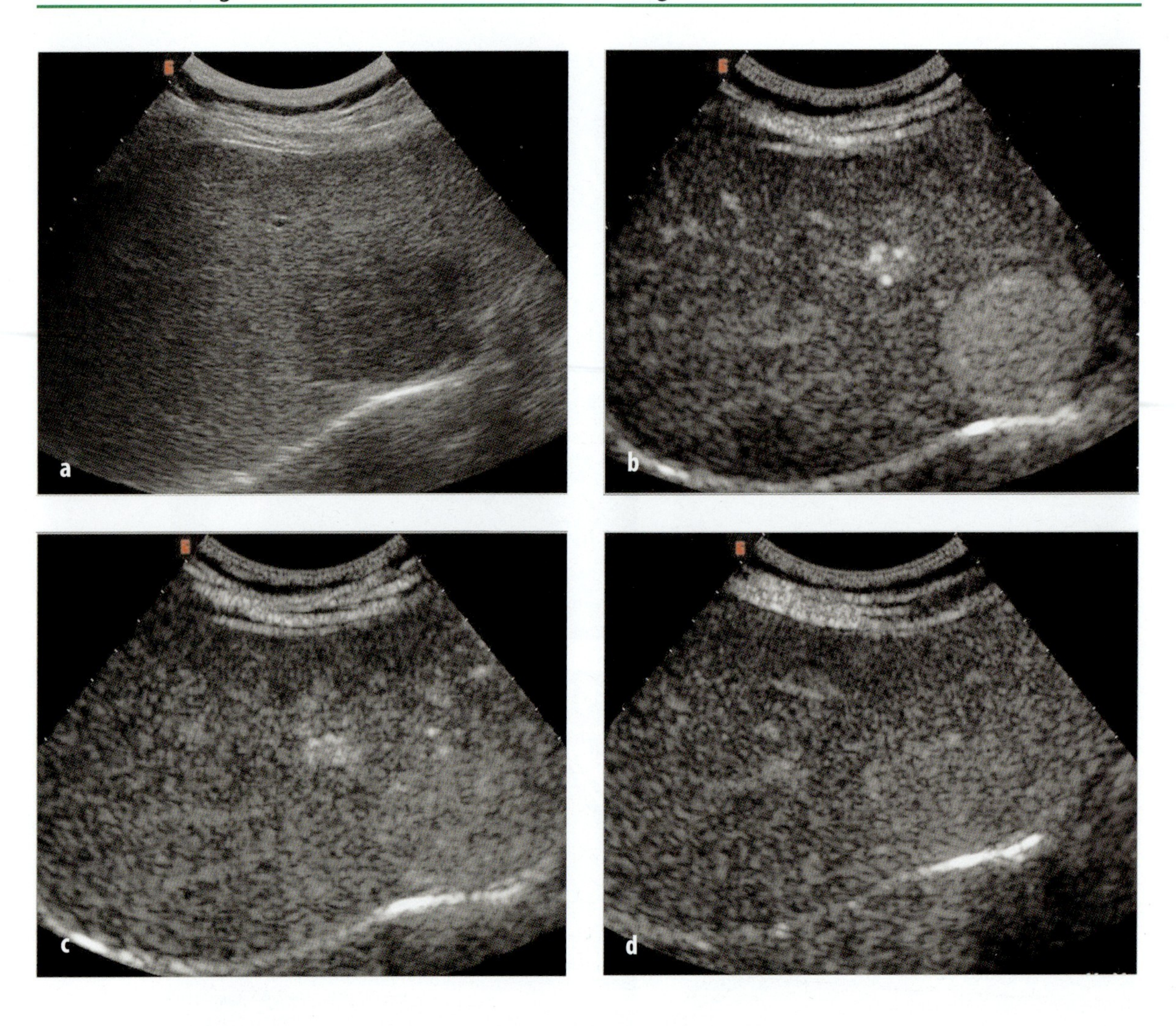

Diagnosis of Hepatocellular Carcinoma in Cirrhosis

The second clinical scenario is represented by patients with hepatic cirrhosis. In view of the high risk of developing HCC, these patients are carefully followed with US examinations repeated at six month intervals [9]. While the detection of a focal lesion in cirrhosis should always raise the suspicion of HCC, it is well established that the pathologic changes inherent to cirrhosis may simulate HCC in a variety of ways, especially because non-malignant hepatocellular lesions, such as regenerative and dysplastic nodules, may be indistinguishable from a small tumor. One of the key pathologic factors for differential diagnosis that is reflected in imaging appearances is the vascular supply to the nodule. Through the progression from regenerative nodule to dysplastic nodule to frank HCC, one sees loss of visualization of portal tracts and development of new arterial vessels, termed non-triadal arteries, which become the dominant blood supply in overt HCC. It is this neovascularity that allows HCC to be diagnosed with contrast-enhanced CT or dynamic MR imaging [10].

According to EFSUMB guidelines, a contrast-enhanced US study is recommended to characterize any lesion or suspect lesion detected at baseline US in the setting of liver cirrhosis [4]. Owing to the ability to display contrast-enhancement in real-time, contrast US appears to be a tool to show arterial neoangiogenesis associated with a malignant change, and, therefore, to help establish the diagnosis of HCC [11, 12]. HCC typically shows strong intratumoral enhancement in the arterial phase (i.e., within 25-35 seconds of the start of contrast injection) followed by rapid wash-out with isoechoic or hypoechoic appearance in the portal venous and delayed phases (Fig. 3). In contrast, large regenerative nodules and dysplastic nodules usually do not show any early contrast uptake, and resemble the enhancement pattern of liver parenchyma. Selective arterial enhancement at contrast US has been observed in 91-96% of HCC lesions, confirming

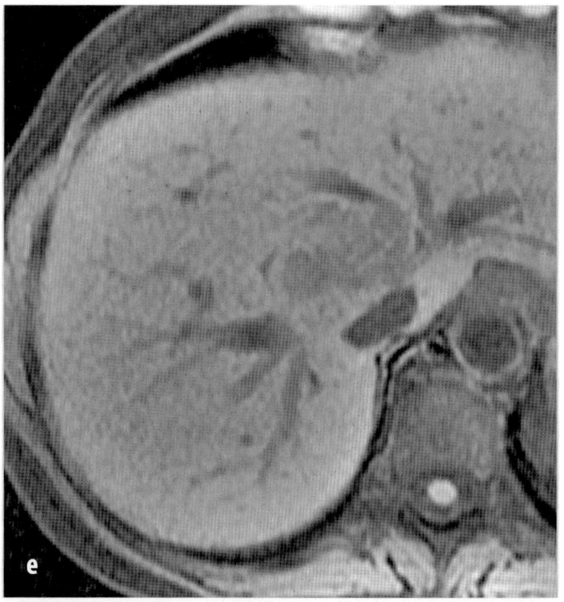

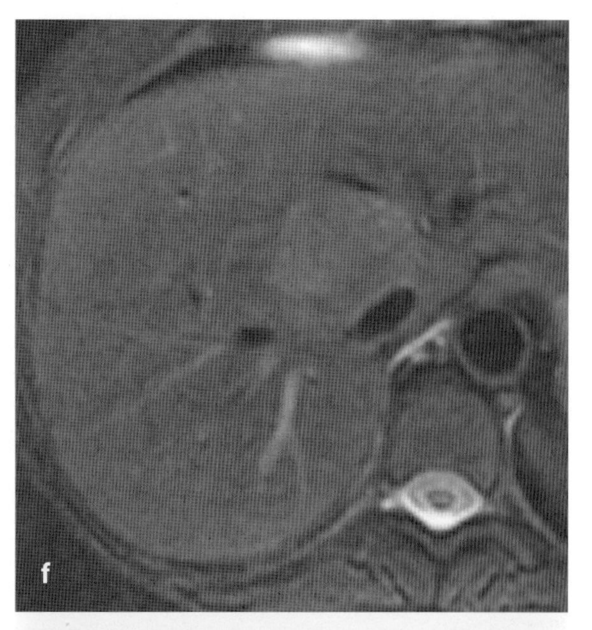

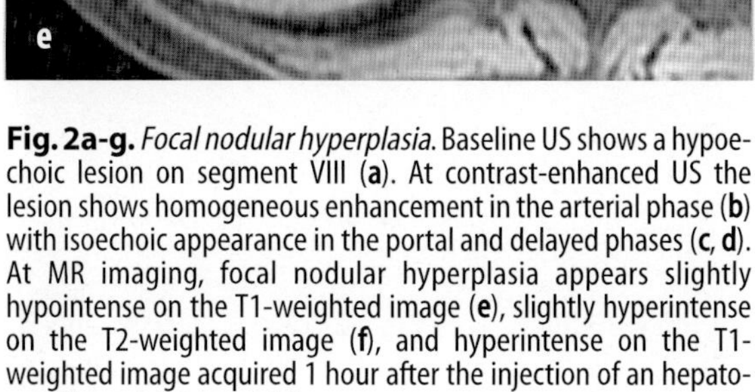

Fig. 2a-g. *Focal nodular hyperplasia.* Baseline US shows a hypoechoic lesion on segment VIII (**a**). At contrast-enhanced US the lesion shows homogeneous enhancement in the arterial phase (**b**) with isoechoic appearance in the portal and delayed phases (**c**, **d**). At MR imaging, focal nodular hyperplasia appears slightly hypointense on the T1-weighted image (**e**), slightly hyperintense on the T2-weighted image (**f**), and hyperintense on the T1-weighted image acquired 1 hour after the injection of an hepatospecific contrast agent (**g**)

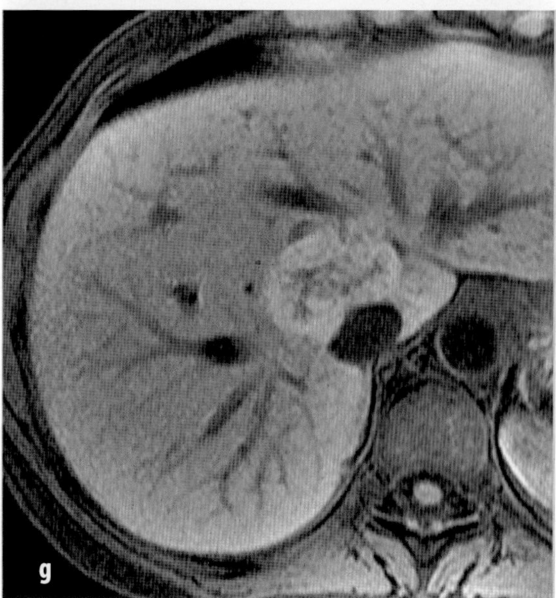

that contrast US may be a useful tool to show arterial neoangiogenesis of HCC [11, 12]. In a recent study, in which findings at spiral CT were assumed as the gold standard, the sensitivity of contrast US in the detection of arterial hypervascularity was 97% in lesions larger than 3 cm, 92% in lesions ranging 2-3 cm, 87% in lesions ranging 1-2 cm, and 67% in lesions smaller than 1 cm [12]. Hence, performing a contrast-enhanced study may be recommended in all lesions or suspected lesions - 1 cm or larger in diameter - detected at baseline US in patients with cirrhosis or chronic hepatitis undergoing surveillance programs.

The use of contrast US as a reliable alternative to CT or MR imaging for characterizing nodular lesions detected by US surveillance has been recently endorsed by the American Association for the Study of Liver Diseases [13]. The diagnostic protocol is structured according to the actual risk of malignancy and the possibility of achieving a reliable diagnosis. Since the prevalence of HCC among US-detected nodules is strongly related to the size of the lesion, the work-up depends on the size of the lesion (Fig. 4) [13]. Lesions smaller than 1 cm in diameter have a low likelihood of being HCC, and only need to be followed-up in order to detect growth suggestive of malignant transformation. When the nodule exceeds 1 cm in size, the lesion is more likely to

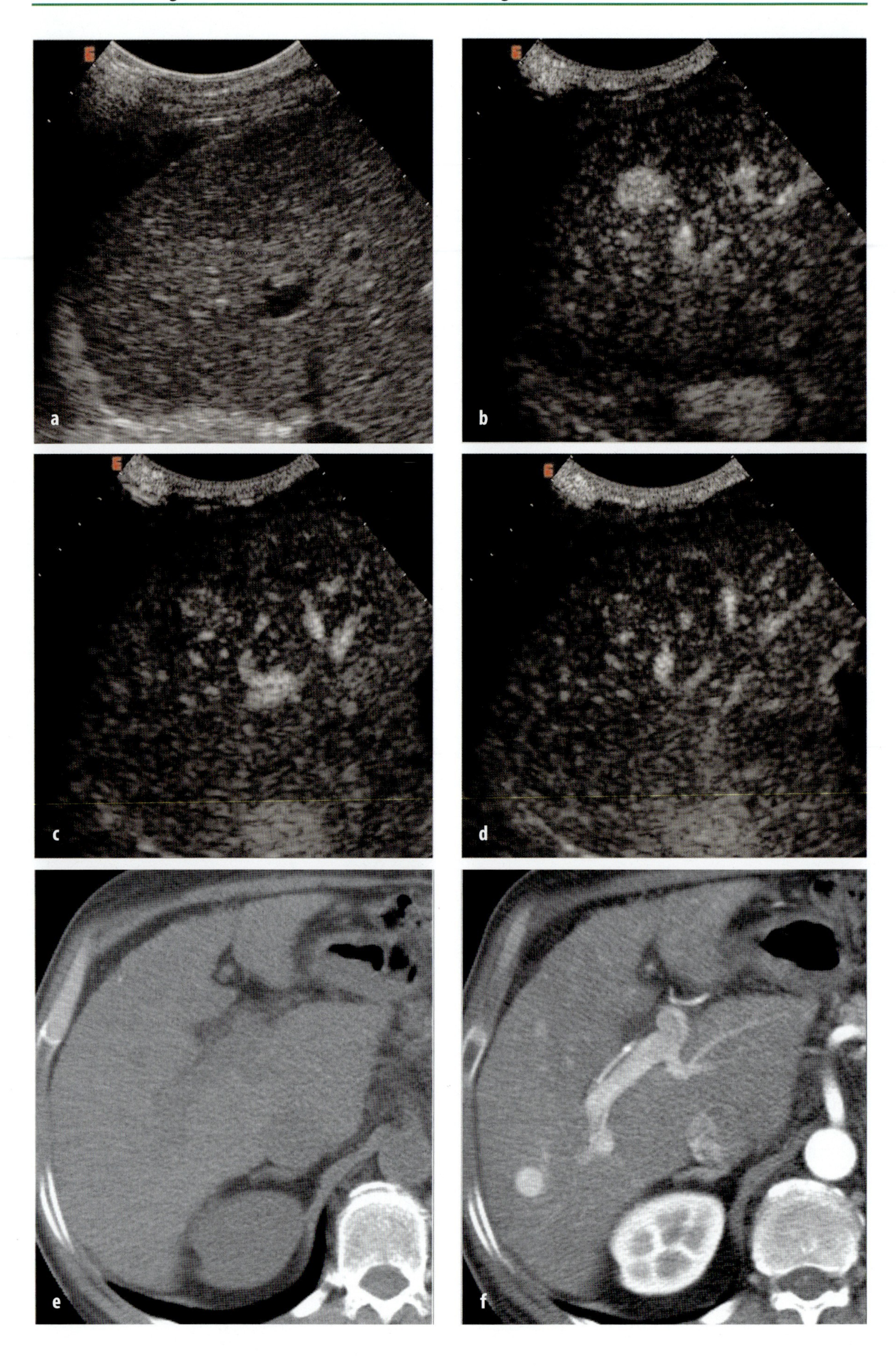
a
b
c
d
e
f

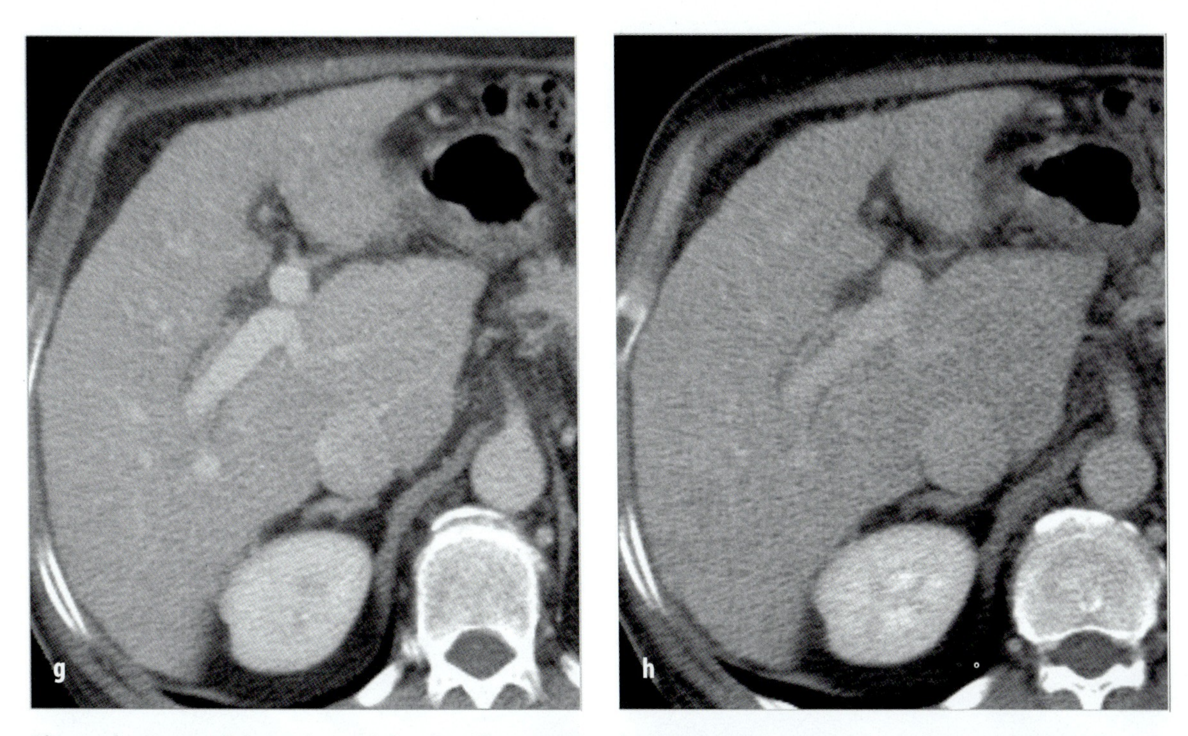

Fig. 3a-h. *Hepatocellular carcinoma.* At baseline US examination the lesion appears as an iso-hypoechoic nodule (**a**). At contrast-enhanced US, the lesion shows early enhancement in the arterial phase (**b**) with rapid wash-out in the portal-venous and delayed phases (**c**, **d**). At multidetector CT (**e**, baseline; **f**, arterial phase; **g**, portal-venous phase; **h**, delayed phase) the same enhancement pattern is observed

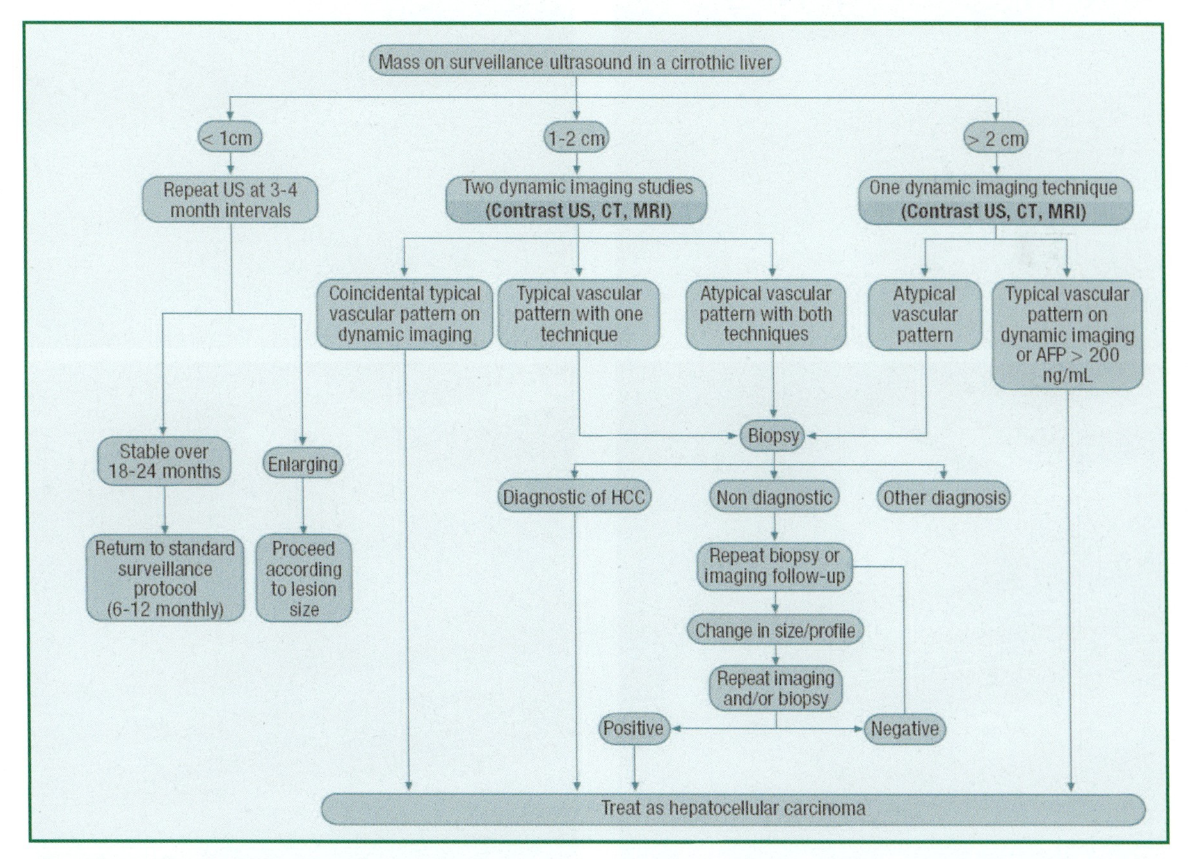

Fig. 4. Suggested algorithm for investigation of a nodule found on US during screening or surveillance. The typical vascular pattern means that the lesion is hypervascular in the arterial phase, and washes out in the portal/venous phase (Modified from [13])

be HCC and diagnostic confirmation should be pursued. It is accepted that the diagnosis of HCC in cirrhosis can be made without biopsy in a nodule larger than 1 cm that shows characteristic vascular features of HCC – i.e., arterial hypervascularization with wash-out in the portal venous or delayed phase - even in patients with normal alpha-fetoprotein values. For lesions ranging 1-2 cm, current guidelines require typical imaging findings to be confirmed by two coincident dynamic imaging modalities – out of contrast-enhanced US, contrast-enhanced multidetector CT, and contrast-enhanced MRI – to allow a non-invasive diagnosis [13]. If the imaging findings are not characteristic or the vascular profile is not coincidental among techniques, biopsy is recommended [13].

Detection of Hepatic Metastases in Oncology Patients

Metastatic disease involving the liver is one of the most common issues in oncology. CT and positron emission tomography (PET) are used in oncology protocols to provide objective documentation of the extent of the liver tumor burden and to effectively assess extrahepatic disease. Nevertheless, US is widely used in post-treatment follow-up to monitor tumor response and to detect the emergence of new hepatic metastatic lesions. One of the major points addressed by the EFSUMB document is the use of contrast agents in this patient population. In fact, the use of contrast agents is recommended

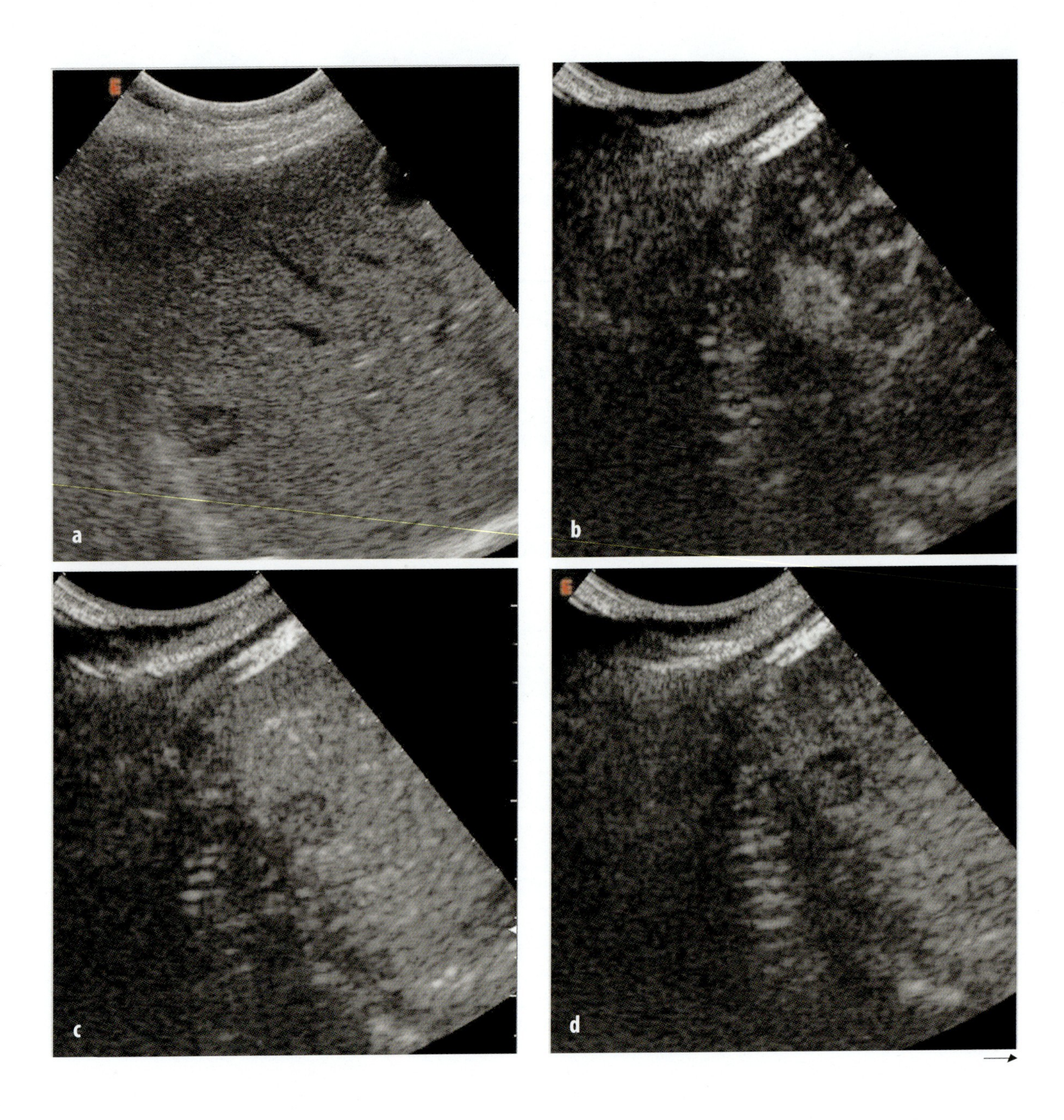

→

not only to clarify a questionable lesion detected at baseline examination. Performing a contrast-enhanced ultrasound study is recommended in every oncology patient referred for liver ultrasound, unless a clear-cut disseminated disease is detected at the baseline study. This means that all liver US examinations performed to rule out liver metastases should include a contrast-enhanced study, even if the baseline scans do not show any abnormality. This strong statement is based on a substantial increase in the ability to detect liver metastases in contrast-enhanced studies compared to baseline [14]. Even small metastases stand out as markedly hypoechoic lesions against the enhanced liver parenchyma throughout the portal venous and delayed phases (Fig. 5). The earlier the detection of liver metastatic disease, the earlier the therapeutic intervention.

Guidance and Monitoring of Tumor Ablation Procedures

Several percutaneous techniques have been developed to treat non-surgical patients with liver malignancies. These minimally invasive procedures can achieve effective and reproducible tumor destruction with acceptable morbidity. Radio-frequency ablation is increasingly accepted as the best therapeutic choice for

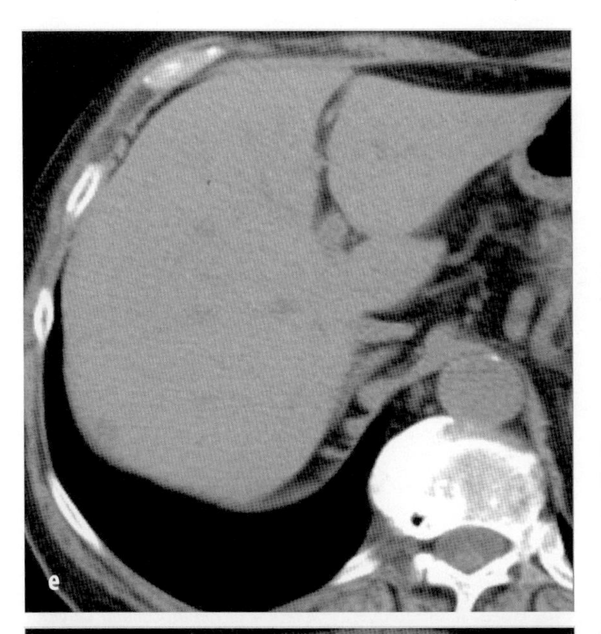

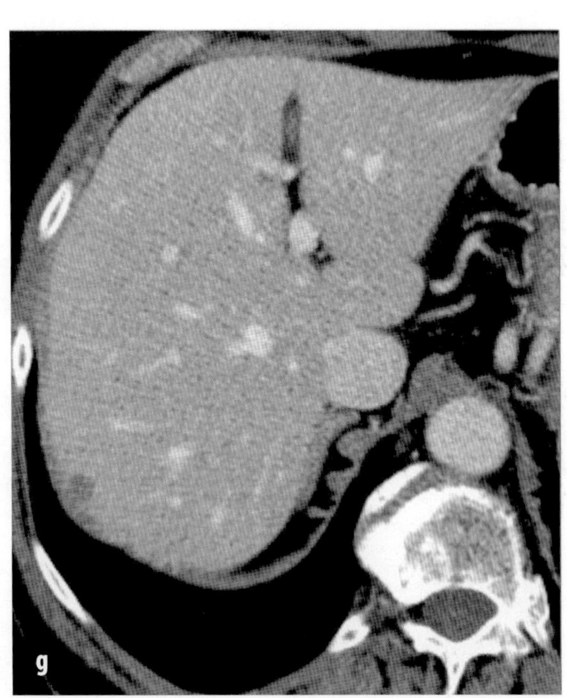

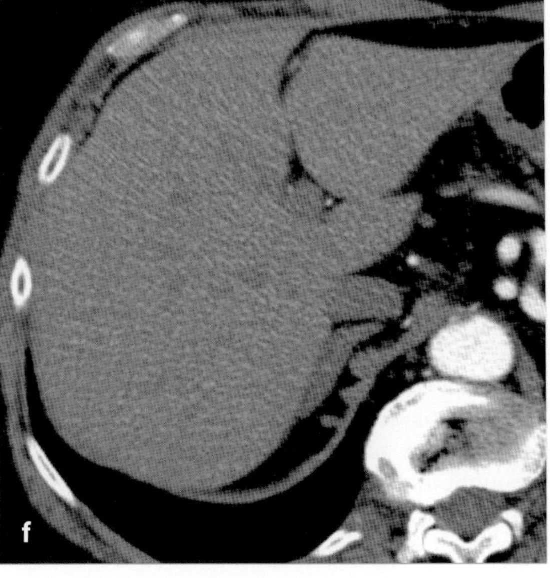

Fig. 5a-g. *Metastasis.* Baseline US examination shows a subcapsular hypoechoic nodule (**a**). At contrast-enhanced US the lesion shows rim enhancement during the arterial phase (**b**) with hypoechoic appearance in the portal-venous and delayed phases (**c**, **d**). At multidetector CT, the metastatic nodule appears hypodense in the baseline scan (**e**) as well as in the arterial (**f**) and the delayed phases (**g**)

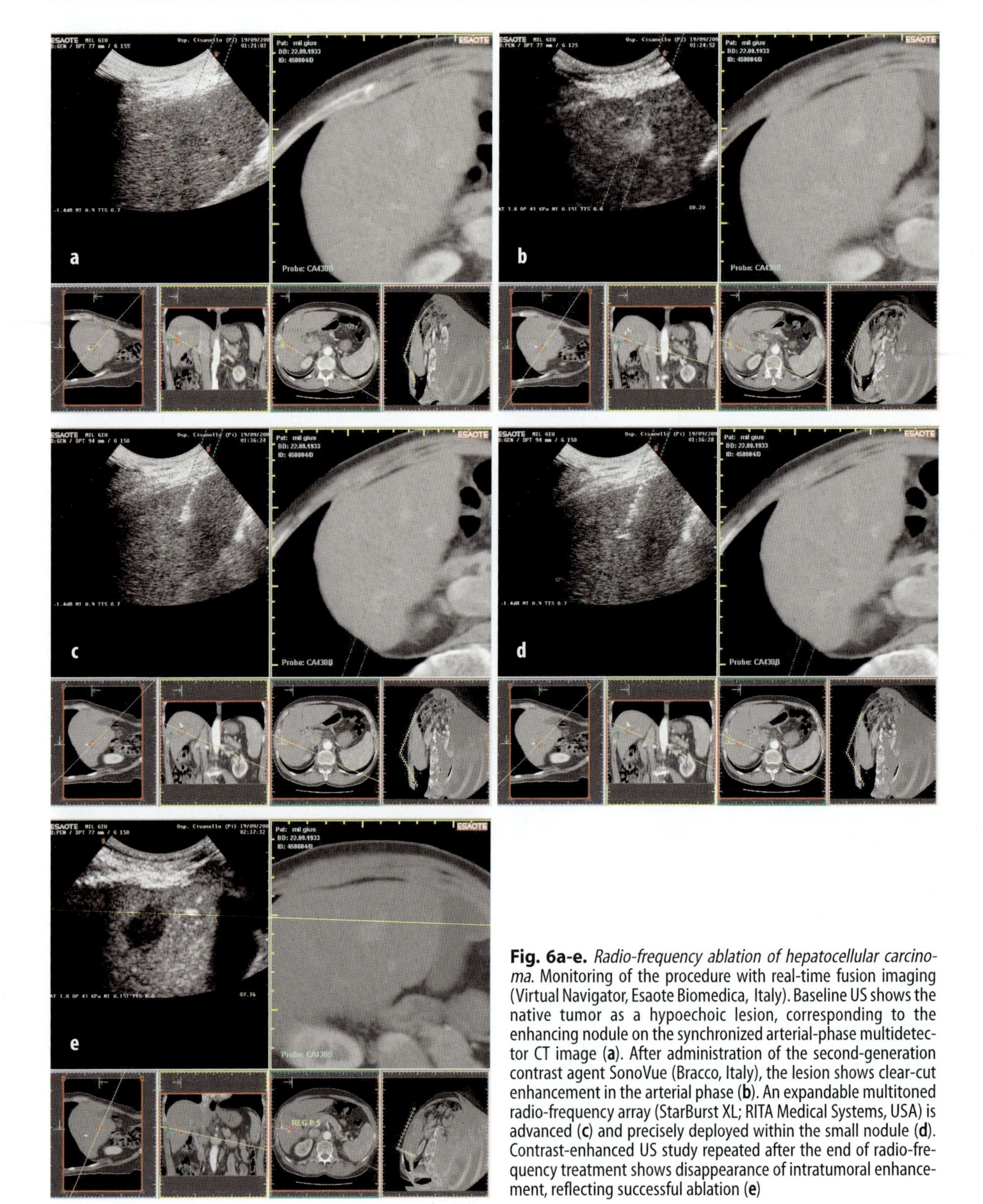

Fig. 6a-e. *Radio-frequency ablation of hepatocellular carcinoma.* Monitoring of the procedure with real-time fusion imaging (Virtual Navigator, Esaote Biomedica, Italy). Baseline US shows the native tumor as a hypoechoic lesion, corresponding to the enhancing nodule on the synchronized arterial-phase multidetector CT image (**a**). After administration of the second-generation contrast agent SonoVue (Bracco, Italy), the lesion shows clear-cut enhancement in the arterial phase (**b**). An expandable multitoned radio-frequency array (StarBurst XL; RITA Medical Systems, USA) is advanced (**c**) and precisely deployed within the small nodule (**d**). Contrast-enhanced US study repeated after the end of radio-frequency treatment shows disappearance of intratumoral enhancement, reflecting successful ablation (**e**)

patients with early-stage HCC when resection or transplantation are precluded and has also become a viable treatment method for patients with limited hepatic metastatic disease from colorectal cancer who are not eligible for surgical resection [15, 16].

When US is used as the imaging modality for guiding ablations, the addition of contrast agent can provide additional important information throughout all the procedural steps: it improves delineation and conspicuity of lesions poorly visualized on baseline scans, facilitating targeting; it allows the immediate assessment of the outcome of treatment by showing the disappearance of any previously visualized intralesional enhancement (Fig. 6); and it may be useful in the follow-up protocols for early detection of tumor recurrence [17].

Conclusions

Despite the improvement in detection and characterization of focal liver lesions that can be achieved using contrast-enhanced US, several issues are still open. First, contrast US will hardly replace CT or MR imaging for preoperative assessment of patients with liver tumors, as these techniques still offer a more comprehensive assessment of the liver parenchyma, which is mandatory to properly plan any kind of surgical or interventional procedure. Second, the daily schedule of each US laboratory doing liver examinations will have to be reformulated, and many US laboratories will have to update their equipment and to provide proper training for their doctors. Last but not least, the cost of the introduction of contrast-enhanced US into daily practice will have to be taken into account. It can be argued that cost saving associated with patients who will no longer need a CT or MR imaging of the liver after contrast-enhanced US could largely counterbalance the cost of the examination. However, an optimal use of contrast-enhanced US will require the definition of precise diagnostic flow charts for each clinical situation. Nevertheless, contrast-enhanced US has the potential to become the primary liver imaging modality for early detection and characterization of focal lesions. Early diagnosis of primary and secondary liver malignancies greatly enhances the possibility of curative surgical resection or successful percutaneous ablation, resulting in better patient care and eventually in improved patient survival.

Key Points

- Several reports have shown that real-time contrast-enhanced US substantially improves detection and characterisation of focal liver lesions with respect to baseline US.
- The European Federation of Societies for Ultrasound in Medicine and Biology (EFSUMB) has issued guidelines that define the indications and recommendations for the use of contrast agents in liver US.
- EFSUMB guidelines are producing a major impact on diagnostic protocols for all the main clinical situations: (1) characterisation of focal liver lesions of incidental detection; (2) diagnosis of hepatocellular carcinoma in patients with cirrhosis; (3) detection of hepatic metastases in oncology patients; and (4) guidance and assessment of the outcome of percutaneous tumor ablation procedures.
- The use of contrast US as a reliable alternative to CT and MR imaging in characterising nodular lesions detected by US surveillance in patients with cirrhosis as hepatocellular carcinoma has been recently endorsed by the American Association for the Study of Liver Diseases.

References

1. Llovet JM, Burroughs A, Bruix J (2003) Hepatocellular carcinoma. Lancet 362:1907-1917
2. Lencioni R, Cioni D, Bartolozzi C (2002) Tissue harmonic and contrast-specific imaging: back to gray scale in ultrasound. Eur Radiol 12:151-165
3. Lencioni R, Cioni D, Crocetti L et al (2002) Ultrasound imaging of focal liver lesions with a second-generation contrast agent. Acad Radiol 9 Suppl 2:S371-374
4. Albrecht T, Blomley M, Bolondi L et al; EFSUMB Study Group (2004) Guidelines for the use of contrast agents in ultrasound. January 2004. Ultraschall Med 25:249-256
5. Lencioni R, Cioni D, Crocetti L et al (2004) Magnetic resonance imaging of liver tumors. J Hepatol 40:162-171
6. Wen YL, Kudo M, Zheng RQ et al (2004) Characterization of hepatic tumors: value of contrast-enhanced coded phase-inversion harmonic angio. AJR Am J Roentgenol 182:1019-1026
7. Quaia E, Calliada F, Bertolotto M et al (2004) Characterization of focal liver lesions with contrast-specific US modes and a sulfur hexafluoride-filled microbubble contrast agent: diagnostic performance and confidence. Radiology 232:420-430

8. Kim MJ, Lim HK, Kim SH et al (2004) Evaluation of hepatic focal nodular hyperplasia with contrast-enhanced gray scale harmonic sonography: initial experience. J Ultrasound Med 23:297-305
9. Bruix J, Sherman M, Llovet JM et al; EASL Panel of Experts on HCC (2001) Clinical management of hepatocellular carcinoma. Conclusions of the Barcelona-2000 EASL conference. European Association for the Study of the Liver. J Hepatol 35:421-430
10. Lencioni R, Cioni D, Della Pina C et al (2005) Imaging diagnosis. Semin Liver Dis 25:162-170
11. Nicolau C, Catala V, Vilana R et al (2004) Evaluation of hepatocellular carcinoma using SonoVue, a second generation ultrasound contrast agent: correlation with cellular differentiation. Eur Radiol 14:1092-1099
12. Gaiani S, Celli N, Piscaglia F et al (2004) Usefulness of contrast-enhanced perfusional sonography in the assessment of hepatocellular carcinoma hypervascular at spiral computed tomography. J Hepatol 41:421-426
13. Bruix J, Sherman M. Management of hepatocellular carcinoma (2005) Hepatology 42:1208-1236
14. Oldenburg A, Hohmann J, Foert E et al (2005) Detection of hepatic metastases with low MI real time contrast-enhanced sonography and SonoVue. Ultraschall Med 26:277-284
15. Lencioni R, Crocetti L, Cioni D et al (2004) Percutaneous radiofrequency ablation of hepatic colorectal metastases. Technique, indications, results, and new promises. Invest Radiol 39:689-697
16. Lencioni R, Cioni D, Crocetti L et al (2005) Early-stage hepatocellular carcinoma in patients with cirrhosis: long-term results of percutaneous image-guided radiofrequency ablation. Radiology 234:961-967
17. Solbiati L, Ierace T, Tonolini M, Cova L (2004) Guidance and monitoring of radiofrequency liver tumor ablation with contrast-enhanced ultrasound. Eur J Radiol 51 Suppl:S19-23

Section III

Clinical Application of Contrast Ultrasound in Vascular Diseases

III.1

Transcranial Doppler

Dirk W. Droste

Introduction

Stroke is the third cause of death and the most frequent cause of acquired handicap in the western world. Its consequences include hemiparesis, hemisensory loss, dysarthria, dysphasia and other cognitive disorders, disorders of vision, and depression. Stroke is thus a major human and socioeconomic burden in our society. The key issue to the understanding of stroke aetiology, and thus to stroke management to reduce the actual deficit and to prevent further deficits, is the assessment of the patients' arterial vascular situation. Neurosonological investigations of the extracranial and intracranial brain-supplying arteries are therefore very helpful in the assessment of stroke and stroke-prone patients. By conventional extracranial and transcranial Doppler sonography (ECD and TCD) and by extracranial and transcranial colour-coded duplex sonography (ECCD, TCCD), stenoses or occlusions, and pathological collateral flow patterns are detected. The following arteries can be evaluated extracranially: common, internal, and external carotid artery, vertebral artery, supratrochlear and subclavian artery. The internal carotid artery, and the middle, anterior and posterior cerebral arteries can be investigated intracranially through the temporal window, and the vertebral and basilar arteries can be investigated through the foramen magnum. Moreover, the ophthalmic artery and the carotid siphon can be insonated through the orbits. Contrast ultrasound is of particular interest in intracranial ultrasound given the poor insonation situation in about 20% of cases.

Baseline Ultrasound

TCCD permits a continuous representation of flowing blood in the arteries and demonstrates their relation to anatomical landmarks, such as bony structures, ventricles, and parenchyma. This allows for a refined spatial orientation compared to conventional TCD, and helps to avoid compression tests. For example, the posterior cerebral artery can unequivocally be identified by its course around the midbrain. Furthermore, several vessels and vessel segments can be assessed simultaneously. However, the individual patient's anatomy and pathology (deep location of arteries, shadowing of the ultrasound beam, low flow, insufficient bone window) may hamper their proper visualisation. Weak Doppler signals due to a large insonation angle, low flow volume, or low flow velocity, are further problems. Our group performed a combined pre-/postmortem study to investigate the influence of the temporal bone on the quality of the ultrasound signal [1]. Thirty-three moribund neurological patients who eventually died were examined by TCCD using the transtemporal approach. The sonographer categorised the quality of the TCCS image. During autopsy, a rectangular sample of the temporal squama was removed, which corresponded to the area of the *in vivo* acoustic window. The thickness of the whole temporal bone, and that of the cortical and cancellous (=diploe) bone, as well as density and homogeneity, were determined by high resolution computed tomography (CT). A significant correlation between the complete bone thickness as well as between the absolute thickness of the diploe and the quality of the acoustic window was found: the thinner the bone/diploe, the better the colour Doppler signal. The thickness of the cortical plates and the homogeneity of the bones were identical in the three image quality categories. Therefore the transtemporal TCCD image quality depends mainly on the thickness of the cancellous (diploe) component of the temporal bone and not on its structure. These limitations to insonation led to the development of echocontrast agents that are able to survive pulmonary and capillary transit and increase the echogenecity of the flowing blood. All the Doppler modalities, i.e., spectral Doppler, colour-Doppler and power mode, show an increased signal with the use of echocontrast agents (Figs. 1, 2).

Contrast Ultrasound Features

Principles

Echocontrast agents are microbubble preparations for intravenous administration that provide useful and reproducible enhancement on ultrasound scans. These microbubbles increase the intensity of the Doppler signal by 10 to 30 dB. The high stability and low diameter (< 8 μm) of the contrast microbubbles provide enough signal to image over several capillary passages. Echocontrast agents with a low stability that are used for the detection of cardiac and extracardiac shunts (e.g. Echovist) will not be discussed

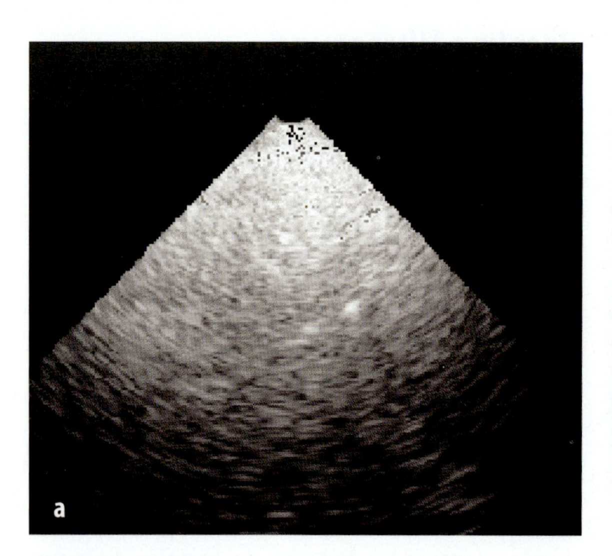

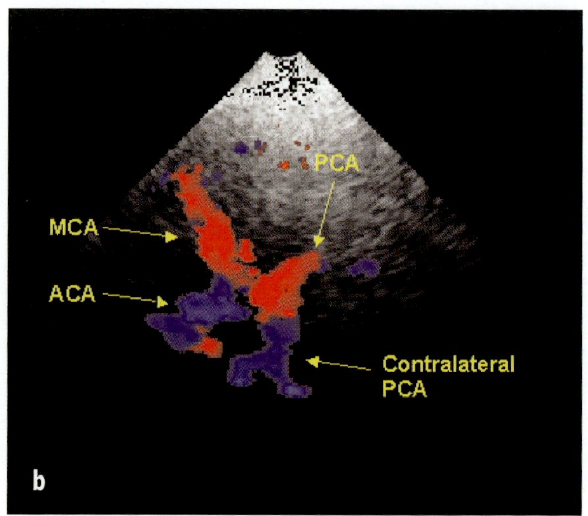

Fig. 1a, b. A patient with an insufficient temporal bone window before (**a**) and after (**b**) application of SonoVue. Colour mode, normal finding. MCA = middle cerebral artery, ACA = anterior cerebral artery, PCA = posterior cerebral artery (Reprinted with permission from [26])

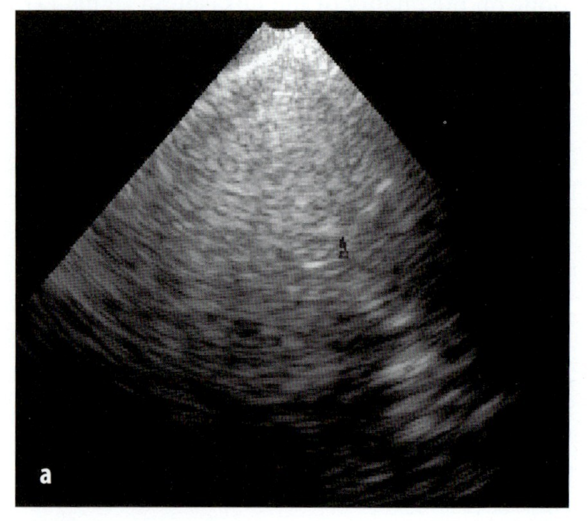

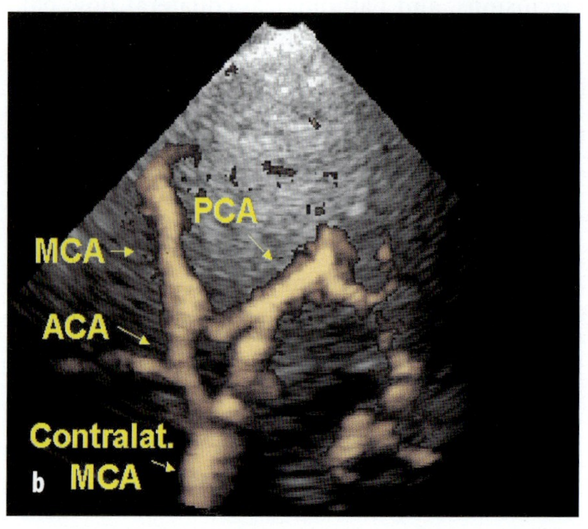

Fig. 2a, b. A patient with an insufficient temporal bone window before (**a**) and after (**b**) application of SonoVue. Power mode, normal finding. MCA = middle cerebral artery, ACA = anterior cerebral artery, PCA = posterior cerebral artery, Contralat = contralateral (Reprinted with permission from [26])

in this context. By injecting the contrast agent into the circulating blood, the propagation of ultrasound is modified in a characteristic manner. For echocontrast-enhancement, the phenomenon of scattering and not of reflection is crucial. There is a much stronger ultrasound scattering at the interface between blood and contrast medium as compared to the interface between erythrocytes and serum.

Products

In many European countries two contrast agents are currently licensed for use in neurosonology: Levovist and SonoVue. The *in vivo* stability of echocontrast agents is related to their shell characteristics and the solubility in blood of the gas used in their preparation. Since second-generation echocontrast agents contain poorly soluble gases such as fluorocarbons or sulfur hexafluoride, agents such as SonoVue have a longer duration of effect than air-containing agents like Levovist.

Levovist (Schering, Germany) is a galactose/palmitic acid-based agent which, on dissolution and agitation in sterile water, generates a suspension of air-filled microbubbles attached to the galactose crystals with a palmitic acid coating and a median diameter of 3 μm. These lipid-coated microbubbles are sufficiently stable and small to survive the capillary circulation. Mean duration of intracranial contrast-enhancement after a single intraveneous (iv) administration was 163-240 seconds [2]. Galactose is metabolised to CO_2, palmitic acid to triglycerides. Only minor transient side effects were observed in a large patient cohort [3]. The short lasting enhancement by echocontrast agents represents a new challenge to the clinical practice of ultrasound. Normally, Doppler interrogations last several minutes. The typical course of an echo-enhancement after administration of a bolus, comprises (1) an initial phase of increasing enhancement, then (2) 'blooming' (overload), followed by (3) a phase ideal for diagnostic use and (4) a phase of decreasing enhancement. Attempts were made to prolong the clinically useful investigation time caused by the echocontrast agent by its continuous iv infusion after bolus injection [4-6]. Giving the contrast agent in fractions (e.g., starting with half the amount followed by a repeated dose of quarter of the amount within a few minutes of each other) can smooth and prolong the enhancing effect as well.

SonoVue (BR1) by Bracco (Italy) is an aqueous suspension of phospholipid-encapsulated sulfur hexafluoride. The agent is prepared by injecting 5 ml of normal saline into vials containing 25 mg of sterile lyophilised powder in a gaseous atmosphere of sulfur hexafluoride. The vial is gently shaken until complete dissolution of the lyophilisate in the suspension. The concentration is approximately $2*10^8$ bubbles/ml, the bubble diameter is about 2.5 μm, and 90% of the bubbles are smaller than 8 μm. In a phase I pharmacokinetic study conducted on 12 healthy volunteers who received SonoVue, more than 75% of the dose was eliminated by 11 minutes via the lungs into the expired air [7]. Figure 3 gives the median durations of clinically useful enhancement recorded in a dose finding study [8]. A dose of 1.2-2.4 ml of SonoVue proved to be most useful. With a dose of 2.4 ml, median durations of clinically useful enhancement of 1.9-6.3 minutes were obtained.

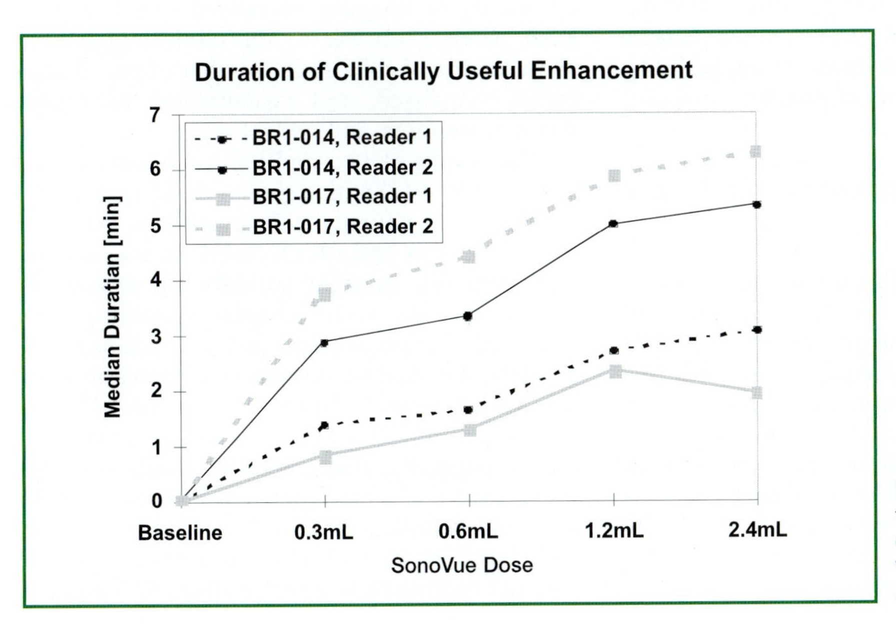

Fig. 3. Duration of clinically useful enhancement of different doses of SonoVue (Reprinted with permission from S. Karger AG, Basel [8])

Safety Issues of SonoVue

In the study reported by Droste et al. [8], which included 113 patients, possible or probable side effects (7.1% of the patients) included heat or pain at the injection site (six patients), headache (one patient) and mild itching (one patient). All these advents were non-serious and resolved without sequelae.

Although in our experience SonoVue has never been associated with side effects worth mentioning, several cases, including heart problems and severe drops in blood pressure and heart rate have been described. Some of the patients who experienced these effects already had severe coronary artery disease. The European Medicines Agency (EMEA) in London therefore defined (besides the usual contra-indications such as pregnancy, lactation and hypersensitivity) specific contraindications. SonoVue is contraindicated for use in patients with recent acute coronary syndrome or clinically unstable ischemic cardiac disease, including: evolving or ongoing myocardial infarction, typical angina at rest within the last seven days, significant worsening of cardiac symptoms within the last seven days, recent coronary artery intervention or other factors suggesting clinical instability (for example, recent deterioration of ECG, laboratory or clinical findings), acute cardiac failure, class III/IV cardiac failure, or severe rhythm disorders. SonoVue is contraindicated in patients known to have right-to-left shunts, severe pulmonary hypertension (pulmonary artery pressure > 90 mmHg), uncontrolled systemic hypertension, and in patients with adult respiratory distress syndrome [9, 10]. Furthermore, patients should be kept under close medical supervision during and for at least 30 minutes following administration. SonoVue is contraindicated in ventilated patients [9, 10]. These restrictions lower its applicability, however, only in a minority of patients.

Practical Considerations of the Machinery Setting

Prerequisite for the sensible use of contrast is an optimal machine setting for the visualisation of the structures of diagnostic interest on native colour mode scans. To visualise flow with low velocity and small intensity, the pulse repetition frequency has to be lowered and the gain has to be increased until colour artefacts appear. Moreover, there should be a favourable insonation angle. The use of echocontrast should be considered only when a proper assessment is not possible under these conditions.

Practical Considerations of the Injection of SonoVue

In general, due to its relatively long effect of 1.9-6.3 minutes, SonoVue can be administered by single injection. This may be of particular importance when only one person is available to do the examination. A second injection, however, is also possible [9, 11].

In our centre, after preparation of one vial, we inject via an indwelling venous catheter either the total amount or half of it as a bolus, depending on the quality of the acoustic window. If the quality is sufficient with half a vial, we inject a quarter of a vial twice, or all the remaining half after 1-2 minutes to prolong the contrast effect. In case of a still insufficient window, following injection of half a vial, we inject a whole vial as a bolus. This allows the investigation to be performed by a single investigator. If no brain structures are seen on B-mode at all, in our experience there is little effect of contrast concerning arterial imaging.

Comparisons of Pre- and Post-Contrast Imaging

The use of echocontrast agents is indicated in about 20% of all transcranial colour-coded duplex investigations in Europe [5, 12, 13]. The number is higher in patients with Asian or African ethnic background [14]. Gas-filled microbubble contrast agents can also be used during conventional continuous wave and transcranial Doppler ultrasound [14], but are of particular benefit in TCCD investigations. The target parameters of the studies mentioned included quality of imaging, visualised vessel length, stent patency, answer to the clinical question, visualisation of collaterals, number of vessel segments visualised, and visualisation of vessel patency, stenoses, and occlusions.

The results of two multicentre studies (BR1-014 and BR1-017) with a similar design involving a total of 113 patients with insufficient acoustic windows before and after SonoVue injection were published [8]. In eight patients, the region of interest was the vertebrobasilar system via the transnuchal approach and in the remaining 105 patients, the anterior or posterior circulation via the transtemporal approach. In 66-74% of patients, a non-diagnostic study was converted into a diagnostic study. SonoVue facilitated the visualisation of vessel patency, stenosis, occlusion, and collateral flow, decreased the need for additional tests, and had an impact on the patient's treatment. In a recent study, 67 temporal bones were insonated before and after application of SonoVue [15]. As compared to the pre-contrast scans, echocontrast allowed for more segments to be evaluated by pulsed Doppler sonography ($p < 0.0001$) and for longer lumen segments to be displayed on colour mode ($p < 0.0001$). With the help of contrast medium, flow velocity in the middle cerebral artery could be measured through 65 windows as compared to only 26 windows before the application of contrast ($p < 0.0001$). Table 1 gives details of the results for the individual vessels.

Table 1. Colour-coded Doppler signals and visualisation of pulsed-wave Doppler spectra before and after contrast application [15]

Before contrast	After contrast (mean ± SD; median, range)	(mean ± SD; median, range)
Length of the artery on colour mode		
Ipsilateral MCA	4.6 ± 0.62mm (0; 0-17.8mm)	23.9 ± 7.4mm (26.0; 0-35.4mm)
Ipsilateral ACA	0.1 ± 0.9mm (0; 0-7.9mm)	7.5 ± 3.4mm (8.0; 0-16.2mm)
Contralateral ACA	0.0 ± 0mm (0; 0-0mm)	7.5 ± 4.0mm (8.0; 0-12.9mm)
Ipsilateral PCA (P1)	0.3 ± 1.2mm (0; 0-5.7mm)	8.1 ± 4.2mm (9.1; 0-14.5mm)
Ipsilateral PCA (P2)	2.3 ± 4.2mm (0; 0-15.7mm)	20.0 ± 8.4mm (22.2; 0-33.2mm)
Ipsilateral PCoA	0 ± 0mm (0; 0-0mm)	4.9 ± 2.7mm (5.5; 0-8.4mm)
Contralateral PCA (P1)	0 ± 0mm (0; 0-0mm)	5.5 ± 4.4mm (7.7; 0-13.6mm)
Number of MCA branches visualised on colour mode	0.0 ± 0 (0; 0-0)	0.68 ± 0.97 (0; 0-3)
Possibility of obtaining a Doppler spectrum		
Ipsilateral MCA	39 ± 49% (0; 0-100%)	97 ± 17% (100; 0-100%)
Ipsilateral ACA	1 ± 12% (0; 0-100%)	91 ± 29% (100; 0-100%)
Contralateral ACA	0 ± 0% (0; 0-0%)	64 ± 48% (100; 0-100%)
AcoA	0 ± 0% (0; 0-100%)	54 ± 50% (100; 0-100%)
Ipsilateral PCA (P1)	6 ± 24% (0; 0-100%)	85 ± 36% (100; 0-100%)
Ipsilateral PCA (P2)	27 ± 45% (0; 0-100%)	90 ± 31% (100; 0-100%)
Ipsilateral PCoA	0 ± 0% (0; 0-0%)	84 ± 37% (100; 0-100%)
Contralateral PCA (P1)	0 ± 0%	64 ± 47%

The benefits of native echocontrast-enhanced neurovascular ultrasound in the literature are summarised in Table 2. In general, the success rate of the enhanced investigation was in the range of two thirds to three quarters of the investigations.

Three examples further illustrate the benefit of echocontrast in the anterior and posterior cerebral circulation (Figs. 4-6).

Role of Contrast Ultrasound in Clinical Practice

General Considerations

Neurovascular ultrasound is a cheap and easy-to-perform bedside procedure. Echocontrast provides effective Doppler signal enhancement and

Table 2. Diagnostic benefit of echocontrast agents in different vessel areas in neurosonology

Vessel	Diagnostic benefit	Literature
Middle, anterior and posterior cerebral artery main stems, middle cerebral artery branches	excellent	[5;8;12-15;29-34]
Intracranial collaterals	excellent	[5;8;12;35]
Vertebrobasilar junction	excellent	[13;28;36;37]
Extracranial carotid arteries	medium	[4;33;38-42]
Distal basilar artery (transnuchal approach)	medium	[13;28;36;37]
Dural arteriovenous fistulae	excellent	[18]

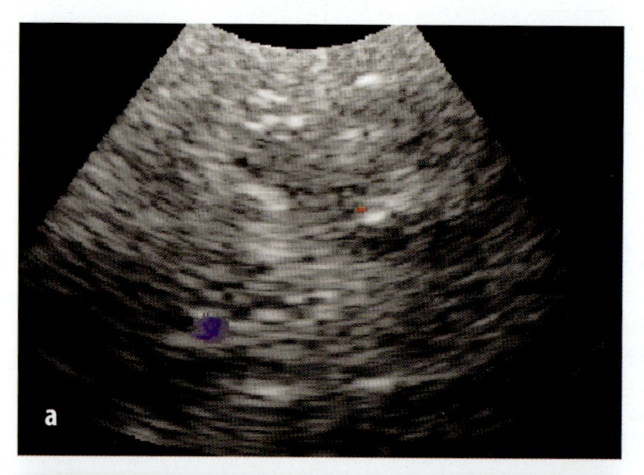

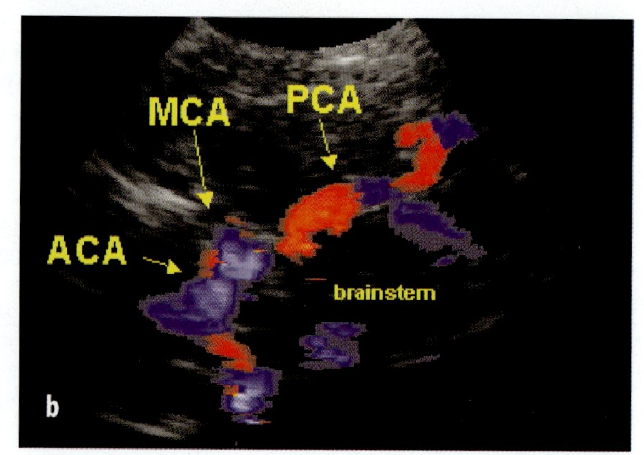

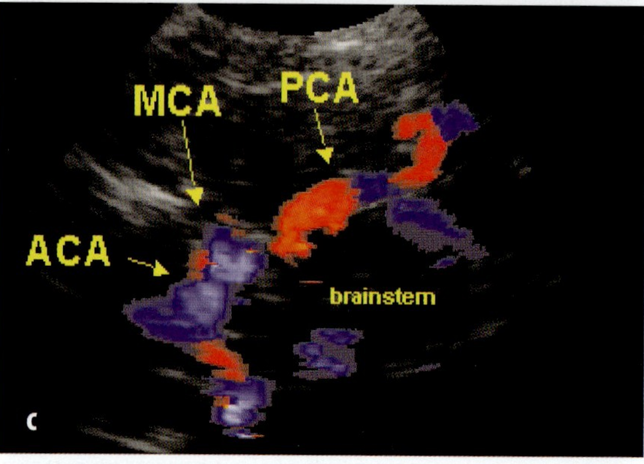

Fig. 4a-c. A patient with an insufficient temporal bone window before (**a**) and after (**c**) application of SonoVue®. Colour mode. The patient had suffered an acute stroke in the middle cerebral artery territory. The upper template demonstrates the unenhanced investigation before application of SonoVue. **b** shows the investigation using SonoVue. A middle cerebral artery main stem occlusion is detected with compensatory flow increase in the anterior cerebral artery. Intravenous thrombolysis is started under colour-coded duplex monitoring. The lower template shows the enhanced investigation following thrombolysis with restored flow in the middle cerebral artery. MCA = middle cerebral artery, ACA = anterior cerebral artery, PCA = posterior cerebral artery (Reprinted with permission from [26])

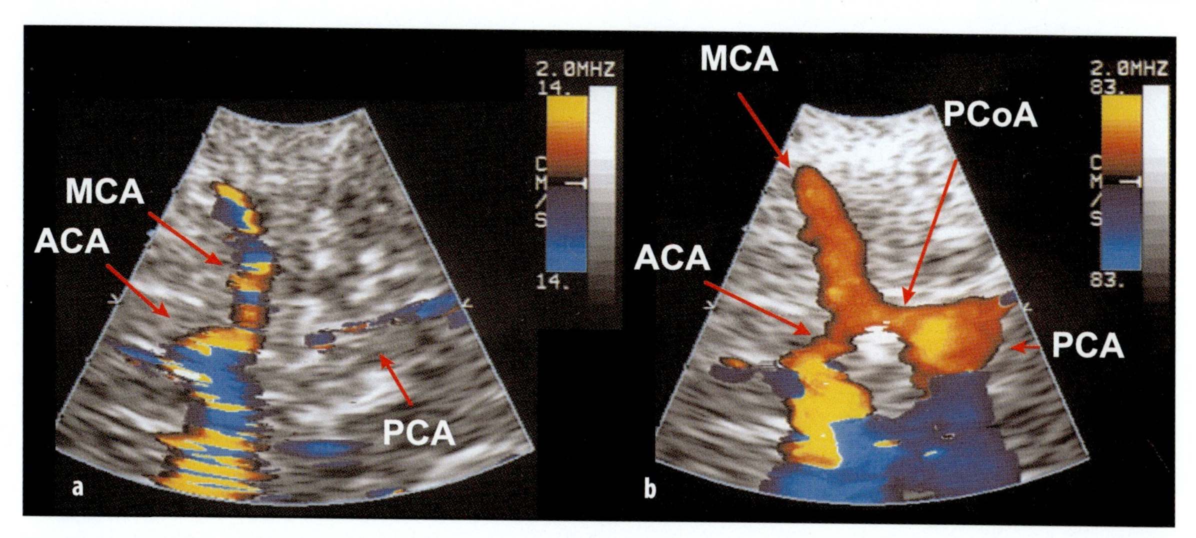

Fig. 5a, b. Transtemporal TCCD investigation in a patient with ipsilateral ICA occlusion. In the pre-contrast investigation (**a**) only with a low pulse repetition frequency (cf. the colour scale) a colour-coded Doppler signal can be obtained in the MCA, the ipsilateral and contralateral ACA, and the ipsilateral PCA. The information of flow direction is lost due to aliasing. The echocontrast investigation (**b**) allows the identification of the PCoA and of the contralateral P1-segment. As the pulse repetition frequency can be increased, proper identification of flow direction in the different arteries under investigation is now possible (cf. the colour scale) (Reprinted with permission from [27])

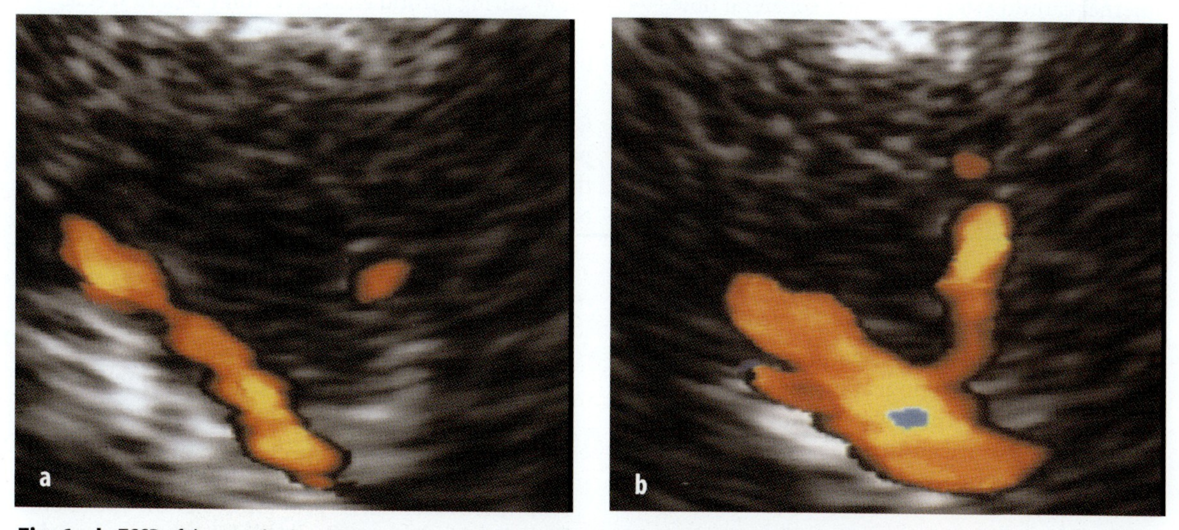

Fig. 6a, b. TCCD of the vertebral arteries and the basilar artery in a patient where intracranial stenosis due to a dissection was presumed. Before echocontrast (**a**) only the right vertebral artery and the presumed proximal basilar artery are visible. After echocontrast (**b**) the vertebrobasilar junction is clearly discernible without evidence of a stenosis (Reprinted with permission from [28])

considerably increases the diagnostic gain of TCCD in the intracranial anterior and vertebrobasilar vasculature. Besides increasing the diagnostic success rate of the examination, echocontrast agents reduce examination time and allow for colour imaging and pulsed Doppler detection of a greater number of vessels. The use of echocontrast can have direct diagnostic and therapeutic consequences (Table 3). Additional investigations like magnetic resonance imaging (MRI), MR-angiography, CT-angiography, or intra-arterial angiography are potentially harmful. Out of 415 patients who underwent intra-arterial angiography following randomisation in the ACAS trial (Asymptomatic Carotid Artery Study), three patients suffered a disabling stroke under the investigation or between the investigation and surgery, and one patient died (1.0%) [16].

A review of eight prospective studies revealed 1% of arteriography-related disabling strokes and 0.06% of deaths in a total of 2227 cerebral arteriographies [17].

Table 3. The benefits of neurovascular imaging

Diagnosis	Consequences
Normal finding	Avoidance of expensive and potentially harmful additional investigations (angiography, MR-angiography, CT-angiography),
Symptomatic extracranial internal carotid artery occlusion without post-occlusional alternating flow	No endarterectomy [43-46]
Aymptomatic extracranial internal carotid artery pseudo-occlusion	Endarterectomy [47]
Arterial stenosis or occlusion, pathological collateral flow	Localisation of stroke and embolic source, differentiation of macro- or microvascular aetiology, differentiation of hemodynamic and embolic stroke
Acute basilar artery occlusion	Intra-arterial thrombolysis [48]
Recanalisation during intravenous thrombolysis	Discontinuation of lysis [49, 50]
Symptomatic stenosis of the intracranial internal carotid artery with poor collateral flow	Knowledge of this situation may lead to the use of a shunt during carotid endarterectomy and to special attention by the anesthesiologist to avoid drops in blood pressure during any surgical intervention [51-53]
Occlusion of the intracranial internal carotid artery or the middle cerebral artery main stem with poor collateral flow	Close-meshed clinical and CT follow-up to guide possible hemicraniotomy, special benefit of intravenous thrombolysis, EC-IC bypass in selected cases, rise in arterial blood pressure [54-56]

Apart from this, investigations like MRI, MR-angiography, CT-angiography, or intra-arterial angiography are expensive and not yet generally available. These are additional arguments for the use of echocontrast in neurosonology.

Future Applications

Vascular ultrasound remains the predominant application of echocontrast agents in neurology. However, these products have an enormous potential for additional applications in the future. The improving quality of ultrasound devices works hand-in-hand with contrast media. In the past, we were lucky to find the middle cerebral artery main stem. Nowadays, we see smaller arteries, branches and veins, we can reconstruct three-dimensional pictures and in the future we will probably be able to assess brain perfusion in a routine procedure or to deliver drugs by microbubbles to their target organ [18-20].

Brain perfusion in stroke patients using ultrasound would help to choose the appropriate blood pressure to maintain perfusion within the penumbra without unnecessarily increasing the risk of bleeding and brain edema. The major principles of contrast-ultrasound-based perfusion measurements are analysis of the bolus kinetics, analysis of the refill kinetics, and analysis of diminution kinetics. Using the bolus method, where the contrast is injected as a bolus, hypoperfused areas in stroke patients can be visualised and parameter images of wash-in and wash-out curves can be generated off-line. Basically, the hypoperfused area will show lower and slower contrast agent filling. The theory on the refill kinetics is based on the destruction of the contrast agent bubbles and the measurement of its reappearance during constant infusion. This technique enables the investigator to calculate quantitative parameters for the description of the cerebral microcirculation, being less affected by the depth dependence of the contrast effect. These parameters, too, can be visualised as parameter images [21, 22]. The opposite of refill kinetics analysis is the analysis of diminution kinetics caused by destruction of the microbubbles [21]. In the context of assessment of brain perfusion, non-harmonic imaging techniques and harmonic imaging techniques are used. Harmonic imaging relies on the following principles: with increasing ultrasound pressure the gas bubbles start to swing in resonance, thus producing harmonics. Microbubbles from contrast-media produce more harmonics than solid tissue. The combination of harmonic imaging with echocontrast permits a very effective suppression of tissue-related artifacts and as well as the detection of blood flow in very tiny vessels [22-24]. Pulse-inversion harmonic imaging is a technique where two ultrasound pulses with a phase shift are emitted. This causes extinction when thrown back from normal tissue. However, contrast agent bubbles cause harmonics that do not lead to extinction [25].

Another potential application of microbubble technology in the cerebral circulation is ultrasound-mediated drug delivery. In this application, microbubbles can be loaded with drugs and then burst by ultrasound energy in the target vessel or organ. This could allow for the local delivery of thrombolytic agents, such as delivery directly to a thrombus in the middle cerebral artery main stem [20]. The process of lysis could concomitantly be monitored by TCCD.

Key Points

- Neurosonological investigations of the extracranial and intracranial brain-supplying arteries are helpful for the assessment of stroke and stroke-prone patients.
- Gas-filled microbubbles have a strong echo-enhancing effect and produce enhancement for several minutes, enabling the sonographer to perform the investigation with a single injection or 2-3 repeated injections without use of an injection. Echocontrast agents provide better delineation of normal blood flow, occlusions, pseudo-occlusions, stenoses, and collaterals in the extracranial and intracranial vascular beds. They are of particular value during transcranial colour-coded duplex investigations via the temporal and occipital window and help to avoid unnecessary, expensive and potentially harmful additional investigations such as intra-arterial digital subtraction angiography (DSA).

References

1. Kollar J, Schulte-Altedorneburg G, Sikula J et al (2004) Image Quality of the Temporal Bone Window Examined by Transcranial Doppler Sonography and Correlation with Postmortem Computed Tomography Measurements. Cerebrovasc Dis 17:61-65
2. Rosenkranz K, Zendel W, Langer R et al (1993) Contrast-enhanced transcranial Doppler US with a new transpulmonary echo contrast agent based on saccharide microparticles. Radiology 187:439-443
3. Gebel M, Caselitz M, Bowen-Davies PE, Weber S (1998) A multicenter, prospective, open label, randomized, controlled phase IIIb study of SH U 508 A (Levovist) for Doppler signal enhancement in the portal vascular system. Ultraschall in Med 19:148-156.
4. Droste DW, Jürgens R, Nabavi DG et al (1999) Echocontrast-enhanced ultrasound of extracranial internal carotid artery high-grade stenosis and occlusion. Stroke 30:2302-2306
5. Droste DW, Jürgens R, Weber S et al (2000) Benefit of echocontrast-enhanced transcranial color-coded duplex ultrasound in the assessment of intracranial collateral pathways. Stroke 31:920-923
6. Schminke U, Motsch L, Bleiss A (2001) Continuous administration of contrast medium for transcranial colour-coded sonography. Neuroradiology 43:24-28
7. Bokor D (2000) Diagnostic efficacy of SonoVue. Am J Cardiol 86:19G-24G
8. Droste DW, Llull JB, Pezzoli C et al (2002) SonoVue((R)) (BR1), a New Long-Acting Echocontrast Agent, Improves Transcranial Colour-Coded Duplex Ultrasonic Imaging. Cerebrovasc Dis14:27-32
9. The European Agency for the Evaluation of Medicinal Products (2004) Public Statement on SONOVUE (Sulphur hexafluoride): New contraindication in patients with heart disease; restriction of use to non-cardiac imaging. http://www.emea.eu.int/pdfs/human/press/pus/021204en.pdf. Ref Type: Data File
10. The European Agency for the Evaluation of Medicinal Products (2004) Questions and answers on SonoVue. http://www.emea.eu.int/humandocs/Humans/EPAR/sonovue/list.htm.
 Ref Type: Data File
11. Correas JM, Burns PN, Lai X, Qi X (2000) Infusion versus bolus of an ultrasound contrast agent: in vivo dose-response measurements of BR1. Invest Radiol 35:72-79

12. Gahn G, Gerber J, Hallmeyer S, Hahn G et al (2000) Contrast-enhanced transcranial color-coded duplex-sonography in stroke patients with limited bone windows. A J N R21:509-514
13. Zunker P, Wilms H, Brossmann J (2003) Echo contrast-enhanced transcranial ultrasound: frequency of use, diagnostic benefit, and validity of results compared with MRA. Stroke 33:2600-2603
14. Hansberg T, Wong KS, Droste DW, Ringelstein EB (2003) Effects of the ultrasound contrast-enhancing agent Levovist on the detection of intracranial arteries and stenoses in chinese by transcranial Doppler ultrasound. Cerebrovasc Dis 14:105-108
15. Droste DW, Boehm T, Ritter MA et al (2005) Benefit of Echocontrast-Enhanced Transcranial Arterial Color-Coded Duplex Ultrasound. Cerebrovasc Dis 20:332-336
16. Young B, Moore WS, Robertson JT et al (1996) An analysis of perioperative surgical mortality and morbidity in the asymptomatic carotid atherosclerosis study. Stroke 27:2216-2224
17. Hankey GJ, Warlow C, Sellar RJ (1990) Cerebral angiographic risk in mild cerebrovascular disease. Stroke 21:209-222
18. Harrer JU, Popescu O, Henkes HH, Klotzsch C (2005) Assessment of dural arteriovenous fistulae by transcranial color-coded duplex sonography. Stroke; 36:976-979
19. Wessels T, Bozzato A, Mull M, Klotzsch C (2004) Intracranial collateral pathways assessed by contrast-enhanced three-dimensional transcranial color-coded sonography. Ultrasound Med Biol 30:1435-1440
20. Della MA, Meyer-Wiethe K, Allemann E, Seidel G (2005) Ultrasound contrast agents for brain perfusion imaging and ischemic stroke therapy. J Neuroimaging; 15:217-232
21. Eyding J, Wilkening W, Postert T (2002) Brain perfusion and ultrasonic imaging techniques. Eur J Ultrasound 16:91-104
22. Seidel G, Meyer K (2001) Harmonic imaging-a new method for the sonographic assessment of cerebral perfusion. Eur J Ultrasound 14:103-113
23. Stolz E, Allendorfer J, Jauss M (2002) Sonographic harmonic grey scale imaging of brain perfusion: scope of a new method demonstrated in selected cases. Ultraschall Med 23:320-324
24. Wiesmann M, Seidel G (2000) Ultrasound perfusion imaging of the human brain. Stroke 31:2421-2425
25. Meairs S, Daffertshofer M, Neff W (2000) Pulse-inversion contrast harmonic imaging: ultrasonographic assessment of cerebral perfusion. Lancet 355:550-551
26. Droste DW, Metz RJ (2004) Clinical utility of echocontrast agents in neurosonology. Neurol Res; 26:754-759
27. Droste DW, Jurgens R, Weber S (2000) Benefit of echocontrast-enhanced transcranial color-coded duplex ultrasound in the assessment of intracranial collateral pathways. Stroke 31:920-923
28. Droste DW, Nabavi DG, Kemény V et al (1998) Echocontrast-enhanced transcranial color-coded duplex offers improved visualization of the vertebrobasilar system in patients with bad examination conditions. Acta Neurol Scand 98:193-199
29. Baumgartner RW, Arnold M, Gonner F et al (1997) Contrast-enhanced transcranial color-coded duplex sonography in ischemic cerebrovascular disease. Stroke 28:2473-2478
30. Gerriets T, Seidel G, Fiss I (1999) Contrast-enhanced transcranial color-coded duplex sonography: efficiency and validity. Neurology 52:1133-1137
31. Gerriets T, Goertler M, Stolz E et al (2002) Feasibility and validity of transcranial duplex sonography in patients with acute stroke. J Neurol Neurosurg Psychiatr 73:17-20
32. Goertler M, Kross R, Baeumer M et al (1998) Diagnostic impact and prognostic relevance of early contrast- enhanced transcranial color-coded duplex sonography in acute stroke. Stroke 29:955-962
33. Nabavi DG, Droste DW, Kemény V et al (1998) Potential and limitations of echocontrast-enhanced ultrasonography in acute stroke patients: a pilot study. Stroke 29:949-954
34. Postert T, Braun B, Meves S et al (1999) Contrast-enhanced transcranial color-coded sonography in acute hemispheric brain infarction. Stroke 30:1819-1826
35. Wessels T, Bozzato A, Mull M, Klotzsch C (2004) Intracranial collateral pathways assessed by contrast-enhanced three-dimensional transcranial color-coded sonography. Ultrasound Med Biol 30:1435-1440
36. Becker G, Lindner A, Bogdahn U (1993) Imaging of the vertebrobasilar system by transcranial color-coded real-time sonography. J Ultrasound Med 12:395-401
37. Stolz E, Nuckel M, Mendes I et al (2002) Vertebrobasilar transcranial color-coded duplex ultrasonography: improvement with echo enhancement. A J N R 23:1051-1054
38. Fürst G, Sitzer M, Hofer M et al (1995) Kontrastmittelverstärkte farbkodierte Duplexsonographie hochgradiger Karotisstenosen. Ultraschall Med 16:140-144
39. Gahn G, Hahn G, Hallmeyer-Elgner S et al (2002) Echo-enhanced transcranial color-coded duplex-sonography to study collateral blood flow in patients with symptomatic obstructions of the internal carotid artery and limited acoustic bone windows. Cerebrovasc Dis 11:107-112
40. Giannoni MF, Bilotta F, Fiorani L et al (1999) Ultrasound echo-enhancers in the evaluation of endovascular prostheses. Cardiovasc Surg 7:532-538
41. Hofstee DJ, Hoogland PH, Schimsheimer RJ, de Weerd AW (2000) contrast-enhanced color duplex for diagnosis of subtotal stenosis or occlusion of the internal carotid artery. Clin Neurol Neurosurg 102:9-12
42. Sitzer M, Rose G, Fürst G et al (1997) Characteristics and clinical value of an intravenous echo- enhancement agent in evaluation of high-grade internal carotid stenosis. J Neuroimaging 7[Suppl 1]:22-25
43. Kniemeyer HW, Aulich A, Schlachetzki F (1996) Pseudo- and segmental occlusion of the internal carotid artery: a new classification, surgical treatment and results. Eur J Vasc Endovasc Surg 12:310-320
44. McCormick PW, Spetzler RF, Bailes JE (1992) Thromboendarterectomy of the symptomatic occluded internal carotid artery. J Neurosurg 76:752-758
45. Meyer FB, Sundt TM, Jr., Piepgras DG et al (1986) Emergency carotid endarterectomy for patients with acute carotid occlusion and profound neurological deficits. Ann Surg 203:82-89
46. Sterpetti AV, Feldhaus RJ, Schultz RD, Farina C (1989) Operative strategies in patients with symptomatic internal carotid artery occlusion. Surgery 105:632-637
47. Barnett HJ, Meldrum HE (2001) Endarterectomy for

carotid stenosis: new approaches in patient selection. Cerebrovasc Dis 11[Suppl 1]:105-111

48. Hacke W, Zeumer H, Ferbert A et al (1988) Intra-arterial thrombolytic therapy improves outcome in patients with acute vertebrobasilar occlusive disease. Stroke 19:1216-1222
49. Kaps M, Link A (1998) Transcranial sonographic monitoring during thrombolytic therapy [see comments]. Am J Neuroradiol 19:758-760
50. Karnik R, Stelzer P, Slany J (1992) Transcranial Doppler sonography monitoring of local intra- arterial thrombolysis in acute occlusion of the middle cerebral artery. Stroke 23(2):284-287
51) Doblar DD, Plyushcheva NV, Jordan W, McDowell H (1998) Predicting the effect of carotid artery occlusion during carotid endarterectomy: Comparing transcranial Doppler measurements and cerebral angiography. Stroke 29:2038-2042
52. Lopez Bresnahan MV, Kearse LA, Jr., Yanez P, Young TI (1993) Anterior communicating artery collateral flow protection against ischemic change during carotid endarterectomy. J Neurosurg 79:379-382
53. Schneider PA, Ringelstein EB, Rossman ME et al (1988) Importance of cerebral collateral pathways during carotid endarterectomy. Stroke 19:1328-1334
54. Berrouschot J, Barthel H, vonKummer R (1998) 99(m)technetium-ethyl-cysteinate-dimer single-photon emission CT can predict fatal ischemic brain edema. Stroke 29:2556-2562
55. Berrouschot J, Sterker M, Bettin S et al (1998) Mortality of space-occupying ('malignant') middle cerebral artery infarction under conservative intensive care. Intensive Care Med 24:620-623
56. Schwab S, Steiner T, Aschoff A et al (1998) Early hemicraniectomy in patients with complete middle cerebral artery infarction. Stroke 29:1888-1893

III.2

Contrast Ultrasound in Cerebrovascular Disease and Stroke Management

Eva Bartels

Introduction

Over the past decade there has been a rapid evolution in the development of contrast agents to increase the backscattered ultrasound signal. The effect of ultrasound contrast agents is based on the presence of microscopic particles that enhance and augment ultrasound information. A variety of fluids have been used as conventional contrast agents, from the hand-agitated saline used initially, to the suspension of microair, or microgasbubbles with a diameter of less than 10 micrometers that is used today.

The most substantial advance in the use of contrast agents was the development of stabilized contrast agents capable of crossing the pulmonary vasculature, a specific region of interest (ROI) to be examined - e.g., myocardium, liver, kidney, extra- and intracranial cerebral vessels - following intravenous administration [1-3]. The stability of the bubbles was increased by the introduction of an encapsulating shell to prevent gas loss, and the optimizing of surface tension and viscosity of the agent. Currently available transpulmonary products comprise stabilized microbubbles filled either by air (first-generation contrast agents) or by an inert gas (second-generation contrast agents) [4, 5].

In neurosonology, ultrasound contrast agents can be used to improve the insonation conditions (e.g., in the case of an insufficient temporal bone window in transcranial imaging) and/or to enhance the backscattered signal from the blood vessels in the case of reduced blood flow velocities in pathological situations (e.g., in an occlusive disease of an artery supplying the brain).

The purpose of this chapter is to describe indicative situations in which the application of contrast agents would provide an additional diagnostic benefit for patients with cerebrovascular disease and to illustrate these with typical contrast-enhanced ultrasonographic findings of the extra- and intracranial brain-supplying arteries. The findings were selected with a view to their relevance for routine diagnostics in stroke prevention and in stroke management. The last part of this chapter describes findings in the evaluation of cerebral perfusion deficit in stroke patients using the contrast agent SonoVue.

SonoVue is a novel second-generation ultrasound contrast medium, consisting of microbubbles stabilized by a highly elastic phospholipid-shell. It consists of sulfur hexafluoride (SF6), an innocuous, poorly soluble gas, which is eliminated through the lungs [6, 7]. In the previous chapter of this book, Droste describes the properties of SonoVue and practical considerations regarding its injection. The safety issues involving this substance were also covered. In our experience, SonoVue is well tolerated in all patients and there have been no side effects observed in association with its use.

Contrast-Enhanced Evaluation of the Extracranial Brain-Supplying Arteries

In the contrast-enhanced sonographic evaluation of the extracranial brain-supplying arteries, it is possible to obtain more detailed information about the anatomical course of the cerebral vessels and about the pathological conditions, especially if the native scanning is insufficient. If a low-velocity flow is detected, the technical parameters of the sonographic system should first be adjusted to optimize the examination, as follows:

- Pulse repetition frequency (PRF) should be set to the lowest value.
- The color box should be as small as possible.
- The frame rate and the wall filter have to be adjusted.
- The global gain and intensity threshold need to be optimized.

If a proper assessment of the structures of diagnostic interest is not possible after the system settings have been adjusted, the use of contrast agents should be considered [8].

The origin of the internal carotid artery is the most frequent site of atherosclerosis in cerebrovascular disease. Therefore, in the extracranial sonographic examination, a reliable assessment of the proximal segments of the internal carotid artery is crucial in the management of patients with stroke risk. Ultrasound contrast agents have proven useful in the quantification of high-grade stenoses of the internal carotid artery, which can only be suboptimally imaged - if at all - by means of native sonographic examination [9] (Fig. 1). Additionally, ultrasound agents provide a clear diagnosis, if the distinction between pre-occlusive stenosis and occlusion is difficult (Fig. 2).

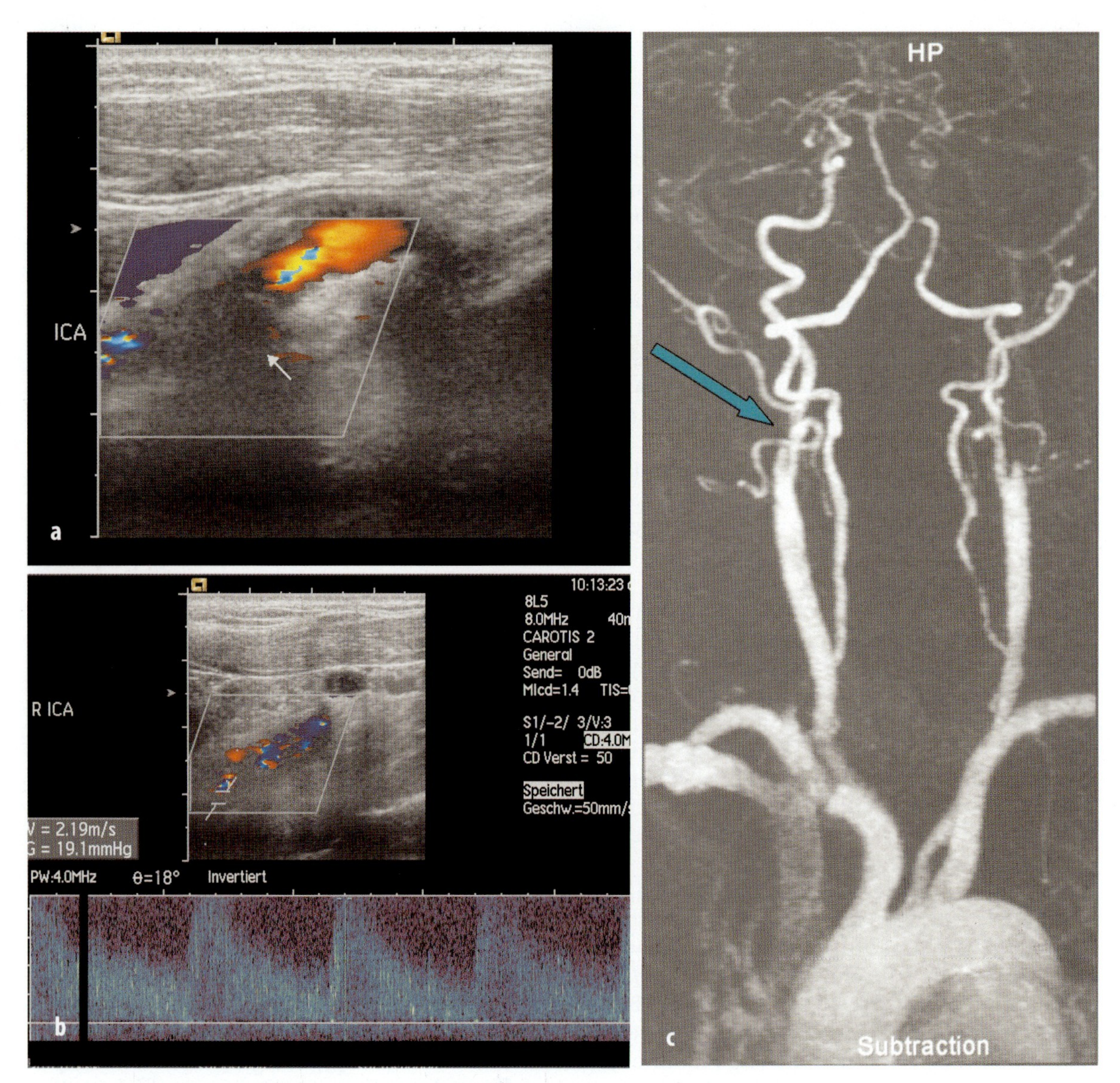

Fig. 1a-c. *Stenosis of the right internal carotid artery in a 60 year old patient with an acute ischemia in the right middle cerebral artery territory.* **a** View of the origin of the right internal carotid artery. Due to acoustic shadowing, an adequate assessment of the area of stenosis (*arrow*) is not possible. **b** After application of SonoVue, color-coded flow signal with an aliasing phenomenon can be registered. In this region, Doppler spectrum shows an increase in angle-corrected maximum systolic flow velocity to 219 cm/s, indicating a moderate stenosis (the white signals in the Doppler spectrum represent the bubbles of the contrast agent SonoVue). **c** MR-angiography shows a stenosis of the right internal carotid artery (*arrow*)

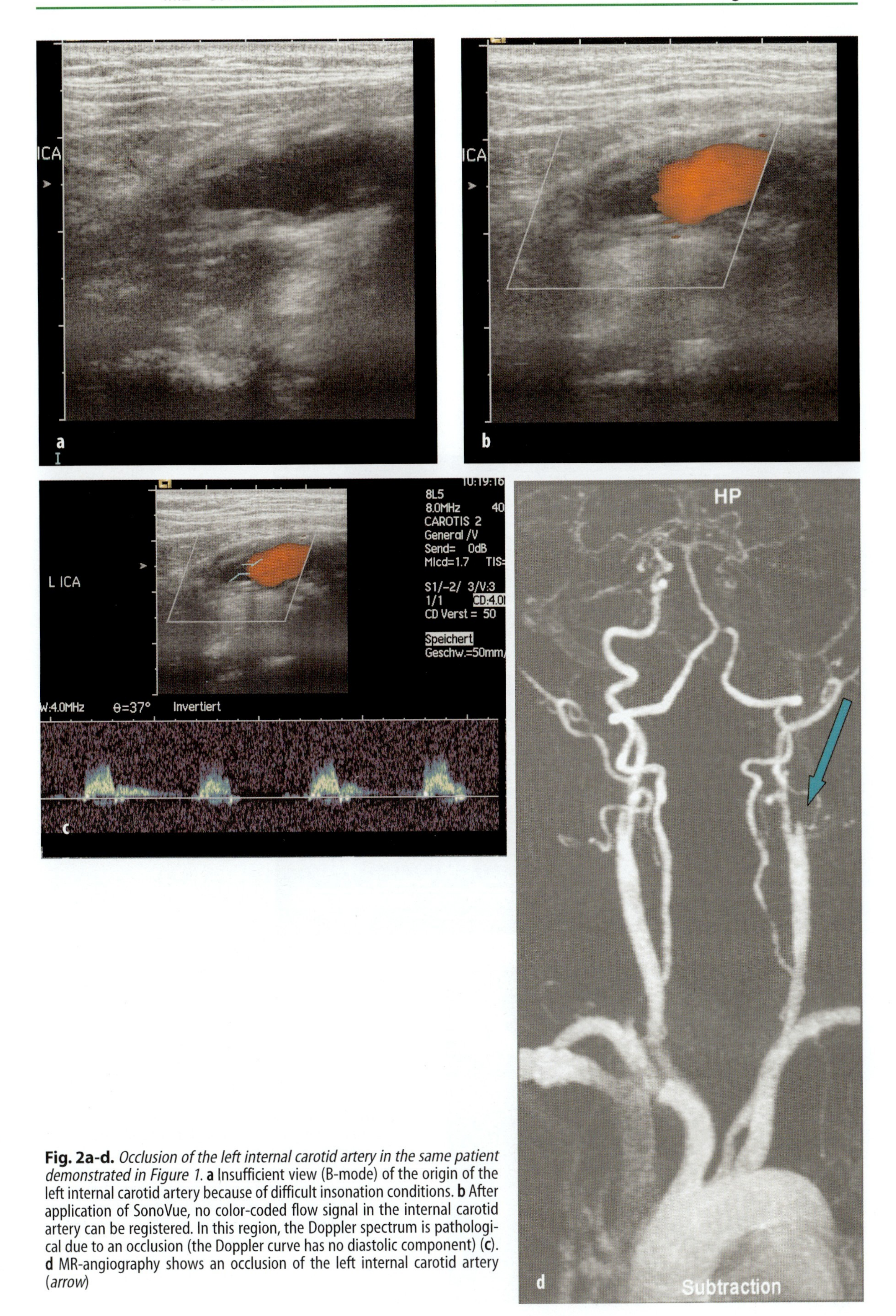

Fig. 2a-d. *Occlusion of the left internal carotid artery in the same patient demonstrated in Figure 1.* **a** Insufficient view (B-mode) of the origin of the left internal carotid artery because of difficult insonation conditions. **b** After application of SonoVue, no color-coded flow signal in the internal carotid artery can be registered. In this region, the Doppler spectrum is pathological due to an occlusion (the Doppler curve has no diastolic component) (**c**). **d** MR-angiography shows an occlusion of the left internal carotid artery (*arrow*)

Detection of low blood flow velocities in cases of dissection is easier using echo-contrast agents in ultrasonography of the extracranial vertebral arteries [10, 11]. Under difficult examination conditions, it is possible to differentiate better between a hypoplastic vertebral artery and an occlusion at the origin (Fig. 3).

Contrast-Enhanced Evaluation of the Intracranial Arteries Supplying the Brain

With the aid of an echo-contrast agent, examination with transcranial Doppler sonography as well as color-coded duplex ultrasonography is possible even in patients with an unfavorable acoustic bone window [1, 12]. Following intravenous injection of the first-generation contrast agent Levovist, the backscattered signal can be enhanced up to 25 dB because of a transient increase in echogenicity of the blood [13]. Figure 4 illustrates a contrast-enhanced study of the posterior circulation, which offers more detailed information about the anatomical course of the basal cerebral arteries. After application of SonoVue, a longer stretch of the basilar artery is visible. Furthermore, the posterior inferior cerebellar artery (PICA), the anterior inferior cerebellar artery (AICA), and the superior cerebellar artery can be displayed. Better visualization of the intracranial arteries facilitates the diagnostic assessment of pathological conditions.

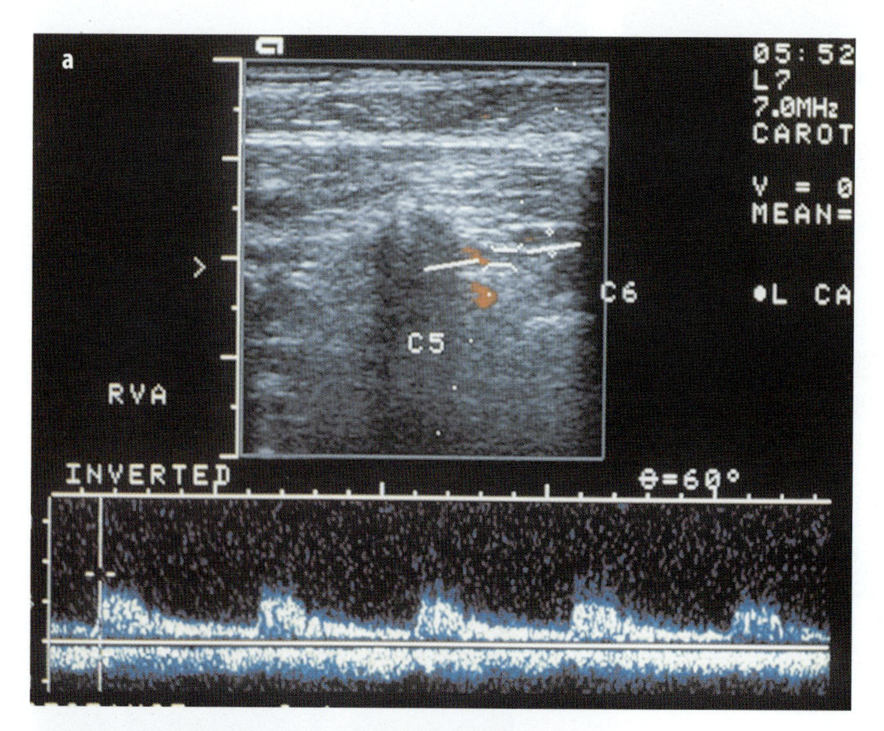

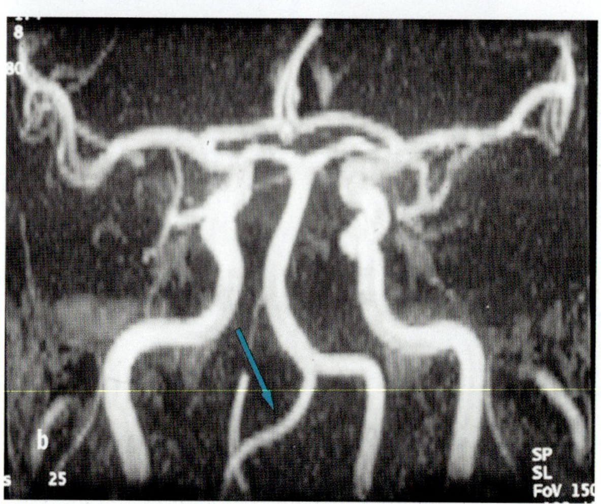

Fig. 3a, b. *Hypoplasia of the right extracranial vertebral artery in a 62 year old patient.* **a** Insufficient B-mode image of the midcervical course of the right extracranial vertebral artery. After application of SonoVue a weak color-coded signal in the vessel lumen can be detected. Under difficult examination conditions, using echo-contrast it is possible to better differentiate between a hypoplastic vertebral artery and an occlusion at the origin. The diameter of the artery is 2.1 mm. **b** MR-angiography shows a hypoplasia of the right vertebral artery. RVA = right vertebral artery, C5 = 5th vertebra, C6 = 6th vertebra

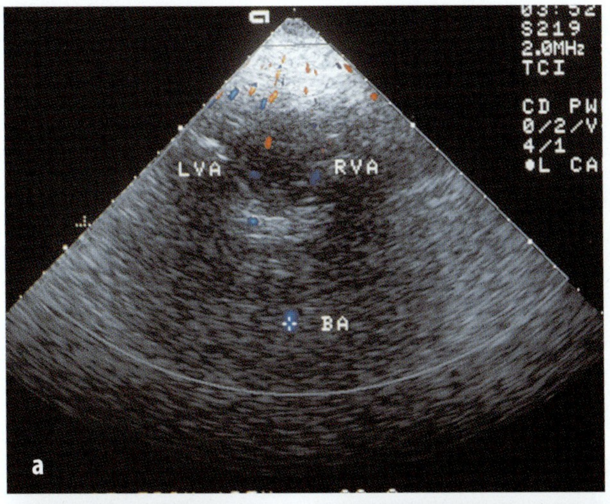

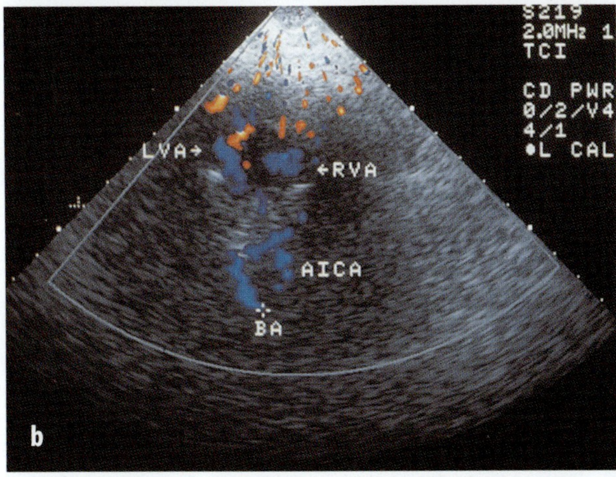

Fig. 4a, b. Patient with an insufficient occipital insonation window before (**a**) and after (**b**) application of SonoVue. Color mode, normal finding. After application of SonoVue, more detailed information about the anatomical course of the basal cerebral arteries can be obtained. BA = basilar artery, RVA = right vertebral artery, LVA = left vertebral artery, AICA = anterior inferior cerebellar artery

The results obtained from a multicenter, open-label, randomized cross-over study investigating the diagnostic potential of SonoVue using transcranial color-coded duplex sonography (TCCS) confirm this clinical observation [14]. In a group of forty patients, echo-enhancement contributed to converting a non-diagnostic study into a diagnostic one in more than half of the indications (in 66%), and increased the confidence of diagnosis in 74%. In a non-trial situation, this would have allowed the diagnosis to be reached more quickly.

In patients with acute stroke, cerebral ischemia is most often due to thromboembolic occlusion of an artery supplying the brain. Using transcranial color-coded duplex sonography as a complementary mobile procedure, the intracranial occlusion can be examined non-invasively at the bedside. The aim of therapeutic intervention is to restore or improve the blood supply. To make good treatment decisions, early, reliable information about the condition of the arteries of the Circle of Willis is necessary [15].

Especially in those patients whose baseline scans are not of good quality, contrast-enhancement is of great value to improve the diagnostic results (Fig. 5). For further diagnostic steps and for therapy in cases of an occlusion in a middle cerebral artery, it is important to know whether failure to visualize a cerebral vessel is due to methodological problems or to a pathological condition. The absence of a color-coded signal for the middle cerebral artery is indicative of an occlusion, if a good contrast-enhanced signal for the ipsilateral posterior cerebral artery can be displayed (Fig. 6). In a posterior circulation, contrast-enhancement is needed in many cases for an unequivocal diagnosis of high-grade stenosis of the intracranial vertebral or basilar arteries, although no data from systematic large series are available [12, 16] (Fig. 7). A further advantage of TCCS lies in the monitoring of stroke patients during and after therapy.

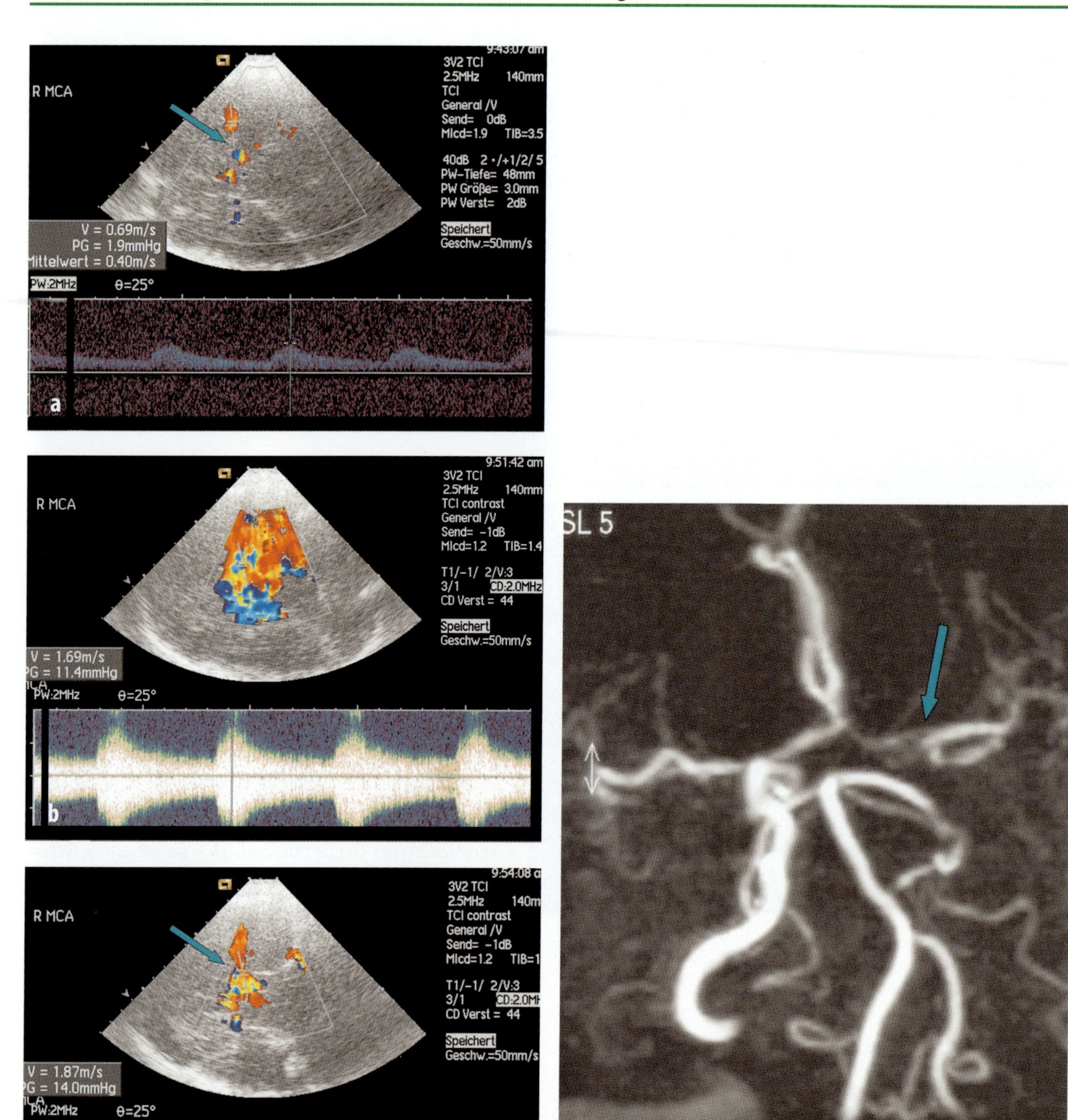

Fig. 5a-d. *Stenosis of the right middle cerebral artery in a 60 year old patient with acute ischemia in the right middle cerebral artery territory. Extracranial ultrasonographic findings are shown in Figure 1 and 2.* **a** Native transcranial color-coded image using a right transtemporal approach. The area of the stenosis of the right middle cerebral artery (MCA) cannot be visualized clearly (*arrow*). **b** Blooming effect after the injection of the contrast agent. **c** The stenotic region can be better displayed after application of the contrast agent SonoVue. The Doppler spectrum at the site of the stenosis shows an increase in angle-corrected maximum systolic flow velocity to 187 cm/s, indicating a moderate stenosis (the white signals in the Doppler spectrum represent the bubbles of the contrast agent SonoVue). **d** Magnetic resonance angiogram of a stenosis of the right MCA. The left MCA is filled by a hypoplastic left anterior cerebral artery (*arrow*) and shows a weak signal due to an extracranial occlusion of the left internal carotid artery at the origin. R MCA = right middle cerebral artery

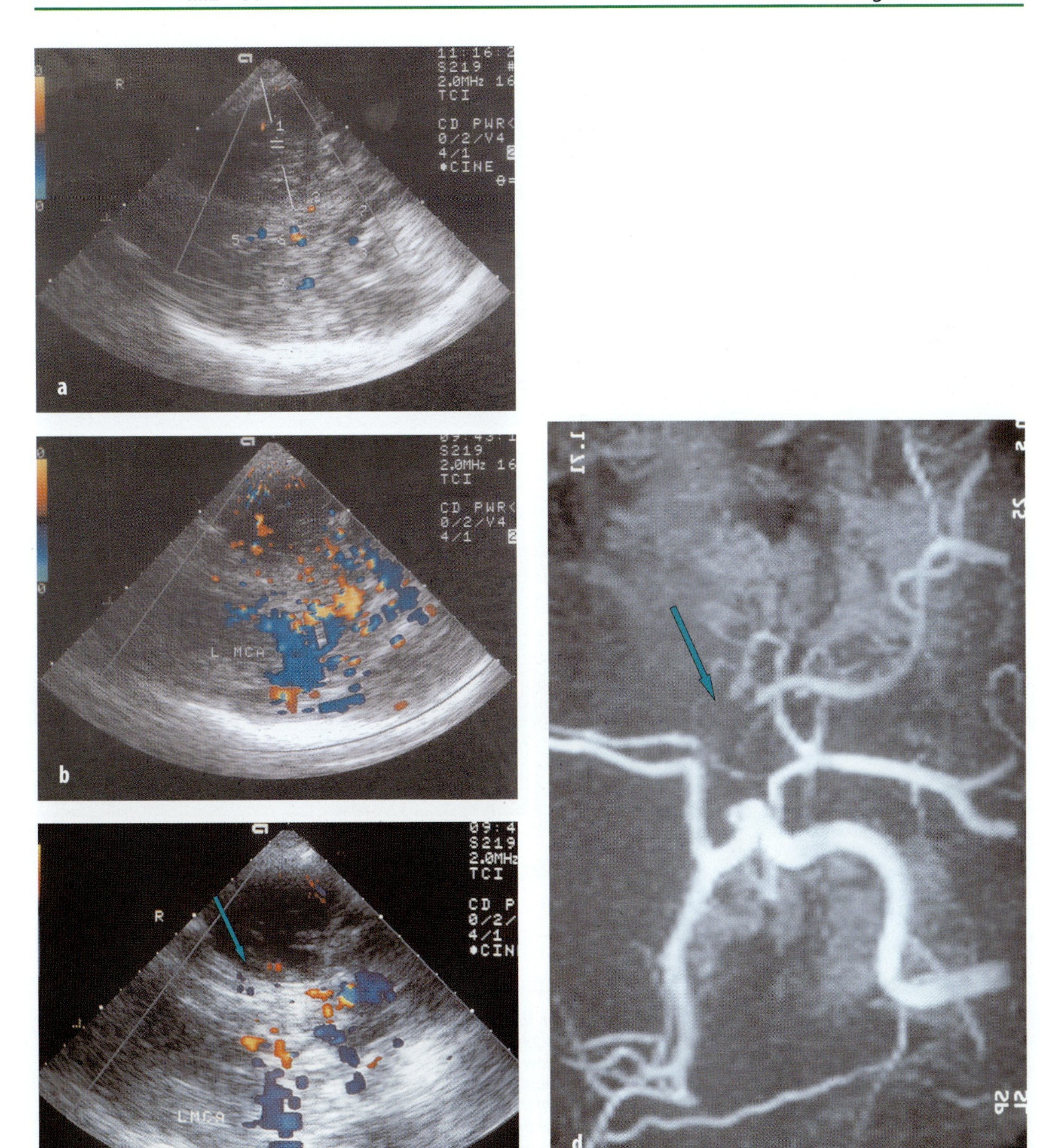

Fig. 6a-d. *Occlusion of the right MCA in 26 year old patient with a dissection of the right internal carotid artery.* **a** Native transcranial color-coded image using a right transtemporal approach with an unfavorable temporal bone window. The visualization of the basal cerebral arteries is of insufficient quality, only fragments of the arteries are visible. (1) No detectable signal of the right middle cerebral artery (MCA); (2) signal of the right posterior communicating artery; (3) left posterior cerebral artery (PCA); (4) left MCA; (5) A2 segment of the left anterior cerebral artery (ACA). **b** Blooming effect after the injection of the contrast agent. **c** After application of an echo-contrast agent, good visualization of the contralateral (*left*) MCA, PCA and ACA and ipsilateral (*right*) PCA. There is no signal registered for the right MCA (*arrow*). MCA, middle cerebral artery; PCA, posterior cerebral artery; ACA, anterior cerebral artery. **d** Magnetic resonance angiogram of an occlusion of the right MCA (*arrow*). The intracranial segment of the right internal carotid artery shows a weak signal due to a dissection at the origin

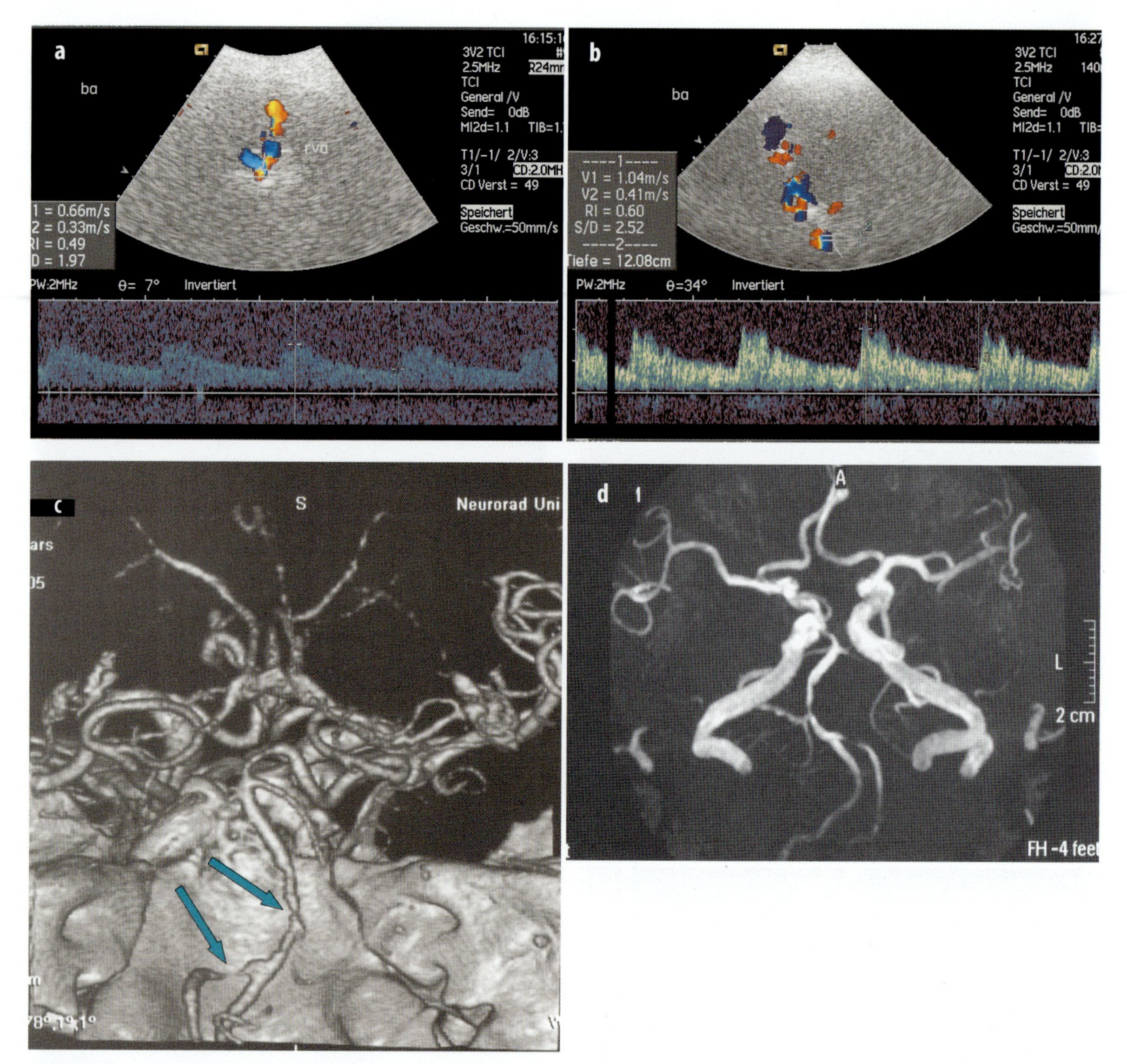

Fig. 7a-d. *Findings in a 72 year old patient with vertebrobasilar TIA. Clinical symptoms: double vision, vertigo, dizziness. The native extracranial sonography revealed non-stenotic heterogeneous plaques at the bifurcation and a difference in the sides regarding flow of the extracranial vertebral artery (right>left). No signs of a distal flow obstruction were found. The transcranial examination showed no pathological findings. The findings of the basilar artery revealed normal signal up to a depth of 90 mm. In response to the pathological MRA findings, which revealed a high-grade, short-length stenosis of the basilar artery and the intracranial left vertebral artery, for further therapeutic decision making, targeted sonographic examination with the contrast agent SonoVue was performed. Using a suboccipital insonation, we recorded a high-frequency Doppler signal at the depth of 120 mm and found an aliasing phenomenon as an indication of a middle-grade stenosis. As a result of the contrast-enhanced intracranial examination, a better assessment of the stenosis was possible, providing a better basis for the consequent therapeutic decision. The patient was treated with antithrombotic agent and his condition has improved.* **a** Suboccipital insonation - native image. Visualization of the vessels is insufficient. The signal of the basilar artery can be recorded only to a depth of 80 mm. The Doppler spectrum at this depth is normal, maximum systolic blood flow velocity is 66 cm/s, and there are no signs of a distal flow obstruction. **b** Suboccipital insonation – contrast-enhanced image. Visualization of the vessels is better, and possible to a greater depth. The signal of the basilar artery can be recorded to a depth of 120.1 mm. The Doppler spectrum shows a low-to-moderate grade stenosis. Maximum systolic blood flow velocity is slightly increased (104 cm/s), and there are no signs of a distal flow obstruction. **c** CT-angiography and (**d**) MR-angiography show a stenosis of the basilar artery and hypoplasia and stenosis in the intracranial V4 segment of the left vertebral artery

Evaluation of Cerebral Perfusion Deficit in Stroke Patients

The use of echo-contrast agents in the color-coded examination of the extra- and intracranial brain-supplying arteries has already become part of the clinical routine for the diagnosis of cerebrovascular disease. At present, further clinical research is focused on the imaging of blood flow in the capillaries of the brain parenchyma and on the evaluation of cerebral perfusion with the aim of imaging the cerebral perfusion deficit in stroke patients. Based on experience from myocardial perfusion imaging, several reports have recently been published on the imaging of cerebral perfusion [17, 18].

The catalyst for further progress in contrast ultrasound was the advent of harmonic imaging technology during the second half of the 1990s [19-21]. When exposed to the ultrasound beam, microbubble contrast agents oscillate. These oscillations have a strong tendency to produce resonance, and the resonant frequency of microbubbles happens to be within the range of diagnostic ultrasound. With increasing transmission power, the bubbles show an increasingly non-linear response (i.e., the backscattered signal contains frequencies that differ from the insonating frequency and the returned signal is thus distorted). The non-linear signals contain overtones or harmonic and subharmonic signals at multiples and fractions of the insonating frequency. The second harmonic signal, which occurs at twice the incidence frequency, is used in a new ultrasound technique known as second harmonic imaging [22-25]. When the energy of the insonating beam is further increased to mechanical indexes (MI) greater than approximately 0.3, there is a corresponding rise in the destruction of the microbubbles. This destructive process is very fast, taking place during a single or a few ultrasound pulses during which a strong and highly non-linear signal is returned from the bubble. It is called 'stimulated acoustic emission (SAE)' or 'loss of correlation (LOC) -imaging' and is a specific *high MI imaging modality.*

In the applications where the microbubbles need to be preserved (e.g., in imaging of very low blood flow velocities in the capillaries of the brain parenchyma), the *low MI imaging modality* is a preferred approach. Different techniques such as pulse-inversion harmonic imaging, power modulation, harmonic power Doppler imaging, and contrast pulse sequencing are described to evaluate perfusion in microcirculation [26]. For quantification of brain tissue perfusion, bolus injection kinetics, refill injection kinetics or diminution kinetics are currently being explored. After a bolus injection of the contrast agent, time intensity curves with wash-in and wash-out phases can be analyzed. Postert and Seidel were able to measure time-intensity curves through the intact skull with transcranial sonography using the bubble response from the contrast agents Levovist and Optison, respectively [27-30]. They showed that the examination is feasible not only in young adults with a good acoustic temporal bone window. The value of this diagnostic method could also be demonstrated in pathological conditions, e.g., in patients with acute hemispheric stroke [31, 32].

In the therapy of acute stroke, an early assessment of the hypoperfused area and the quickest possible treatment and reperfusion of the ischemic deficit is necessary for an optimum clinical outcome. The size of the ischemic area plays an important role in prognosis. With cranial computed tomography, the early ischemic signs may only be visible several hours after the onset of the acute symptoms. For this reason, imaging of the hypoperfused region is preferably performed by magnetic resonance imaging (MRI) techniques. Using perfusion- and diffusion-weighted MRI (PWI, DWI), the permanently damaged tissue as shown in DWI can be distinguished from the potentially salvageable tissue (following the so-called "mismatch theory") within minutes to hours after onset of the first symptoms [33]. However, MRI examination is still not widely accessible in the early management of stroke. Therefore, ultrasound techniques could be considered as a possible diagnostic alternative for the early visualization of the ischemic area. The main advantage in comparison to the MRI techniques is the bedside application and the real-time results of the sonographic examination.

However, at the present time, imaging of cerebral perfusion is limited because of methodological problems, especially if the temporal bone window is not suitable for the insonation [34, 35]. The higher MI needed to penetrate the temporal bone window is one of the key restraints in transcranial sonography. To learn more about cerebral perfusion sonography (and to avoid the temporal bone problem), our group performed a study on the contrast imaging of cerebral perfusion deficits in acute stroke patients following decompressive craniectomy [36] (Figs. 8-10). This study, in which a lower MI was used, demonstrated the capabili-

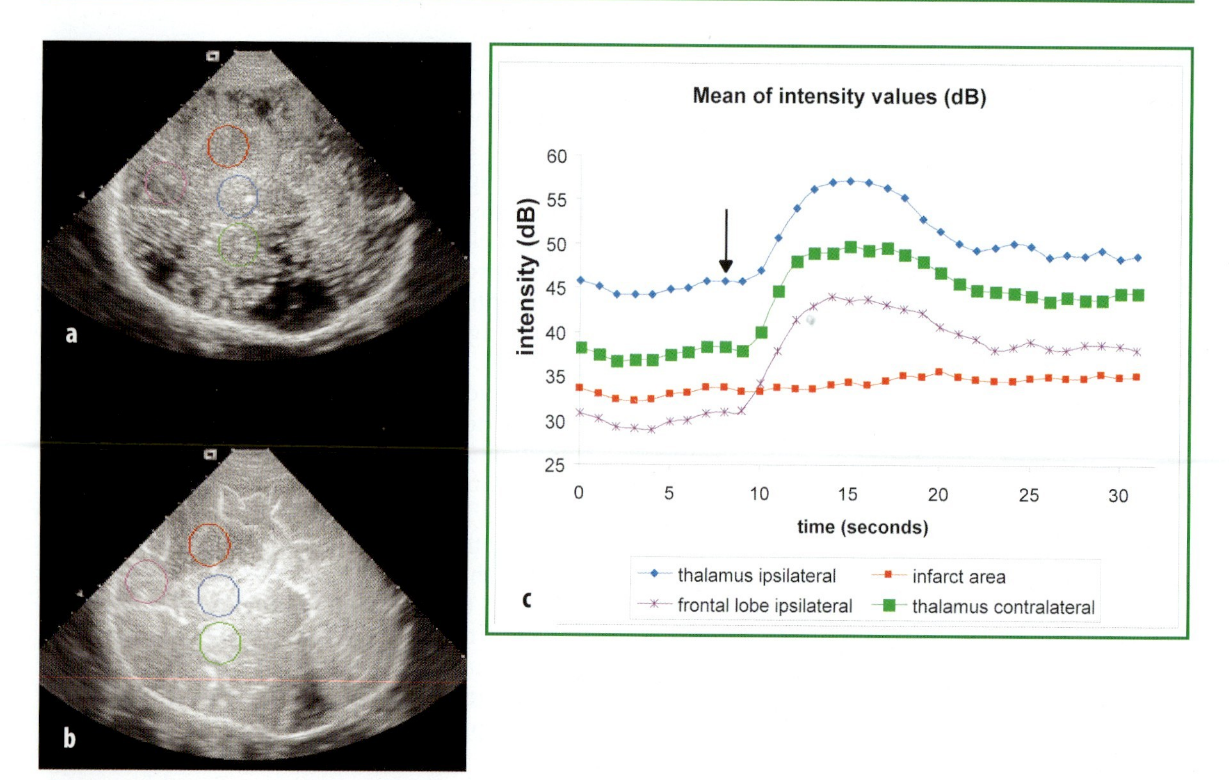

Fig. 8a-c. Transcranial B-mode sonography in the axial diencephalic plane in a 49 year old female patient with malignant MCA infarction following decompressive craniectomy before (**a**) and after (**b**) application of the contrast agent. The region of the perfusion deficit is hypoechoic on both images and is marked by the red circle. After application of the contrast agent, the area of hypoperfusion is clearly delineated. The ipsilateral thalamus and adjacent area of the infarct area near the midline (further from the penumbra) show hyperperfusion. **c** Time intensity curves showing the mean intensity values in the infarct area, thalamus ipsi- and contralaterally and in the frontal lobe ipsilaterally. No increase of intensity in the infarct area (red line), whereas in the ipsilateral thalamus and midline area (blue line) hyperperfusion with a clear increase of intensity can be observed. After the bolus effect of approximately 9 seconds, a steady-state plateau with higher intensities than the baseline intensities can be observed. *Arrow:* injection of the contrast agent (Reprinted with permission from Georg Thieme [36])

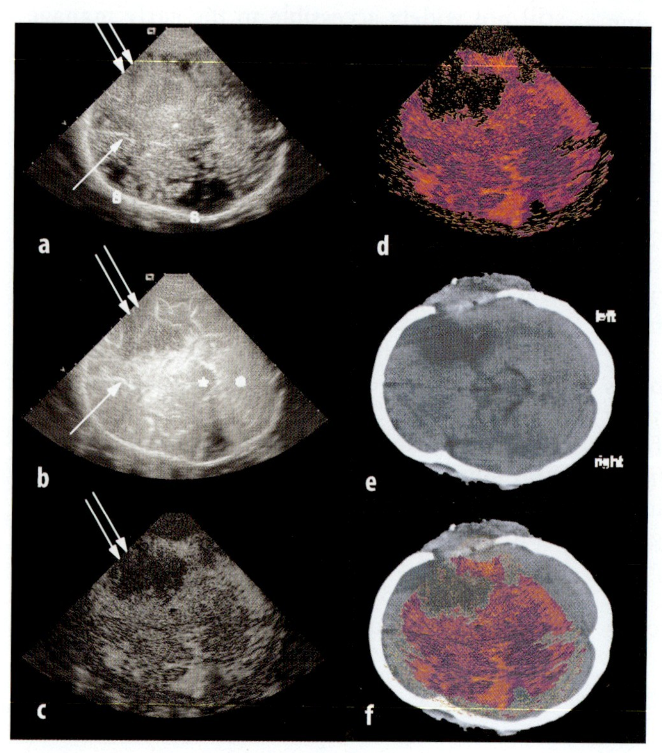

Fig. 9a-f. *Calculation of image parameters demonstrated in the same patient in Figure 8.* **a** View of a background image (before application of the contrast agent) established by averaging six non-enhanced images. *Arrow:* midline shift, *two arrows:* hypoperfusion in the infarction area. **b** Contrast-enhanced B-mode image showing better delineation of the structures of the cerebral parenchyma. *Arrow:* midline shift, *two arrows:* hypoperfusion in the infarction area, *: brain stem, O: cerebellum. **c** View of a difference-image created by subtracting the intensity of the background image from the contrast-enhanced image. **d** View of the difference-image transferred in color. **e** CT scan showing status following decompressive craniectomy and the area of the malignant space-occupying infarction in the left MCA territory. **f** Superimposition of (**d**) and (**e**) demonstrating the good correspondance of the CT and ultrasound findings (Reprinted with permission from Georg Thieme [37])

ty of the contrast agent SonoVue to image cerebral perfusion and the less perfused areas of the brain.

Building on our experience from this report, in our most recent preliminary study we evaluated the feasibility of analyzing cerebral perfusion deficits using a new contrast imaging technology, namely Cadence contrast pulse sequencing technology (CPS), in addition to the contrast agent SonoVue. In this study, continuous and triggered registrations with pulsing intervals of 1000 ms were performed. The MI was set at 1.1 for the triggered registration and at 0.28 for the continuous registration [37].

Using CPS imaging technology in young, healthy volunteers with a good insonation temporal bone window, the distribution of the contrast agent was easier to detect than in previous studies. The contrast-enhanced signal could also be well recognized in the contralateral hemisphere right up to the skull crown, because the depth-dependent attenuation of the backscattered ultrasound waves was less pronounced (Fig.11).

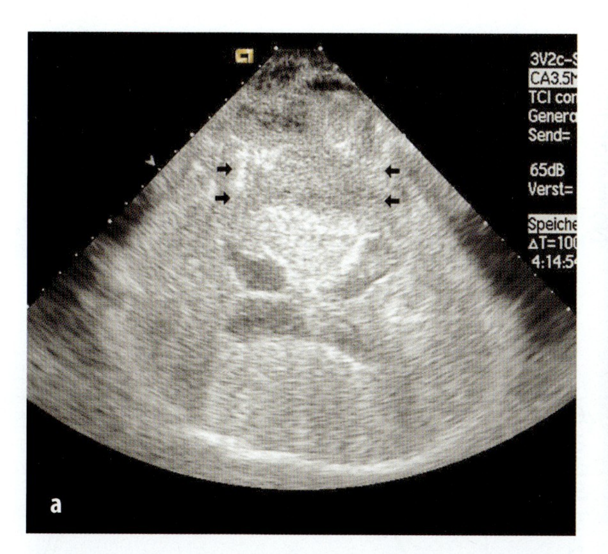

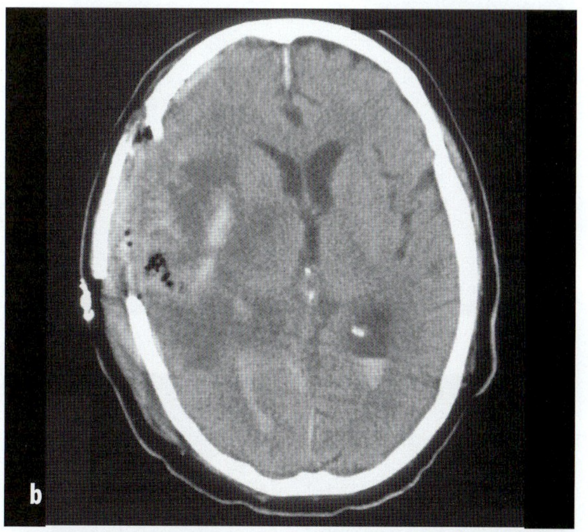

Fig. 10a, b. *Transcranial B-mode sonography in a 69 year old man with malignant MCA infarction and a secondary hemorrhage in the ischemic area, following decompressive craniectomy.* **a** After application of the contrast agent SonoVue, the hypoechoic area of perfusion deficit can be recognized (*black arrows*) in the modified diencephalic insonation plane. **b** CT scan of status following decompressive craniectomy due to malignant MCA infarction showing a secondary hemorrhage in the infarction area

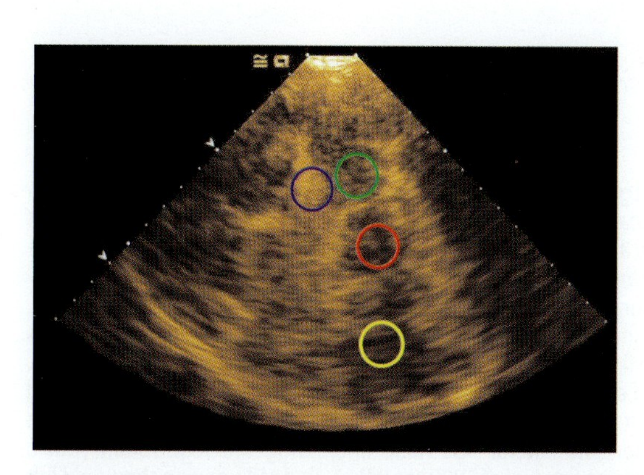

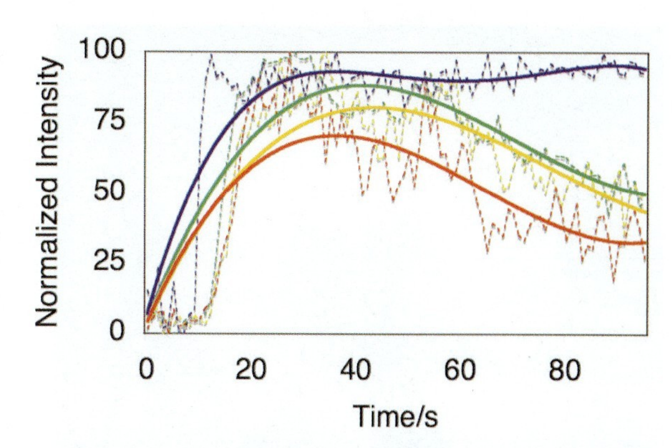

Fig. 11. Contrast-enhanced transcranial B-mode sonography in the axial diencephalic plane in a 23 year old healthy volunteer after intravenous application of the contrast agent SonoVue (*left*), and the time-intensity curves in the ipsi- and contralateral MCA territories (*right*), showing the mean intensity values and a good distribution of the contrast agent after 15 seconds - not only ipsilaterally, but also on the contralateral side. Triggered registration with a pulsing interval of 1000 ms (MI = 1.1). Raw data is shown in dotted lines. The trend lines more clearly depict the perfusion dynamics (the region of interest marked with a blue circle and a blue line shows higher intensity values than those measured in the neighbouring regions, as it was placed in the area of the left middle cerebral artery) (Reprinted with permission from Georg Thieme [37])

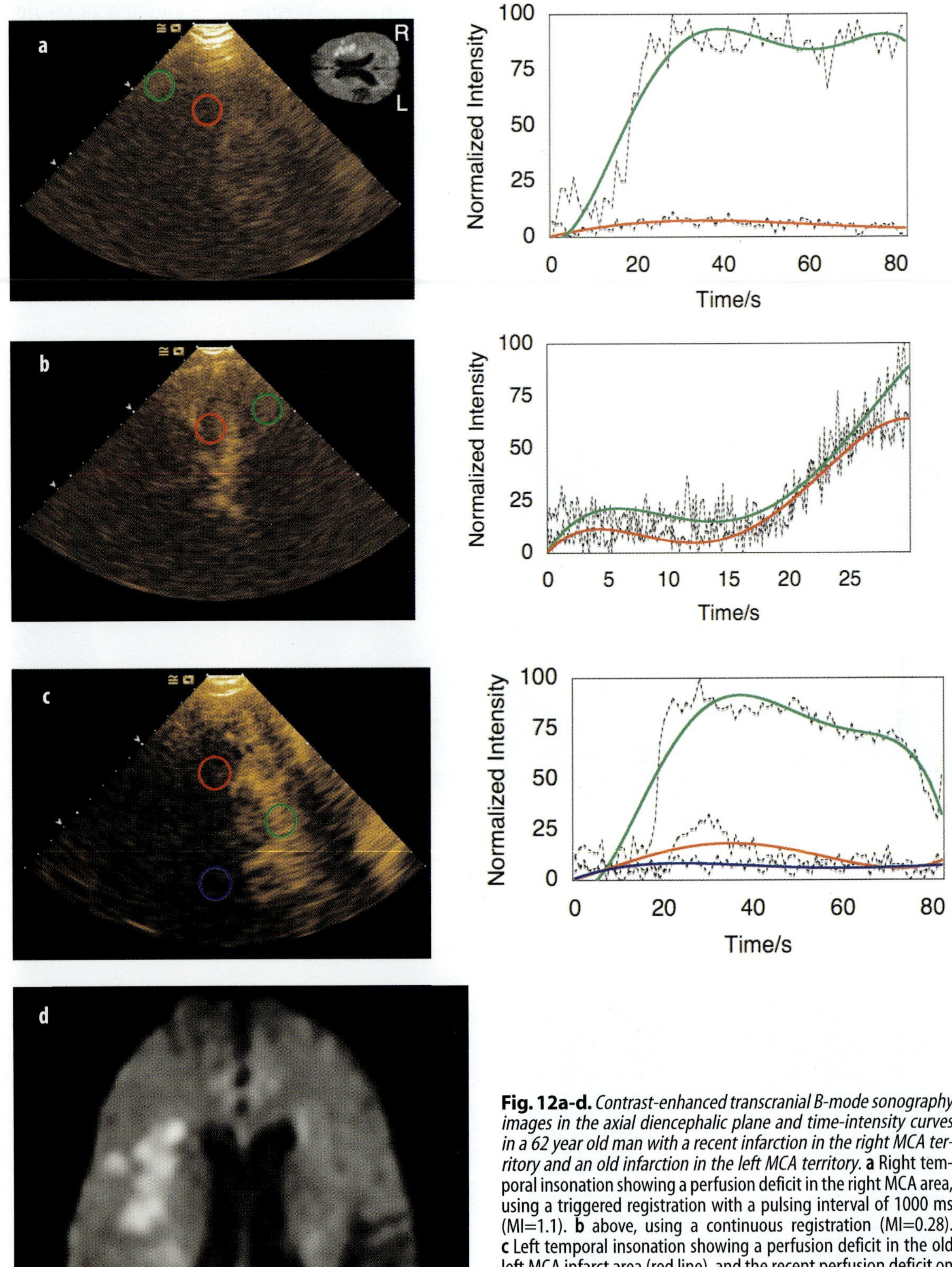

Fig. 12a-d. *Contrast-enhanced transcranial B-mode sonography images in the axial diencephalic plane and time-intensity curves in a 62 year old man with a recent infarction in the right MCA territory and an old infarction in the left MCA territory.* **a** Right temporal insonation showing a perfusion deficit in the right MCA area, using a triggered registration with a pulsing interval of 1000 ms (MI=1.1). **b** above, using a continuous registration (MI=0.28). **c** Left temporal insonation showing a perfusion deficit in the old left MCA infarct area (red line), and the recent perfusion deficit on the contralateral side (blue line). Triggered registration with a pulsing interval of 1000 ms (MI=1.1). **d** MR imaging shows old left temporal infarction and recent right temporal infarction (FLAIR sequence). Raw data is shown in dotted lines. The trend lines more clearly depict the perfusion dynamics. The region of the ipsilateral perfusion deficit is hypoechoic on all three images and is marked by a red circle. Note the acoustic shadowing behind the old infarct zone that can lead to misinterpretation (**c**) (Reprinted with permission from Georg Thieme [37])

In the group of older stroke patients with poorer insonation conditions, the distribution of the contrast agent and the detection of the less perfused areas were possible not only ipsilaterally, but also contralaterally in about one third of the patients (Fig.12).

Pitfalls in the assessment of intensities in ischemic regions occur if the ROI selected is over a vessel (e.g., the branch of a middle cerebral artery). Moreover, in evaluating the intensities of smaller lesions, mistakes can occur due to a limited spatial resolution, if the ROI also covers parts of a non-affected brain region.

Furthermore, careful adjustment of the position of the transducer during the insonation is critical and errors here render the evaluation problematic since slight shifts in transducer placement can make exact calculations of perfusion values and time-intensity curves impossible.

Future Aspects

In clinical practice, recently developed sonographic techniques, such as harmonic power Doppler imaging, or CPS technology, offer new perspectives for the imaging of organ perfusion.

Much effort has been invested in the development of targeted ultrasound contrast agents using ligands (e.g., specific drugs) with the aim of transporting them to a specific site.

Under certain conditions, microbubbles could be used as a therapeutic agent. At present, different research groups are investigating the combination of tissue plasminogen activator (tPa) therapy with application of microbubbles in stroke patients. It has been demonstrated that thrombolysis is potentiated by concomitant ultrasound treatment [38, 39].

In cerebral ischemic disease, another possible therapeutic application of microbubbles is the delivery of genes mediating neuroprotection, nerve regrowth, and revascularization.

Key Points

- In neurosonology, ultrasound contrast agents improve the insonation conditions - e.g., in the case of an insufficient temporal bone window in transcranial imaging. They enhance the backscattered signal from the blood vessels in cases of reduced blood flow velocities in pathological extra- and/or intracranial conditions.
- In extracranial examination, echo-contrast agents allow a clear diagnosis, if the distinction between pre-occlusive stenosis and occlusion is difficult.
- An easier visualization of the intracranial arteries facilitates the diagnostic assessment of the obstruction in the middle cerebral artery and/or basilar artery flow of patients with acute stroke.
- Ultrasonographic imaging of cerebral perfusion is possible using echo-contrast agents. Further improvement in sonographic technology is necessary to increase the diagnostic reliability of contrast-enhanced imaging of cerebral perfusion deficit in stroke patients.

References

1. Bogdahn U, Becker G, Schlief R, Redding J, Hassel W (1993) Contrast-enhanced transcranial color-coded real time sonography. Results of a phase-two study. Stroke 24:676-684
2. Bauer A, Bogdahn U, Haase A, Schlief R (1997) Echo-enhanced transcranial three-dimensional color Doppler imaging. In: Klingelhöfer J, Bartels E, Ringelstein EB (eds) New Trends in Cerebral Hemodynamics and Neurosonology. Elsevier, Amsterdam, pp 509-517
3. Nabavi DG, Droste DW, Kemény V (1998) Potential and limitations of echocontrast-enhanced ultrasonography in acute stroke patients. Stroke 29:949-954
4. Schneider M, Arditi M, Barrau M-B et al (1995) BR1: A new ultrasonographic contrast agent based on sulfur hexafluorid-filled microbubbles. Investigative Radiology. 8:451-457
5. Bokor D (2000) Diagnostic efficacy of SonoVue. Am J Cardiol 86[Suppl]:19G-24G
6. Droste DW, Llull JB, Pezzoli C et al (2002) SonoVue™ (BR1), a new long-acting echocontrast agent, improves transcranial colour-coded duplex ultrasonic imaging. Cerebrovasc Dis 14:27-32
7. Droste DW, Metz RJ (2004) Clinical utility of echocontrast agents in neurosonology. Neurol Res 26(7):754-759
8. Bartels E (1999) Color-Coded Duplex

Ultrasonography of the Cerebral Vessels / Atlas and Manual; Farbduplexsonographie der hirnversorgenden Gefässe / Atlas und Handbuch. Schattauer, Stuttgart, pp195-196
9. Sitzer M, Fürst G, Siebler M, Steinmetz H (1994) Usefulness of an intravenous contrast medium in the characterization of high grade internal carotid stenosis with colour Doppler assisted duplex imaging. Stroke 25:385-389
10. Bartels E, Flügel KA (1996) Evaluation of extracranial vertebral artery dissection with duplex color flow imaging. Stroke 27:290-295
11. Bartels E (2006) Dissection of the extracranial vertebral artery: clinical findings and early noninvasive diagnosis in 24 patients. J Neuroimaging, in press
12. Becker G, Lindner A, Bogdahn U (1993) Imaging of the vertebrobasilar system by transcranial color-coded real-time sonography. J Ultrasound Med 12:395-402
13. Ries F, Honisch C, Lambertz M, Schlief R (1993) A transpulmonary contrast medium enhances the transcranial Doppler signal in humans. Stroke 24:1903-1909
14. Kaps M, Legemate DA, Ries F (2001) SonoVue™ in transcranial Doppler investigations of the cerebral arteries. J Neuroimaging. 11:261-267
15. Bartels E, KA Flügel (1994) Quantitative measurements of blood flow velocity in basal cerebral arteries with transcranial color Doppler imaging. J Neuroimaging 4:77-81
16. Kaps M, Seidel G, Bauer T, Behrmann B (1992) Imaging of the intracranial vertebrobasilar system using colour-coded ultrasound. Stroke 23:1577-1582
17. Postert T, Muhs A, Meves S (1998) Transient response harmonic imaging: An ultrasound technique related to brain perfusion. Stroke 29:1901-1907
18. Seidel G, Greis C, Sonne J, Kaps M (1999) Harmonic grey scale imaging of the human brain. J Neuroimaging 9:171-174
19. Burns P, Powers JE, Hope Simpson D (1996) Harmonic imaging, principles and preliminary results. Angiology 47[Suppl]:S63-S74
20. Schrope BA, Newhouse VL, Uhlendorf V (1992) Simulated capillary blood flow measurement using a nonlinear ultrasonic contrast agent. Ultrason Imag 14:134-139
21. Burns PN (1996) Harmonic imaging with ultrasound contrast agents. Clin Radiol 51[Suppl 1]:50-55
22. Albrecht T, Hoffmann CW, Schettler S et al (2000). B-mode enhancement at phase-inversion US with air-based microbubble contrast agent: Initial experience in humans. Radiology 216:273-278
23. Forsberg F, Goldberg BB, Liu JB (1996) On the feasibility of real-time, in vivo harmonic imaging with proteinaceous microspheres. J Ultrasound Med 15:853-860
24. Mulvagh SL, Foley DA, Aeschbacher BC (1996) Second harmonic imaging of an intravenously administered echocardiographic contrast agent. J Am Coll Cardiol 27:1519-1525
25. Schwarz KQ, Chen X, Steinmetz S, Phillips D (1997) Harmonic imaging with Levovist. J Am Soc Echocardiogr 10:1-10
26. Martina DM, Meyer-Wiethe K, Allémann E, Seidel G (2005) Ultrasound contrast agents for brain perfusion imaging and ischemic stroke therapy. J Neuroimaging 15:217-232
27. Seidel G, Algermissen C, Christoph A et al (2000) Harmonic imaging of the human brain. Visualization of brain perfusion with ultrasound. Stroke 31:151-154
28. Postert T, Federlein J, Rose J et al (2001) Ultrasonic assessment of physiological echo-contrast agent distribution in brain parenchyma with transient response second harmonic imaging. J Neuroimaging 11:18-24
29. Seidel G, Meyer K (2001) Harmonic imaging – a new method for the sonographic assessment of cerebral perfusion. Eur J Ultrasound 14:103-113
30. Wiesmann M, Seidel G (2000) Ultrasound perfusion imaging of the human brain. Stroke 31:2421-2425
31. Postert T, Federlein J, Weber S et al (1999) Second harmonic imaging in acute middle cerebral artery infarction. Preliminary results. Stroke 30:1702-1706
32. Federlein J, Postert T, Meves S et al (2000) Ultrasonic evaluation of pathological brain perfusion in acute stroke using second harmonic imaging. J Neurol Neurosurg Psychiatry 69:616-622
33. Keir SL, Wardlaw JM (2000) Systematic review of diffusion and perfusion imaging in acute stroke. Stroke 31:2723-2731
34. Harrer JU, Klötzsch C, Stracke CP, Möller-Hartmann (2004) Cerebral perfusion sonography in comparison with perfusion MRT: a study with healthy volunteers. Ultraschall in Med 25:263-269
35. Shiogai T, Takayasu N, Mizuno T et al (2004) Comparison of transcranial brain tissue perfusion images between ultraharmonic, second harmonic, and power harmonic imaging. Stroke 35:687-693
36. Bartels E, Bittermann H-J (2004) Transcranial contrast imaging of cerebral perfusion in stroke patients following decompressive craniectomy. Ultraschall in Med 25:206-213
37. Bartels E, Henning S, Wellmer A et al (2005) Evaluation of cerebral perfusion deficit in stroke patients using new transcranial contrast imaging CPS™ technology. Preliminary results. Ultraschall in Med 26:478-486
38. Alexandrov AV, Demchuk AM, Burgin WS et al (2004) Ultrasound-enhanced thrombolysis for acute ischemic stroke: phase I. Findings of the CLOTBUST trial. J Neuroimaging 14:113-117
39. Tsutsui JM, Grayburn PA, Xie F, Porter TR (2004) Drug and gene delivery and enhancement of thrombolysis using ultrasound and microbubbles. Cardiol Clin 22:299-312

III.3

Abdominal Vessels

Alberto Martegani, Luca Aiani and Claudia Borghi

Introduction

Technological development of colour Doppler equipment (CD) has enabled endovascular flow phenomena to be more easily understood, but this imaging technique is still limited by some physical restrictions [1, 2].

In fact, the more haematic flow velocity is reduced, the less CD sampling is able to distinguish colour signals coming from vessel walls and surrounding tissues from those derived from corpuscular haematic components. This difficulty gives rise to an intrinsic CD artefact that remarkably affects its diagnostic efficacy, particularly in physiological or pathological 'slow flow' conditions.

In clinical practice, the less favourable haemodynamic situation occurs in 'stationary' flow conditions, such as aneurysmatic dilations, hypersevere stenoses or peri-vascular hemorrhagic collections. Neither modern technologies such as power Doppler (Energy), nor the grey-scale coding of flow phenomena (B-flow) are able to overcome these limitations [3].

Microbubbles are the corpuscular components of ultrasound contrast agents and are detected and depicted in real-time also in extremely reduced flow, if a dedicated and sufficiently sensitive ultrasound system is used [4, 5].

Low Mechanical Index (MI) techniques, such as contrast-enhanced ultrasound (CEUS) achieve this goal as they obtain a more linear contrast media signal owing to almost absent microbubble destruction and a more proportional ratio between bubble concentration and signal entity. In addition, through a subtraction of the signal coming from steady tissues, it strongly enhances even low concentrations of microbubbles.

For these reasons, it is easy to understand how this approach has recently found many fields of application with a real clinical interest.

Abdominal Aortic, Iliac and Visceral Aneurysmatic Dilatations

Ultrasound diagnosis of abdominal aortic aneurysms (AAA) is based on evaluation of the dimensions of the involved vessel, basically, on its transversal diameter; this information is easily obtained with the bare grey-scale image eventually integrated by CD module morpho-functional evaluations (Fig. 1).

On the other hand, the identification of a peripheral intra-aneurysmatic thrombus is sometimes difficult using B-mode and the CD module in particular, because of the extremely reduced flow velocity inside a dilated lumen; parietal thrombi are also usually variably hypoechoic.

For the same reasons, it is sometimes difficult to detect false flow chambers with the CD module, due to the dissection of endo-aneurysmatic thrombus. On the other hand, some artefactual intrathrombotic CD signals may be depicted erroneously, due to the movement of these structures (Figs. 2, 3).

CEUS permits the correct definition of thrombi profiles, thanks to a 'contrastographic' hyperechoic depiction of blood flow; ulcerations or thrombotic dissections, supplied with blood flow, are easily detectable as well, and are not dependent on blood flow velocity (Fig. 4).

Even if this morphological information is not essential for the evaluation of the seriousness of aneurysmatic disease, it may result in the diagnosis of 'instability' and sometimes be an unfavourable sign, especially in association with abdominal pain.

In the case of a rupturing abdominal aortic aneurysm, when clinical conditions permit an imaging approach, CEUS is able to rapidly diagnose the aneurysm and also any haematic retroperitoneal / para-aortic bleeding (Figs. 5, 6).

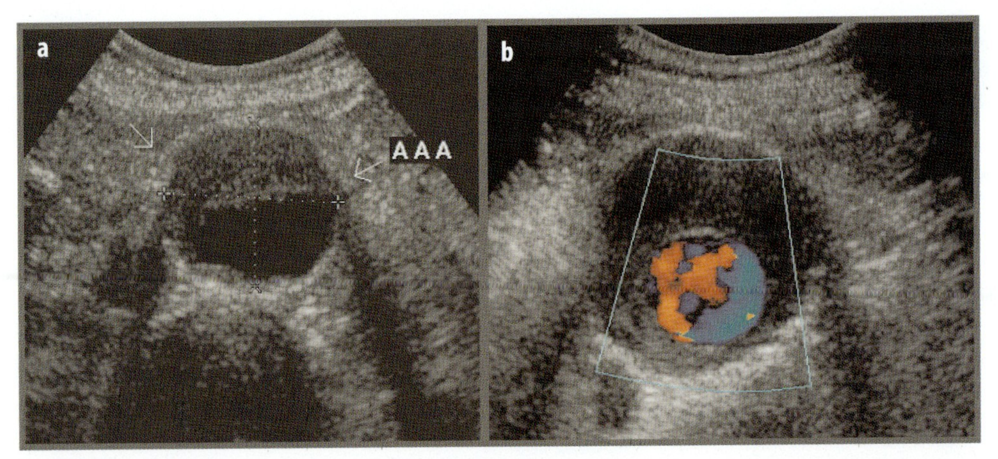

Fig. 1a, b. *Abdominal aortic aneurysms (AAA).* **a, b** Transverse US and CD scans of the aorta. An abdominal aorta aneurysm with anterior parietal thrombus is depicted (**a**). With this approach, the aneurysmatic transversal diameter is detected. **b** A peripheral thrombus, particularly thick in its anterior part, surrounds the flow chamber; CD outlines the smooth and regular thrombus surface

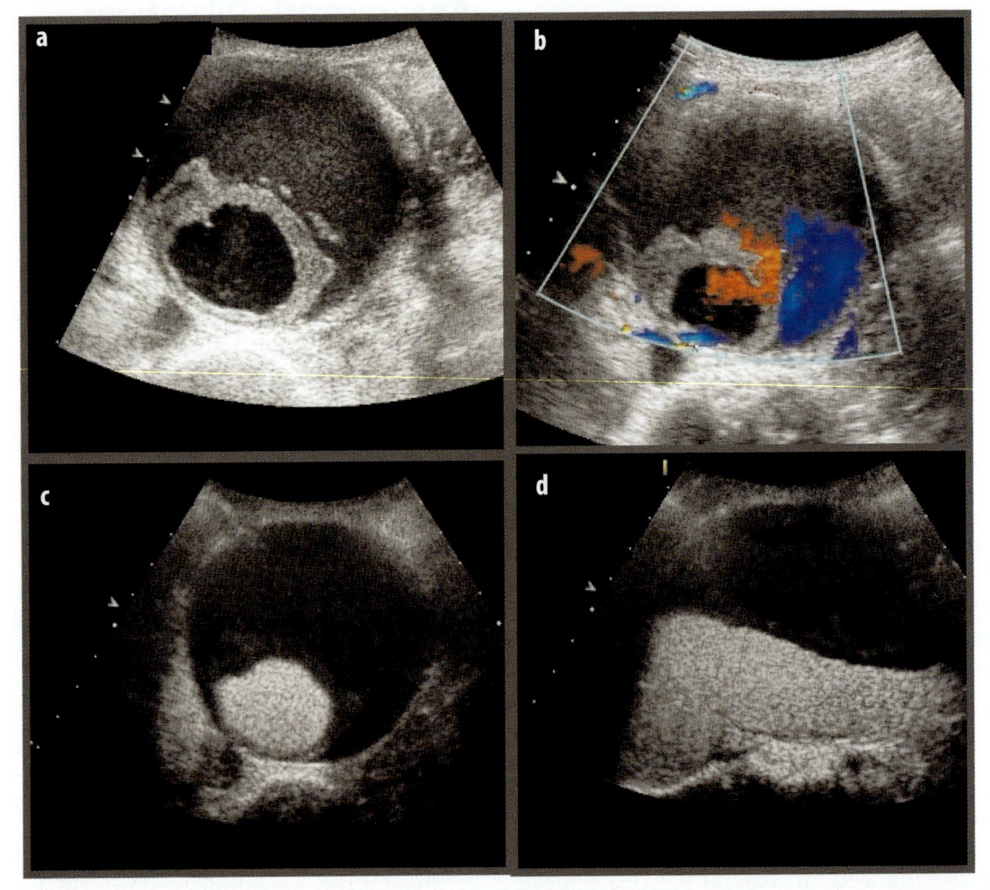

Fig. 2a-d. *Large abdominal aortic aneurysm with inhomogeneous solid and fluid thrombus.* **a, b** Transverse and longitudinal US and CD scans of the aorta. An approximately 5 cm large abdominal aortic aneurysm is presented with a thin, irregular, hyperechoic thrombus, which is 2 cm thick, delimiting the flow chamber. There is a significant, finely corpuscolar, fluid component in the left antero-lateral region, peripheral to the thin hyperechoic thrombus. The colour Doppler image of this fluid shows the presence of some sporadic colour signals (in blue). **c, d** Transverse and longitudinal CEUS scan of the aorta. The use of a contrast-specific harmonic algorithm performed at a low mechanical index nearly completely canceled out the signals derived from the stationary anatomic structures. Only minor signals from the thrombus remain (the thrombus is markedly hyperechogenic in baseline US). Approximately 20 seconds after administration of the contrast medium, hyperechogenic microbubbles appear and remain confined into the flow lumen delimited by the thin thrombus. No vascular phase shows signs of passage of the contrast medium into the fluid component of the thrombus

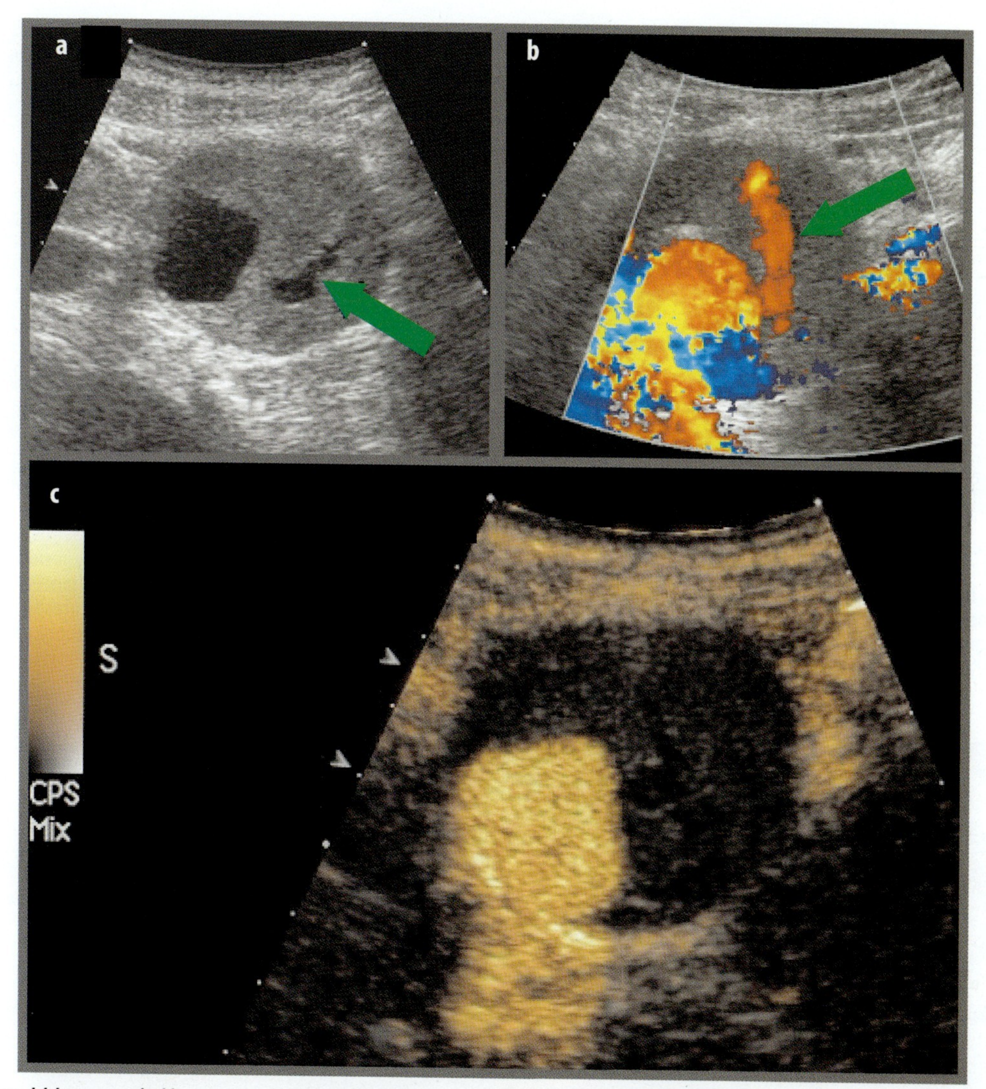

Fig. 3a-c. *AAA surrounded by a parietal layered thrombus, not supplied with blood.* **a** Transversal scan, B-mode. An AAA with homogeneous peripheral thrombus with a layered anechoic appearance (*green arrow*) is detected; the true lumen is located laterally, on the right. **b** Transversal scan, colour Doppler. A chromatic signal is detectable both inside the residual lumen and in the anechoic layer of the thrombus (in red), potentially supplying inflow (*green arrow*). **c** Transversal scan, CEUS. The aortic lumen is enhanced; inside the thrombus and its anechoic portion no signal of contrast agent is demonstrable

Use of CEUS is less common in emergency situations.

In the case of dissecting abdominal aortic aneurysms, both flow lumina are opacified and hyperechoic with CEUS; contrastosonographic kinetics help to differentiate the high flow aortic lumen from the low delivery flow lumen; the precocious enhancement permits correct identification and definition of the true lumen (Fig. 7).

In the case of extra-aortic aneurysmatic disease, involving small calibre or distal vessels (iliac, renal or splanchnic), CEUS rapidly identifies the vascular nature of these lesions; the time of transit and the intensity of contrastographic phenomena distinguishes the arterial from the venous nature (Fig. 8).

Any thrombotic endo-aneurysmatic deposition may be easily diagnosed using contrast agents, for example, in the aorta.

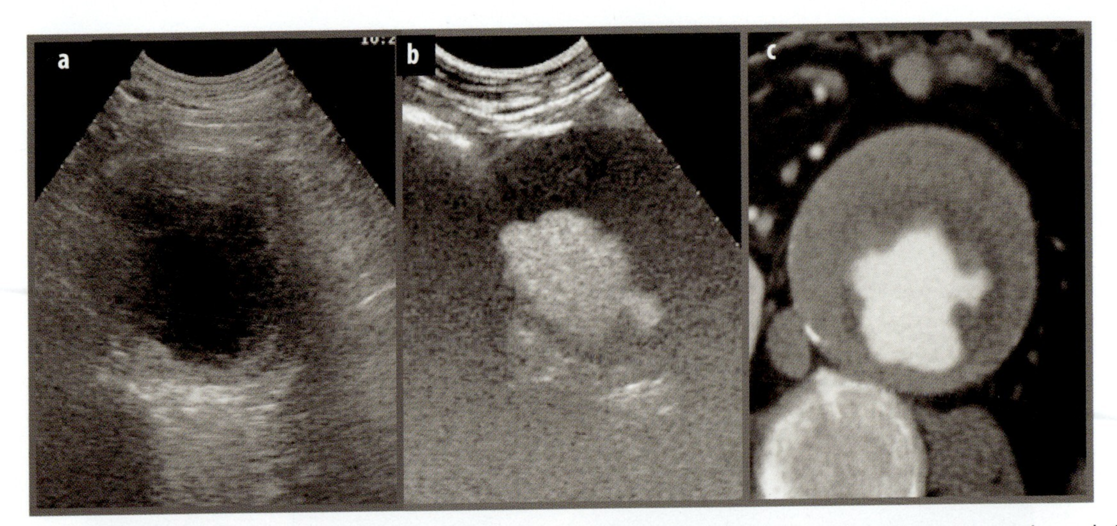

Fig. 4a-c. *Abdominal aorta aneurysm.* **a** Transversal scan, B-mode. An abdominal aortic aneurysm with an inhomogeneous, hypoechoic, peripheral thrombus is detectable; a correct evaluation of the thrombus surface and therefore of the diameter of the residual lumen is prevented, because of its morphological appearance. **b** Transversal scan, CEUS. The aortic lumen is homogeneously enhanced by contrast agent, appearing hyperechoic; the peripheral thrombus inner surface is remarkably irregular. **c** Helical angio-CT corresponding scan. Contrast agent outlines the thrombus profile; in such a situation, the residual lumen is well depicted and so is the presence of large penetrating atheromasic ulcers

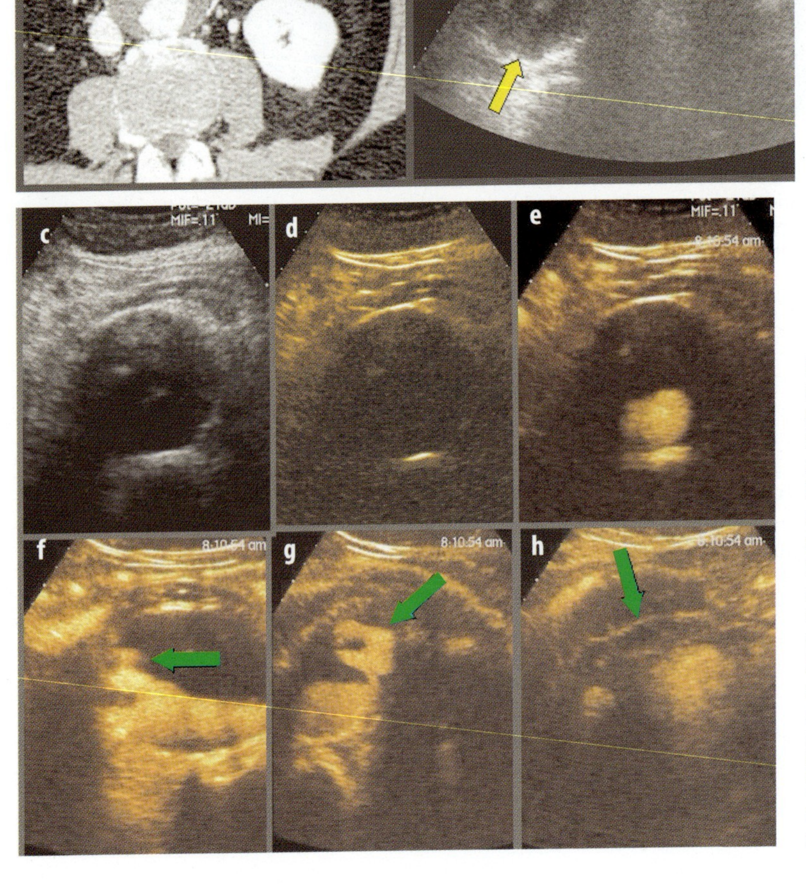

Fig. 5a-h. *Rupturing abdominal aortic aneurysm.* **a** Transversal angio-CT scan. A wide parietal thrombus delimits a small flow chamber posteriorly located in this aneurysmatic sac. **b** Transversal scan, US. Marked inhomogeneous and hypoechoic appearance of peri-aneurysmatic tissues on the left side; the aneurysm has an identical caliber to the previous scan (*yellow arrows*). **c-h** Trasversal scan, CEUS. After contrast injection, the flow lumen enhances; an irregular hyperechoic image branches off the flow lumen into an anterior thrombus (*green arrows*), corresponding to the dissection seat; a small amount of contrast agent is detectable inside the peripheral tissues, which are hypoechoic (**h**) due to the presence of a minimal blood supply in the peri-aneurysmatic haematoma

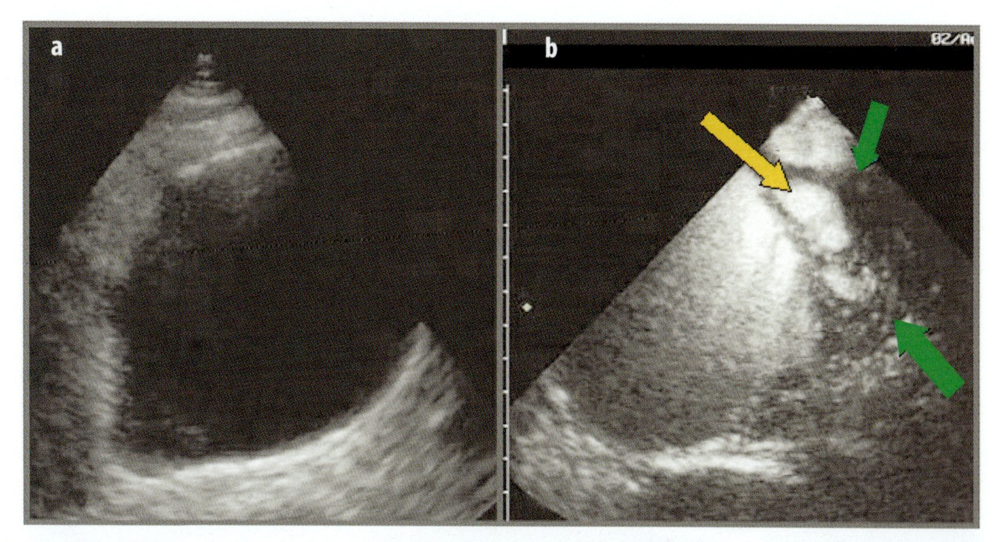

Fig. 6a, b. *Breaking AAA with para-aortic retroperitoneal haematoma supplied with blood flow.* **a** Transversal scan, B-mode. Large AAA. **b** Transversal scans, CEUS. In **b** the aortic lumen is enhanced by contrast agent; in the left retroperitoneal para-aortic space a hypoechoic semilunar mass (*green arrows*) corresponding to haematoma is depicted, in which two hyperechoic, vascularised areas are evident, corresponding to active supply (*yellow arrows*)

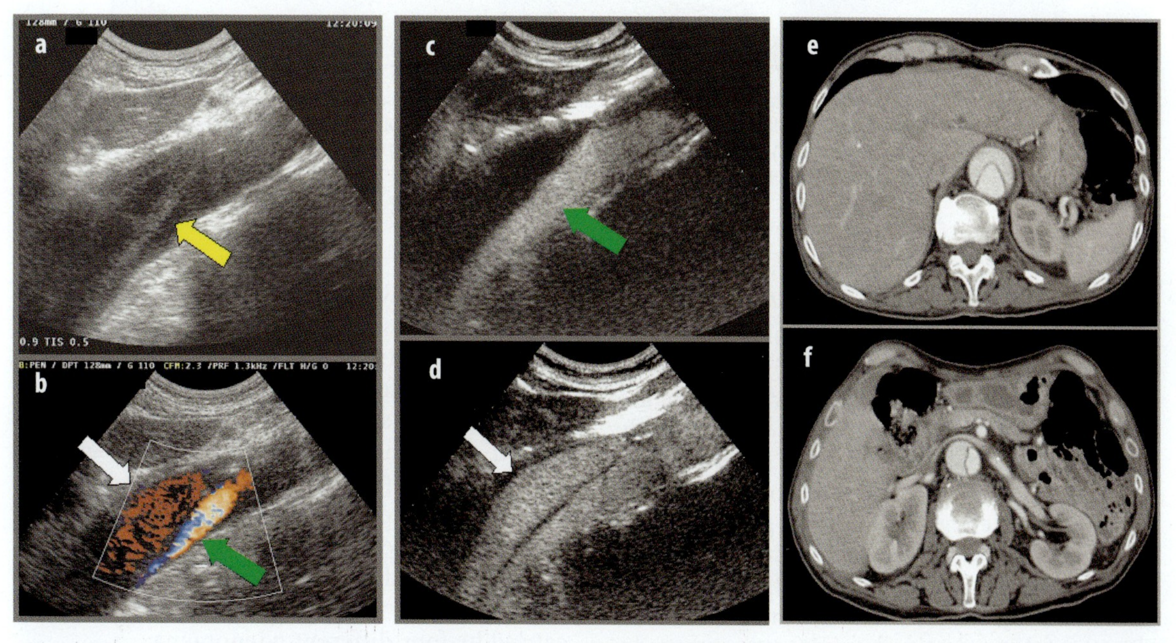

Fig. 7a-f. *Dissecting abdominal aorta aneurysm.* **a** Longitudinal scan, B-mode. The abdominal aorta is slightly enlarged; in its lumen a thin hyperechoic laminar image corresponding to dissected intima is detected (*yellow arrow*). **b** Longitudinal scan, CD. Two flow chambers with different velocity rates are depicted with CD; the posterior lumen has a high flow velocity (true lumen: *green arrow*) while anterior chamber has a slow flow velocity (false lumen: *white arrow*). **c-d** Longitudinal scan, CEUS. After contrast administration (**c**), the posterior lumen (true lumen: *green arrow*) enhances rapidly and homogeneously in early phase; in late phase (**d**) the false lumen (anterior: *white arrow*) enhances homogeneously as well. **e-f** Angio-CT, trasversal plane. The abdominal aorta is slighty enlarged; the dissected flap divides the vessel in two flow lumina

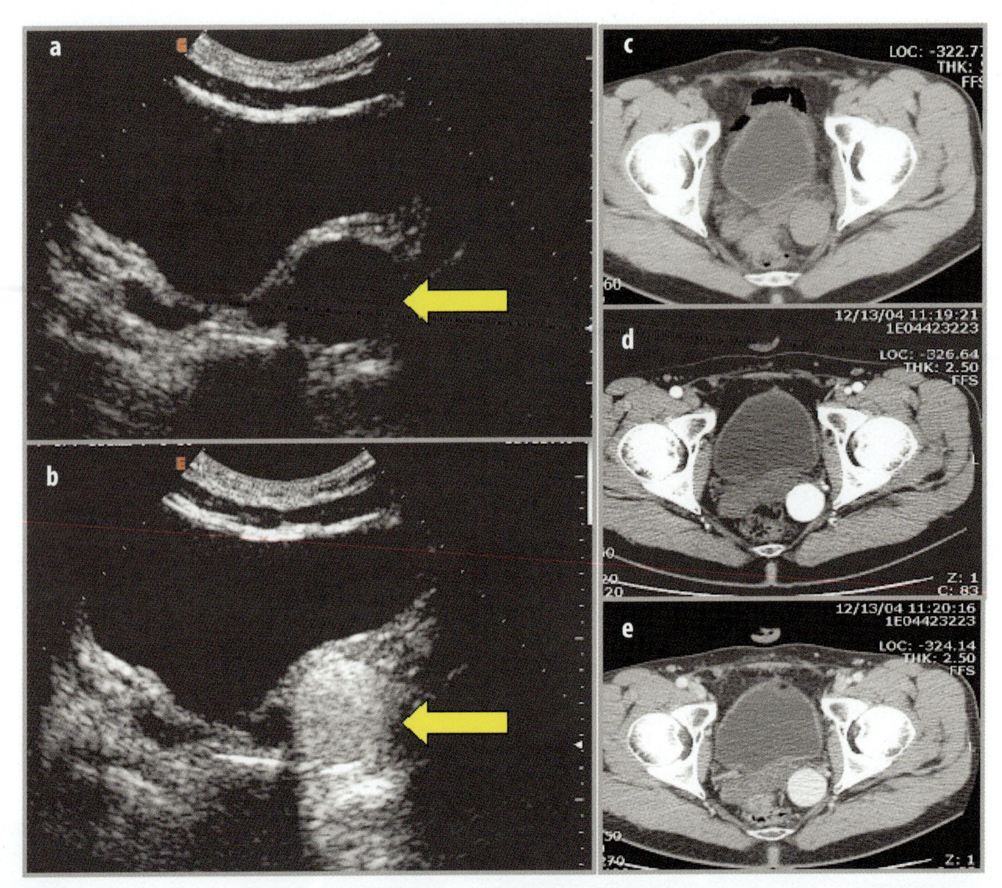

Fig. 8a-e. *Hypogastric aneurysm.* **a** Transversal scan, B-mode. A small anechoic rounded lesion (*yellow arrow*) is detected posteriorly and left laterally to the urinary bladder. **b** Transversal scans, CEUS. After contrast administration, a homogeneous enhancement inside the rounded image is already evident in arterial phase (*yellow arrow*). **c-e** Angio-CT, transversal plane. In baseline scan (**c**) the rounded image is confirmed behind the bladder; it homogeneously enhances in arterial phase (**d**) and more poorly in late vascular phases (**e**)

Follow-up of Aortic Vascular (Percutaneous or Surgical) Grafts

CEUS is a valid and consolidated diagnostic tool with computed tomography angiography (angio-CT) for the follow-up of surgically repaired aneurysms. CEUS is able to demonstrate the patency of vascular grafts and to detect any flow signal inside hypo-anechoic peri-aneurysmatic collections, helping to distinguish fluid collections such as seromas or lymphoceles from pulsating haematomas or pseudoaneurysms (Fig. 9). These last two conditions are potentially unstable, because they are supplied with blood flow, and usually require an individual therapy.

Stenoses of anastomotic seats are easily diagnosed and quantified by CD module; high flow velocities, always associated with these pathologic conditions, do not benefit from CEUS.

On the contrary, the indication of CEUS in early and late follow-up of percutaneous repair of aneurysms is extremely important; morphological and functional follow-up must exclude the presence of recanalisation of the aneurysmatic sac (endoleak) (Fig. 10) [6-9]. By CEUS, this phenomenon appears as a hyperechoic signal (corresponding to contrast agent) inside the peri-prosthetic aneurysmatic sac and may be caused by four different phenomena:

- detachment of any part of the endograft from aneurysmatic necks (type I)
- flow inversion inside a collateral vessel (type II)
- lesion of the endograft covering or rupture (type III)
- abnormal porosity of the graft covering (type IV).

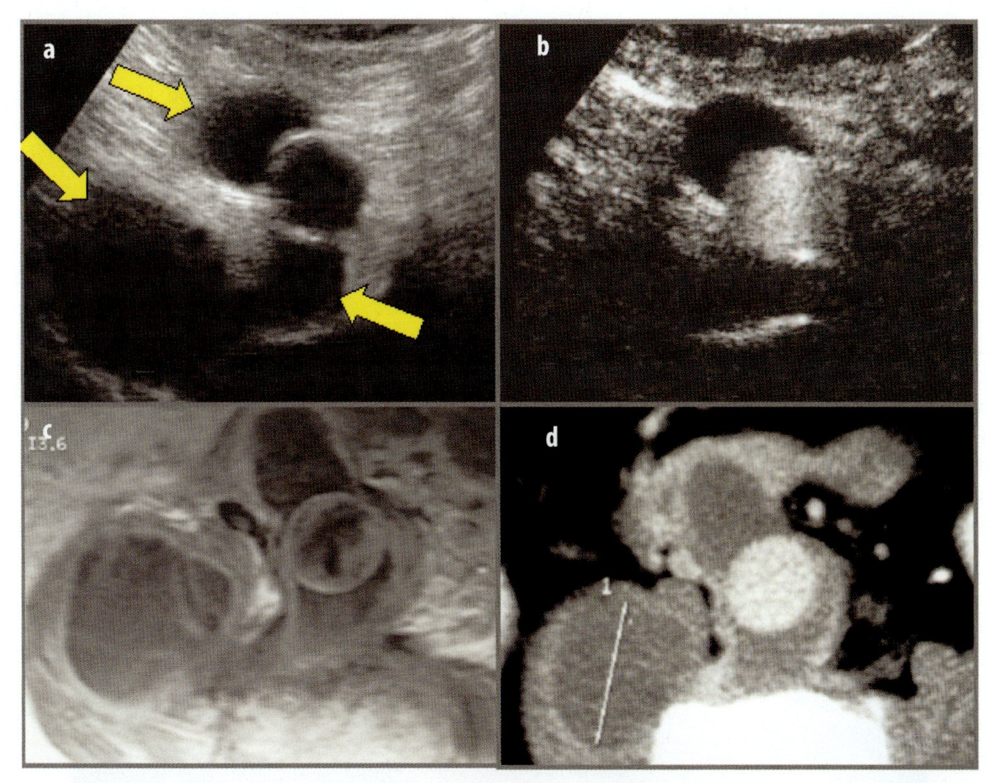

Fig. 9a-d. *Surgical aortic stentgraft with peripheral fluid collections.* **a** Transversal scan, B-mode. A linear hyperechoic rounded structure corresponding to the aortic graft is evident; anteriorly, posteriorly and in right postero-lateral position three anechoic images (*yellow arrows*) are detectable peripheral to the prosthesis, but strictly adherent to the prosthesic wall (possibly peri-prosthesic collections or anastomotic pseudo-aneurysm). **b** Transversal scan, CEUS. The prosthesic lumen is regularly enhanced by contrast agent; none of the three collections is filled with contrast, and therefore they are excluded by vascular bed. Periprosthesic collections. **c-d** Angio-RMN and angio-CT corresponding planes. No vascular supply is detected inside the three collections

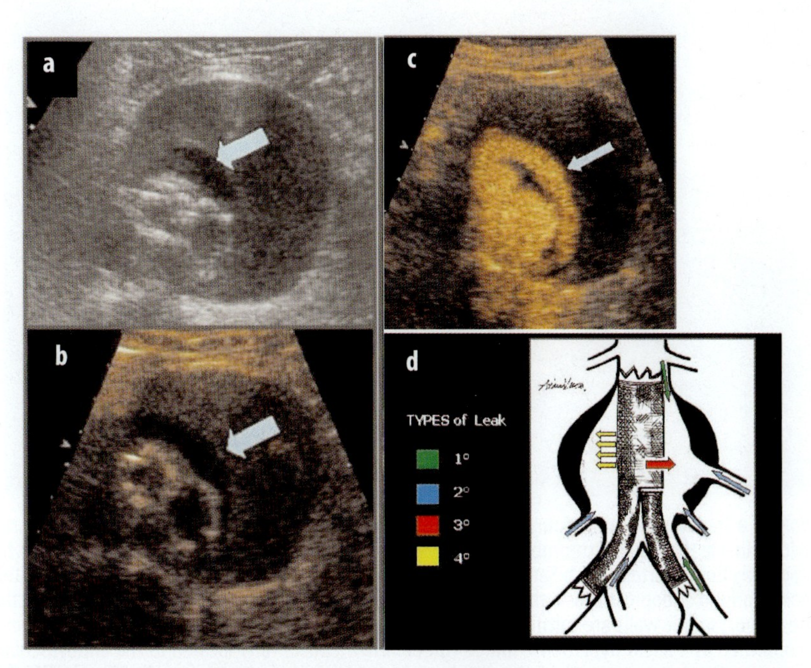

Fig. 10a-d. a B-mode transversal scan. Abdominal aortic aneurysm. Inside the sac, iliac prosthesic branches are detectable. Peripherally, a parietal thrombus with a hypo-anechoic area surrounding the prosthesis is demonstrable (*white arrow*). **b, c** Transversal CEUS scan. After contrast agent administration (**c**), a hyperechoic signal due to microbubbles appears inside the prosthesis lumen and in the fluid peri-prosthesic collection (*white arrow*), in comparison to unenhanced scan (**b**). Schematic drawing of different endoleak types (**d**)

Compared to CEUS, angio-CT, the gold standard technique, is more panoramic in its evaluation of the graft and native aorta; on the other hand, it is burdened with intrinsic limitations mainly due to the use of a potentially nephrotoxic contrast agents, which is dangerous for patients who have impaired renal function [10-13].

CEUS, in the presence of a suitable sonographic window, permits morphological and functional information to be obtained, comparable to that achieved by angio-CT (Figs. 11, 12) [14-18].

Simultaneous application of CEUS and low MI colour Doppler enables the combination of morpho-functional data with the 'direction' information necessary to comprehend the complex means of residual aneurysmatic sac supply; these two imaging modalities may identify the feeding and the efferent artery in the case of type II endoleak (Fig. 13).

CEUS also detects type IV endoleak; endograft porosity allows the filtration of contrast agent through many points of the prosthesis wall (Fig. 14).

A specific type of leakage, known as tensoleak, must be also considered; it appears as a progressive increase in the diameter of the residual aneurysmatic sac in the absence of detectable inflow phenomena. Its cause seems to be related to arterial pressure transmission from the endograft walls to the peripheral thrombus; the large aneurysmatic dimensions and the presence of a inhomogeneous thrombus mixed with fluid intrathrombotic lacunae seem to favour such pressure transmission (Fig. 15).

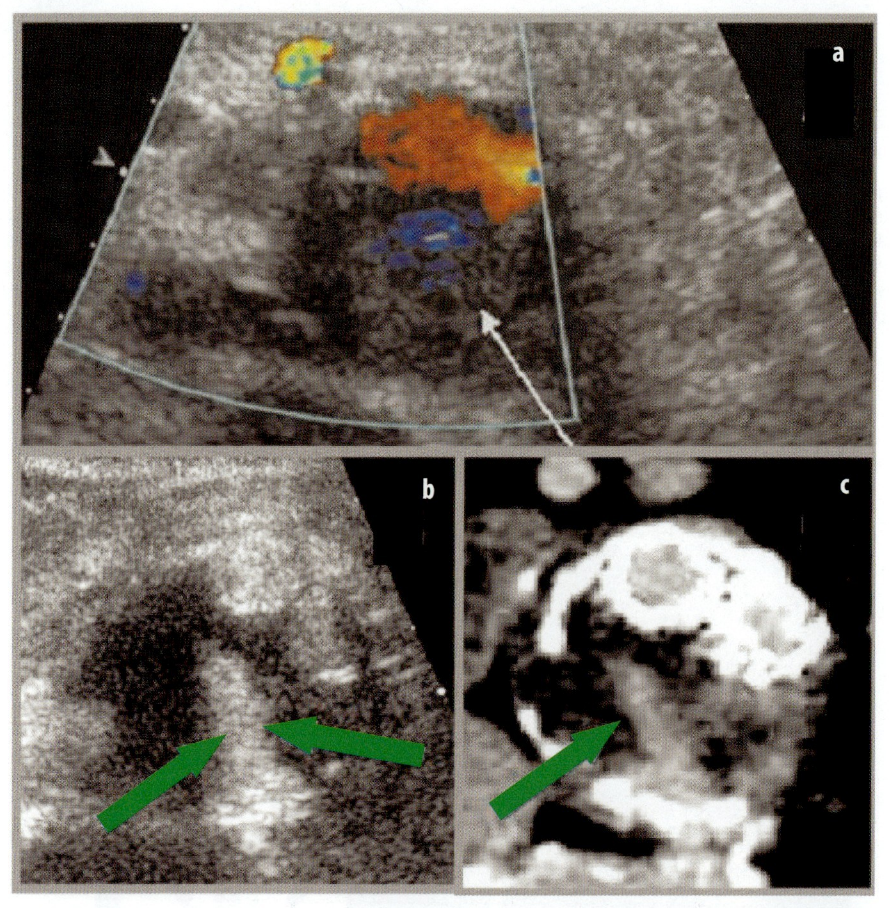

Fig. 11a-c. *Type II Endoleak.* **a** Transversal scan, colour Doppler. The aorto-iliac endovascular graft in the anterior part of the aneurysm is correctly patent; posteriorly, inside the residual thrombosed aneurysmatic sac, there is a chromatic signal (blue) (*white arrow*), which is not easily interpretable (possibly flow or artefact?). **b** Same, CEUS scans. In longitudinal (**c**) scan, the graft lumen is patent (hyperechoic); inside the residual sac, posteriorly to endoprosthesis a thin, hyperechoic, winding flow lumen (*green arrows)* is detectable (endoleak). **c** Angio-CT, trasversal plane. Aneurysmatic walls are calcified. The metallic structure of the graft iliac branches are hyperdense and so are their lumen. The leak is confirmed as a linear hyperdense image (*green arrow*), posteriorly located to the endovascular graft. There is a perfect overlapping between the flow phenomena depiction inside and outside the prosthesis of angio-CT and CEUS (**b**)

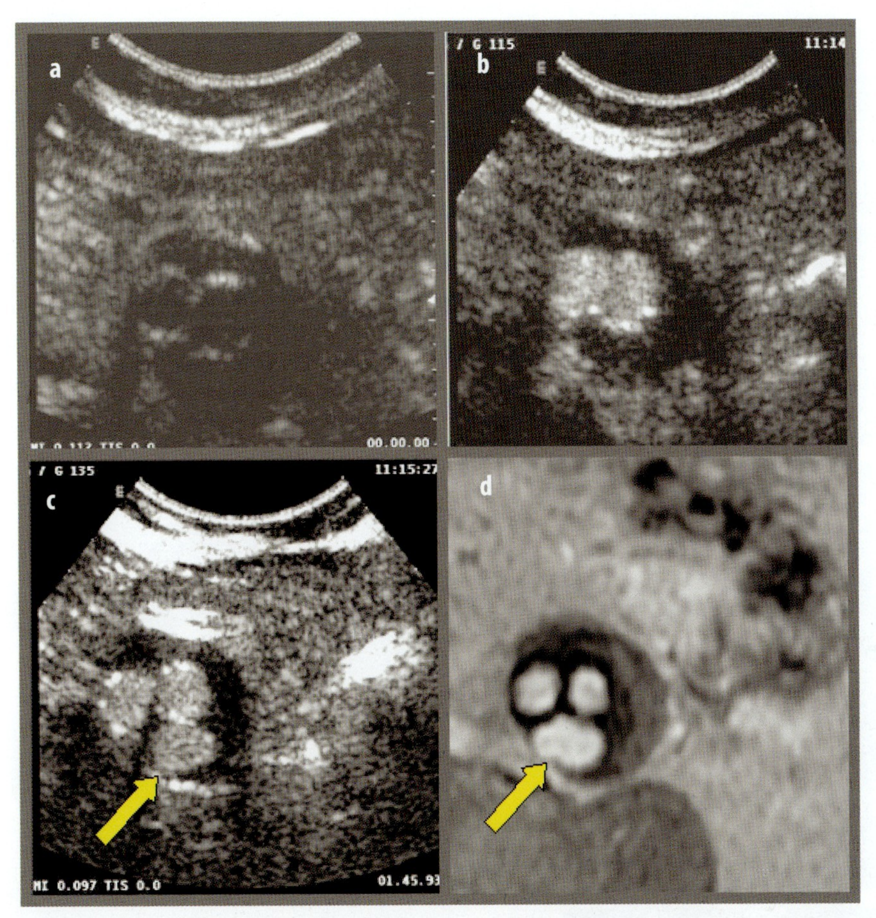

Fig. 12a-d. *Type II Endoleak.* **a-c** Transversal scan, CEUS. Before contrast administration (**a**), two linear rounded images corresponding to iliac branches of the prosthesis are evident: the graft lumen and the aneurysmatic sac are hypoechoic. After contrast injection, in early phase the iliac branches are completely filled with contrast and their lumen appears hyperechoic (**b**); in late phase, an oval-shaped hyperechoic image appears outside the prosthesis, posteriorly to the iliac branches, inside the aneurysmatic sac (*yellow arrow*) - endoleak (**c**). **d** Transversal scan, angio-NMR. Behind the patent iliac branches of the endoprosthesis, a small oval enhancement is detectable, corresponding to the endoleak

Another advantage of CEUS is linked to the opportunity of performing subsequent (also daily) follow-up examinations even at the patient's bedside; in such conditions a precise and non-invasive monitoring of the first post-therapy phases is obtained without patient discomfort.

Finally, the recently gained ability to use dedicated overlapping systems of ultrasound images in real-time, baseline and contrast-enhanced, and CT/magnetic resonance (MR) images should be mentioned. Fusion imaging is achieved using a magnetic field (generated by a transmitter) combined with a small receiver, where positioning information is acquired through second-by-second detection of the US probe.

In these conditions, the dimensions of the residual peri-prosthesic aneurysmatic sac are more precisely and easily detectable (baseline CT image), and at the same time the presence of contrast agent inside the vascular lumen, or inside the peripheral thrombus if a leakage occurs, is identifiable as well (CEUS image) (Figs. 16, 17).

This system enables the advantages of both techniques to be enhanced and their intrinsic limitations to be counterbalanced through information integration.

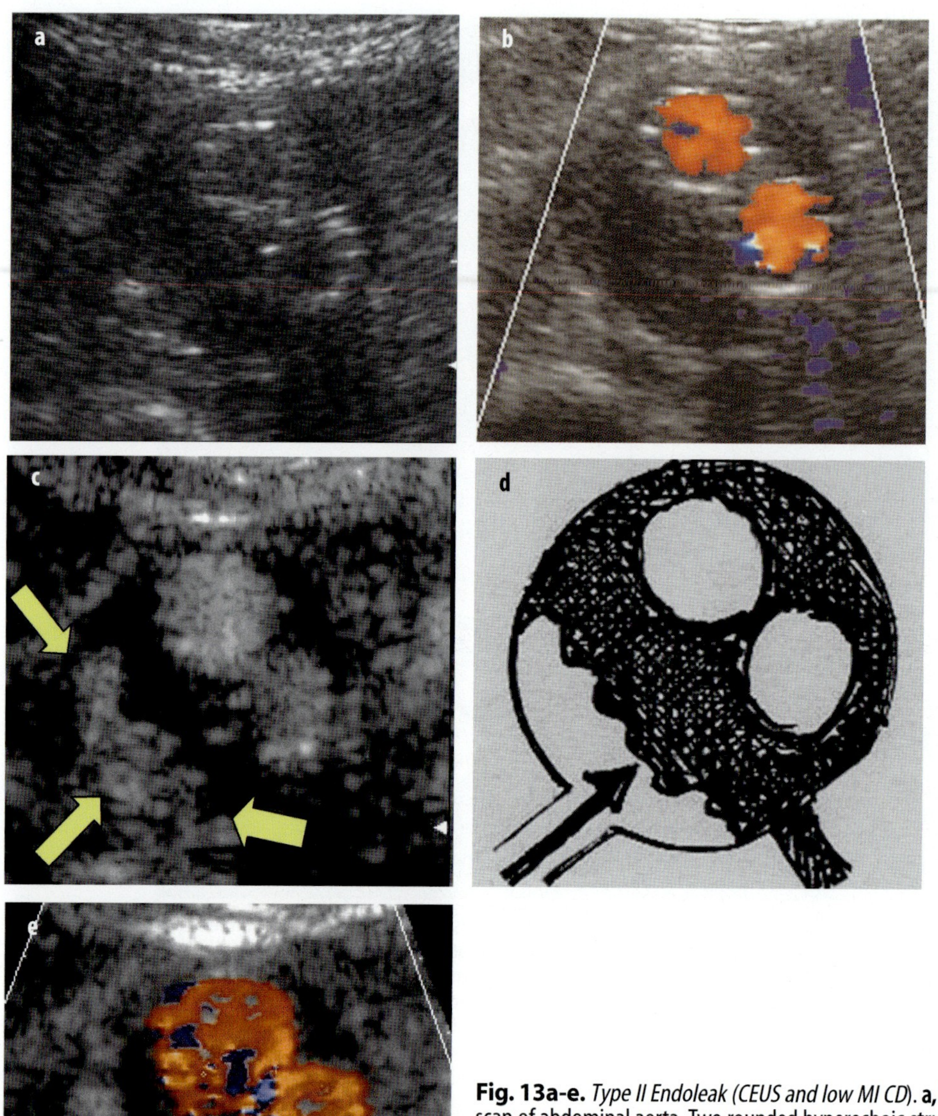

Fig. 13a-e. *Type II Endoleak (CEUS and low MI CD).* **a, b** Transversal US and CD scan of abdominal aorta. Two rounded hyperechoic structures corresponding to the iliac endoprosthesic branches. **c** CEUS transversal scan. The branches are enhanced by contrast bubbles; the hyperechoic area placed in the aneurysmal sac postero-laterally corresponds to the leakage (*yellow arrows*). **d** Drawing depicting the leakage area in the right posterolateral region and the lumbar vessel responsible for the recanalisation. **e** CEUS and low MI colour Doppler in systolic phase. Colour signal inside the iliac branch lumen; flow directed towards the aneurysm corresponding to the lumbar vessel (*green arrow*) that refills the sac (type II endoleak)

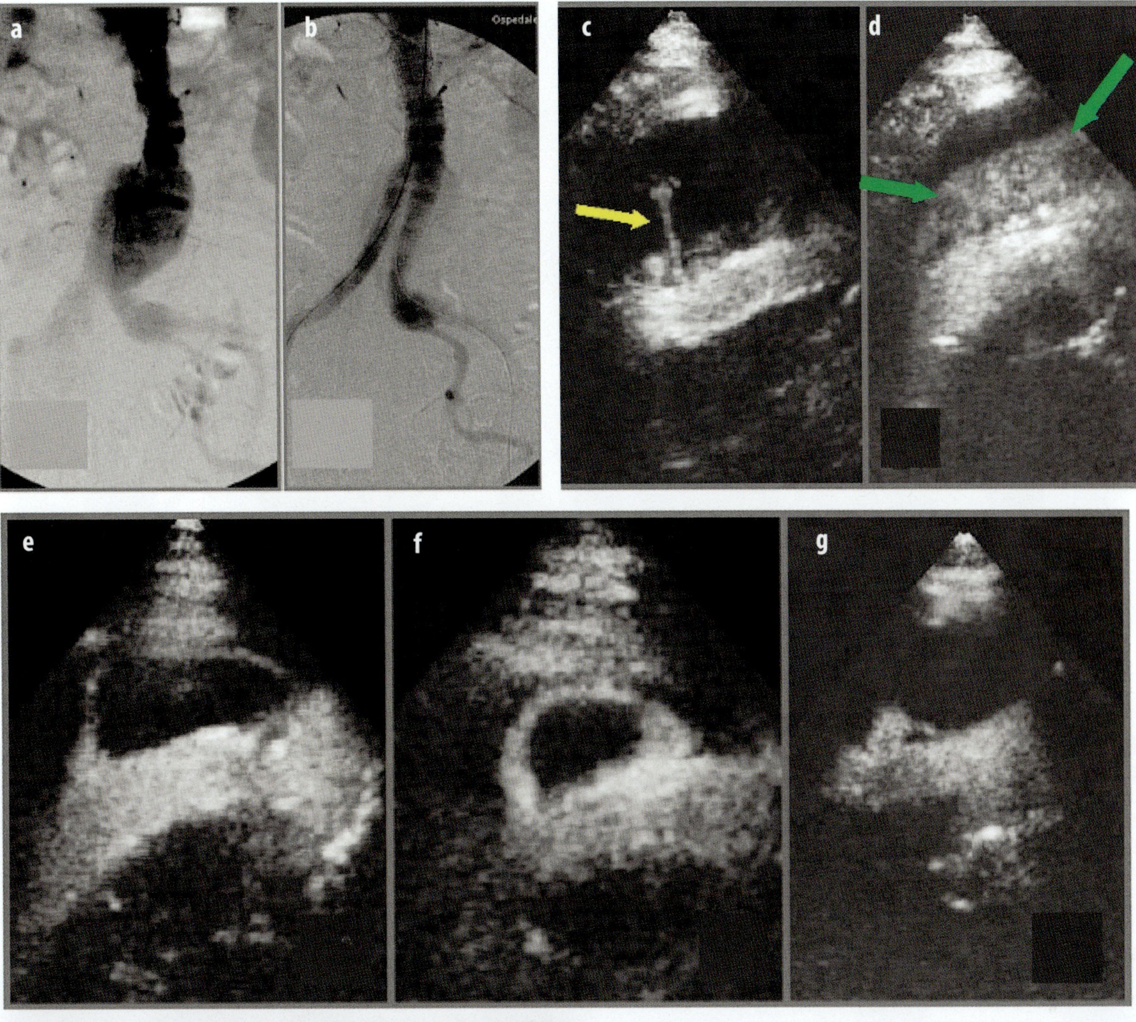

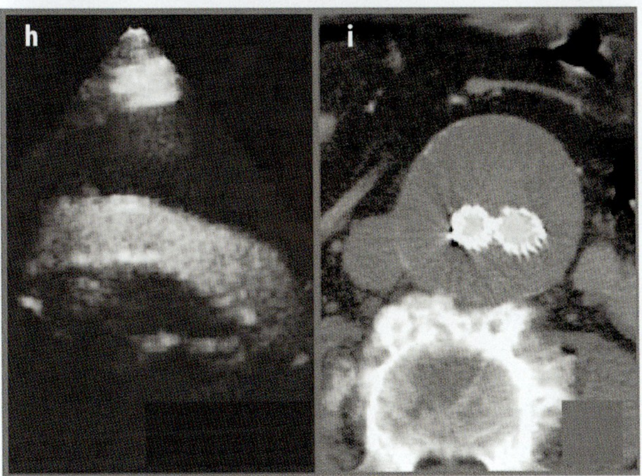

Fig. 14a-i. *Type IV Endoleak (due to abnormal porosity of the prosthesic wall).* **a, b** Digital subtraction angiography. In **a** a dilated aneurysm of the abdominal aorta and a slight dilation of the left common iliac artery are depicted. After endovascular repair (**b**) a minimal quantity of contrast agent is detectable inside the peri-prosthesic sac. **c-h** CEUS. In the first follow-up examination (first day after procedure) after contrast administration, in early phase, a normal canalisation of the prosthesis and multiple filtrations of contrast agent (*yellow arrow*) through the prosthesic wall are diagnosed (**c**); in late phase (**d**) the peri-prosthesic space is hyperechoic because of the contrast amount (*green arrows*). In the second day follow-up examination, there is a remarkable reduction of the endoleak phenomenon and only a small thin flow lumen is detectable in the residual aneurysmatic sac (**e, f**). In the fourth day follow-up examination (**g**), the aortic prosthesis is still patent and the endoleak is progressively less evident. In the sixth day follow-up examination no endoleak phenomena are detectable (**h**). **i** Angio-CT. Before discharge, the iliac branches are normally perfused; outside the graft, no contrast agent is detectable

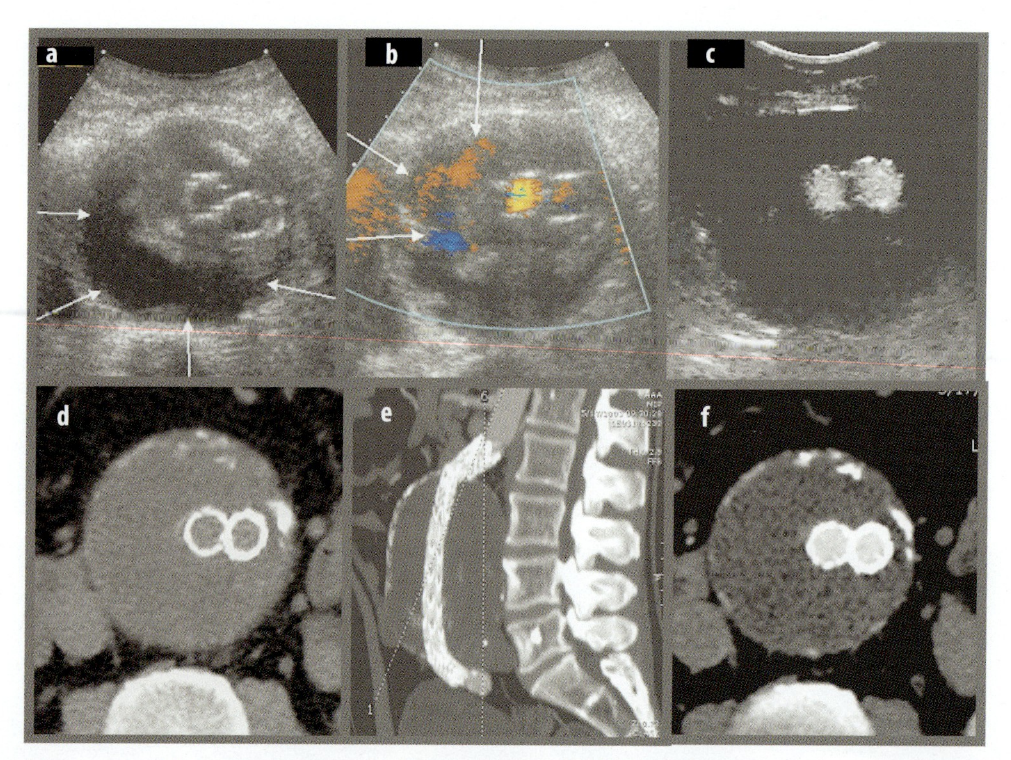

Fig. 15a-f. *Endotension.* **a** US baseline. Large sac with inhomogeneous and 'fluid' thrombus; strong hyperechoic structures correspond to endoprosthesic iliac branches. **b** Colour Doppler scan. Colour signals in iliac prosthesic branches; inside the residual thrombosed aneurysmatic sac, there is a chromatic signal (*white arrows*), not easily interpretable (possible flow or artefact?). **c** CEUS. The iliac branches enhance with contrast microbubbles; in the sac no hyperechoic sign due to contrast bubbles is detectable. **d-f** Spiral CT. Absence of contrast inside the aneurysmatic sac in early and late phase. No endoleak is evident

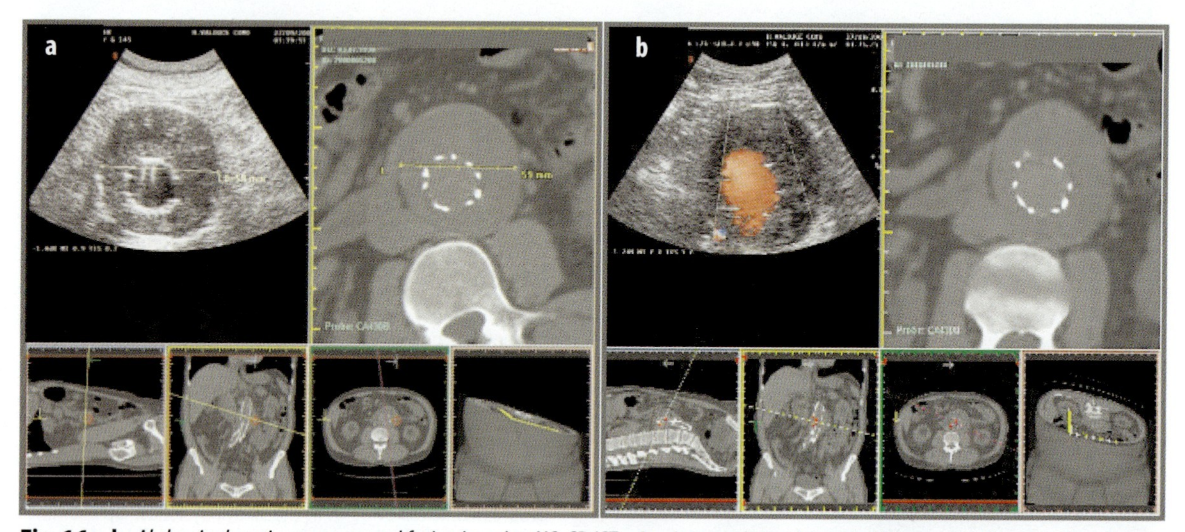

Fig. 16a, b. *Abdominal aortic aneurysm and fusion imaging US-CD/CT.* **a** Precise correlation between US transversal scan and analogous baseline CT transversal scan. **b** Correlation between CD transversal scan and analogous baseline CT transversal scan. The coupling system enables a comparison in the same screen in 'real-time' between US and/or CD images and corresponding CT scan

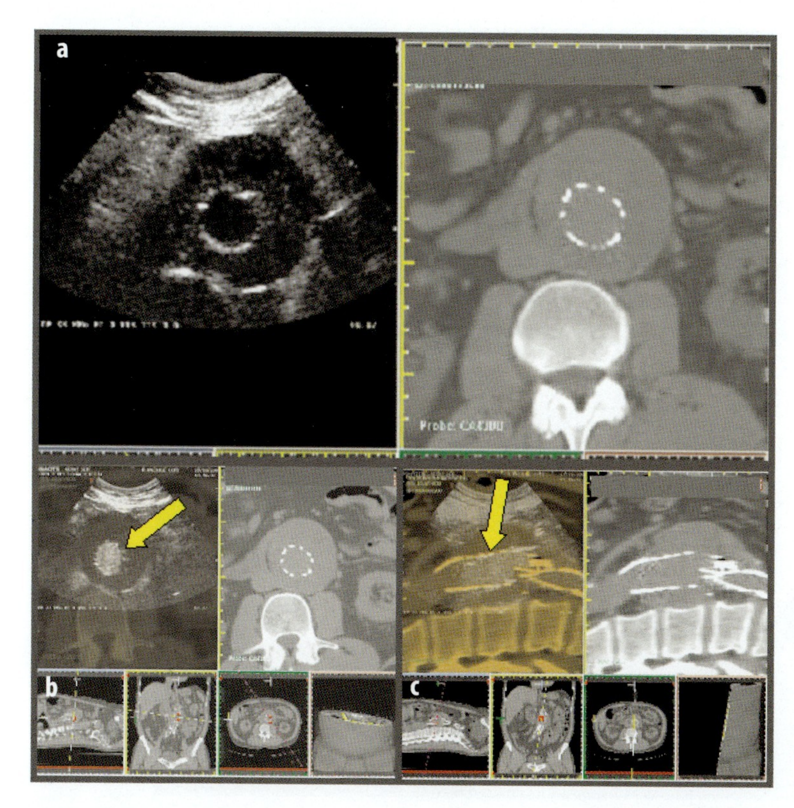

Fig. 17a-c. *Abdominal aortic aneurysm and Fusion Imaging CEUS/CT.* **a** CEUS transversal baseline scan and analogous transversal baseline CT. Transversal (**b**) and longitudinal (**c**) CEUS scan after contrast administration; prosthesis is normally patent (*yellow arrow*) without any signs of endoleak; in the left of the screen there are analogous transversal and longitudinal CT baseline scans

Follow-Up After Embolisation and Guidance for Percutaneous Intervention

Follow-up of percutaneous embolizing treatments of visceral aneurysms is a further interesting field of application for CEUS.

The presence of metallic intravascular coils gives rise to the onset of artefacts in CT and MR images, which may sometimes impair the diagnostic efficacy of these imaging tools. CEUS, on the contrary, is not limited by density artefacts, or by posterior acoustic shadowing artefacts (Fig. 18).

Any persisting flow signal inside the aneurysmatic chamber is detectable with CEUS both in precocious and in late follow-up examinations; the contrast and spatial resolution of the system is high enough to provide a significant diagnostic accurary (Fig. 19).

CEUS may also be used as a guidance tool for interventional procedures in real-time [19].

Once identified and characterised, the type II leakage can be excluded percutaneously through thrombin injection directly into the aneurysmatic sac using an anterior or posterior approach. CEUS permits the entire procedure to be guided in real-time.

In fact, CEUS enables the operator to identify the exact position of the leakage, monitoring of the percutaneous puncture and correct injection of thrombotic agent. Finally, the procedure outcomes are evaluated with CEUS, identifying the persistence of any residual endoleaks and the determination of the timing of subsequent treatments (Fig. 20).

Follow-up of endoleak percutaneous embolisation is facilitated by a fusion imaging system; CT, as a reference technique, demonstrates hyperdense material in place of the previous endoleak, showing the area of maximum interest where CEUS examination should be performed (Fig. 21).

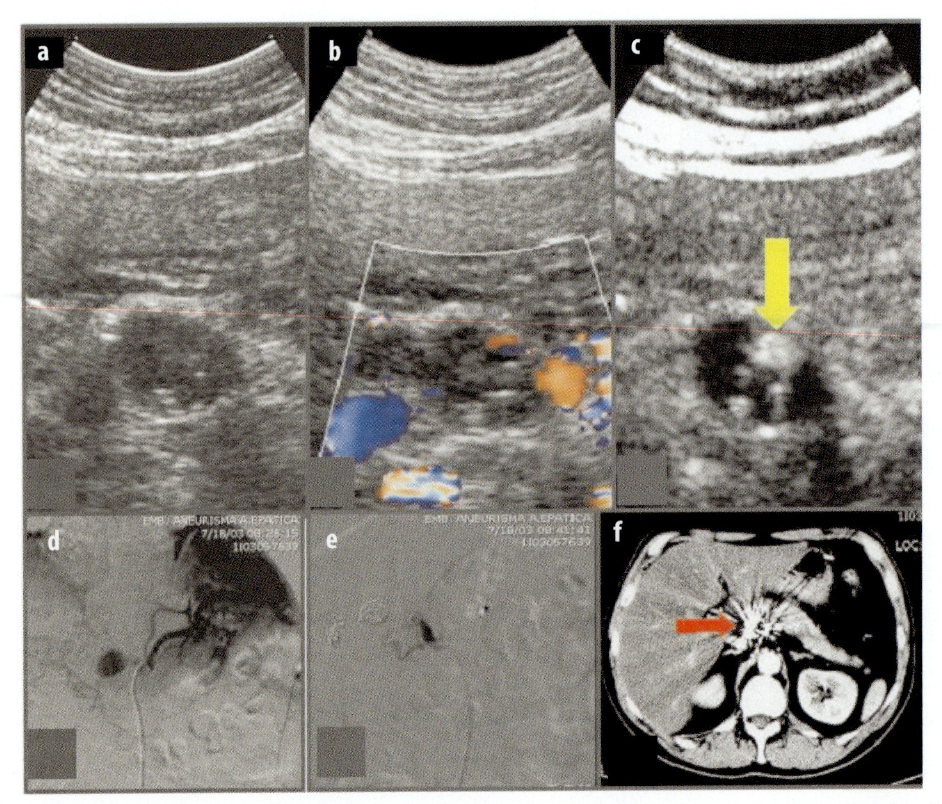

Fig. 18a-f. *Recanalisation of an hepatic artery aneurysm after metallic coil embolisation.* **a, b** Transversal US and CD scan. In B-mode an oval, 2 cm large image, inhomogeneous in echo-texture and with some internal small hyperechoic spots due to metallic coils, is detectable. The corresponding CD scan demonstrates some colour pixels inside the aneurysm (possibly due to artefacts or persisting flow?). **c** CEUS scan. After contrast administration, a small hyperechoic nidus (*yellow arrow*) is detectable inside the aneurysm corresponding to an area of revascularisation. **d-f** DSA and angio-CT. In F, coarse artefacts (*red arrow*) due to metallic coils prevent the correct evaluation of the aneurysm with this technique. DSA: diagnosis (**d**) and post-embolisation control (**e**)

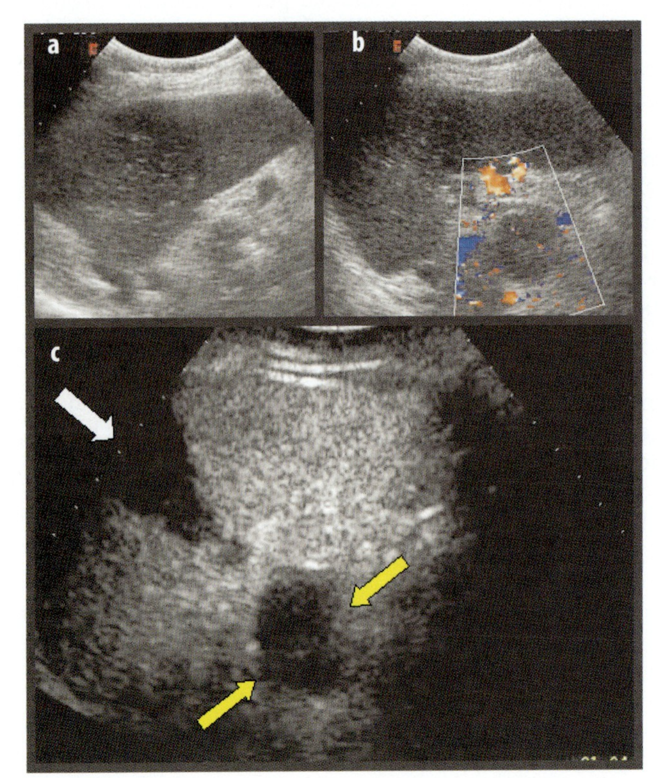

Fig. 19a-c. *Complete embolisation of a splenic artery aneurysm with partial ischemia in the middle third of the spleen.* **a, b** Transversal US and CD scan. In B-mode, an oval image 15 mm large, echo-structured and hypoechoic, is depicted medially to the splenic hilum. **c** CEUS scan. After contrast agent administration, the splenic aneurysm is completely unenhanced because of a complete exclusion (*yellow arrows*); the triangular mesosplenic hypoechoic area with apex directed towards the hilum corresponds to the ischemic lesion (*white arrow*). The remaining splenic parenchyma is homogeneously hyperechoic

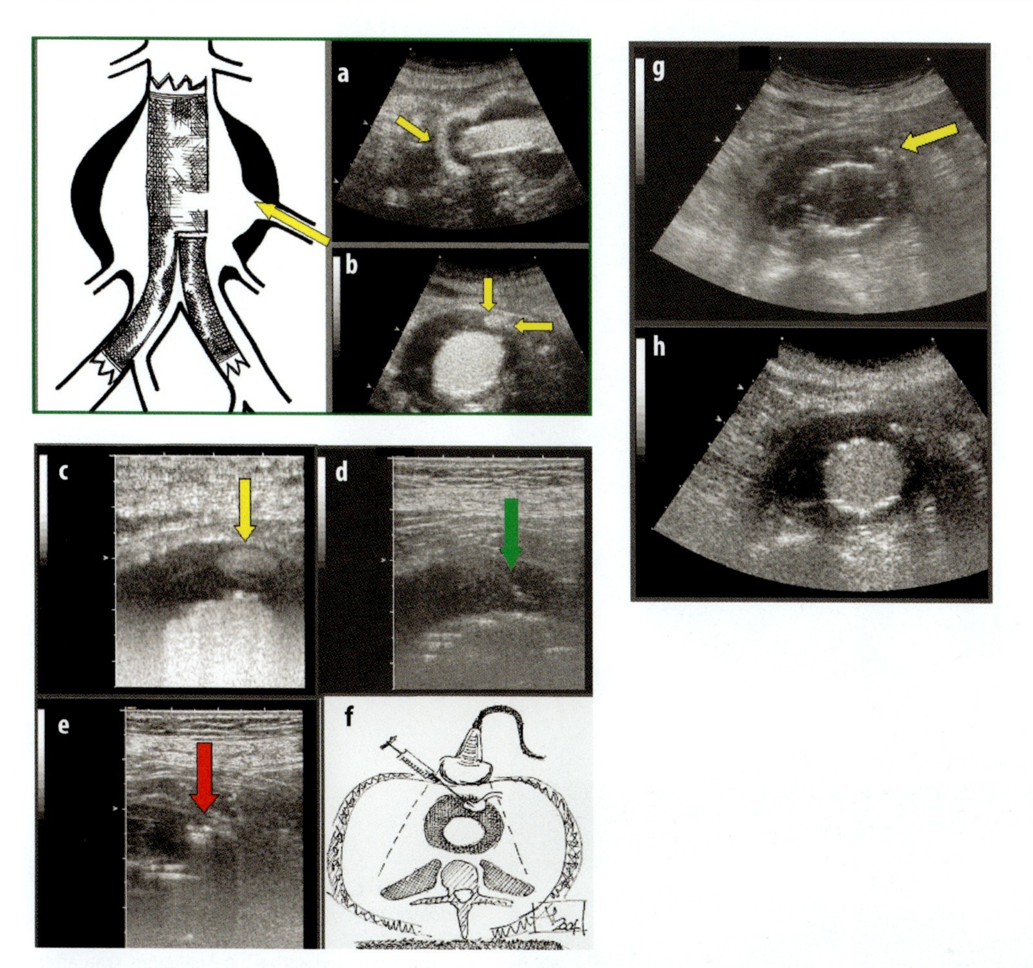

Fig. 20a-h. *CEUS-guided percutaneous exclusion through thrombin injection of a type II endoleak (due to recanalisation of inferior mesenteric artery).* **a, b** Longitudinal and transversal scan, CEUS. A thin flow lumen in the left antero-lateral portion of the thrombus is demonstrated (**a**); in B the site of inflow through the inferior mesenteric artery (*yellow arrows*) is diagnosed. In both scans, the endoprosthesis is normally perfused. **c-f** CEUS combined to B-mode scan (at low MI). In **c**, CEUS shows the precise site of revascularisation characterised by a small hyperechoic area (*yellow arrow*) located in the anterior part of the peripheral thrombus: targeting phase. The prosthesis is normally perfused. Low MI B-mode evaluation (**d**) permits visualisation of the tip of the needle (*green arrow*): puncture phase. Low MI B-mode (**e**) detects multiple hyperechoic spots in the thrombus corresponding to the thrombosing agent selectively injected in the leak (*red arrow*): injection phase. In **f**, the scheme of the procedure performed via an anterior percutaneous approach is depicted. **g, h** Post-procedure B-mode and CEUS examination. B-mode shows some hyperechoic spots (*yellow arrow*) in the left anterior region of the thrombus corresponding to injected thrombin. CEUS (**h**) demonstrates the normal patency of the prosthesis and the absence of contrast agent inside the thrombus, even in the position of the previous endoleak

Particular Situations: Diagnosis of 'Slow' Extraluminal Flows

A particular field of interest is the evaluation of extravascular slow flows in active bleeding [20, 21].

CEUS is less panoramic in comparison to other imaging techniques such as CT, caused by the physical obstacles of air and bone structures; on the other hand, its high spatial and contrast resolution for the representation of contrast agent justifies the important role of the technique in post-traumatic and spontaneous retroperitoneal bleeding, and is thus very frequent nowadays in clinical practice, secondary to antiplatelet and anticoagulant agents (Fig. 22).

In these situations, even at the patient's bedside, CEUS is able to identify any active bleeding and to follow the evolution spontaneously or after embolisation of the collection.

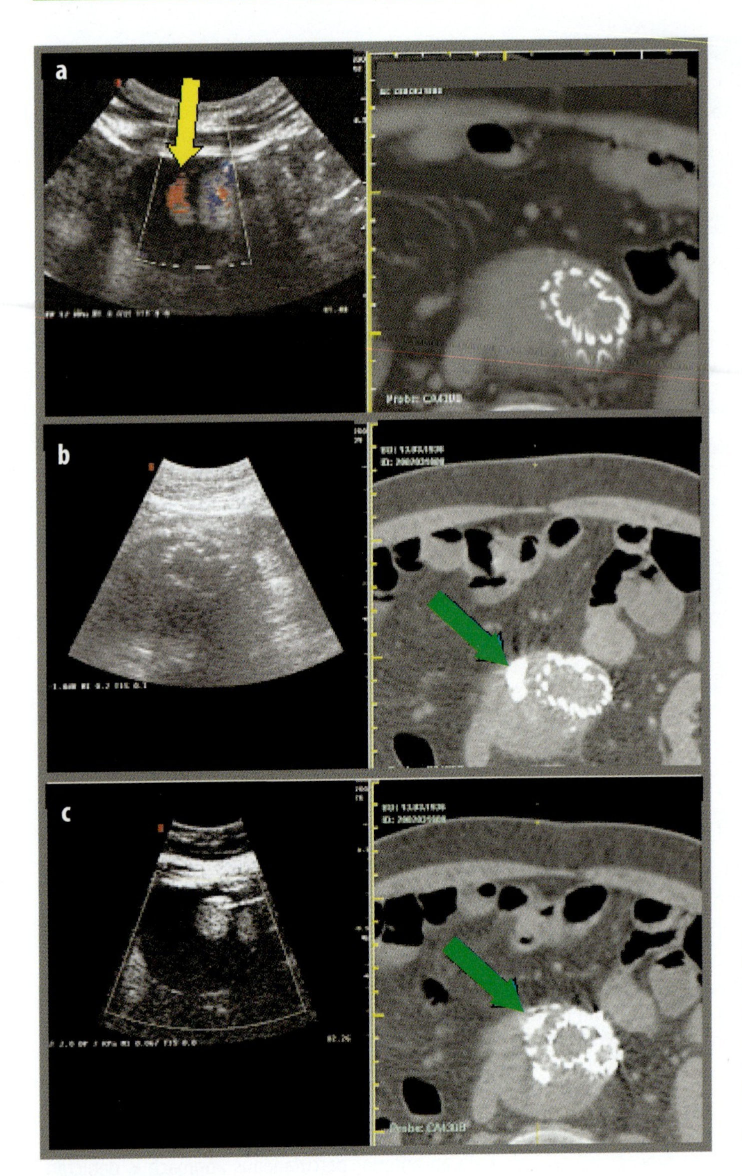

Fig. 21a-c. *Follow-up evaluation after type II endoleak embolisation through CEUS-Low MI CD/CT fusion imaging.* **a** Transversal Fusion CEUS/low MI CD scan combined with CT. **b** Analogous scan after embolisation. CT detects a hyperechoic material corresponding to embolisation materials in the leakage position (*green arrow*); the position corresponds to **a**. **c** Analogous follow-up scan. With CEUS, no sign of leak is detectable; prosthesis is regularly patent. The precision of the follow-up evaluation is guaranteed by the corresponding CT image

Conclusions

The recent introduction of B-mode contrast-specific low MI algorithms (CEUS) has provided a quality of vascular US imaging similar to other imaging techniques such as angio-CT, angio-MR and digital angiography (DSA).

CEUS enables a morphological demonstration of blood flow to be easily obtained, even when the speed of the flow is so reduced as to be undetectable on CD or when movements of anatomical structures around vessels produce colour artefacts.

CEUS is not nephrotoxic or invasive and so it can be performed even at short intervals, in order to help determine the patient's appropriate therapeutic regime.

Patients can be submitted to CEUS not only in a Radiology Department, but anywhere in the hospital (the bedside, Emergency Room, Intensive Care Unit, Surgery).

The diagnostic role of CEUS in vascular studies is limited to a 'segmental' and focused analysis of a specific vascular district, primarily percutaneous aortic prostheses evaluation, because it is burdened with the same limits as US, i.e., a limited panorama.

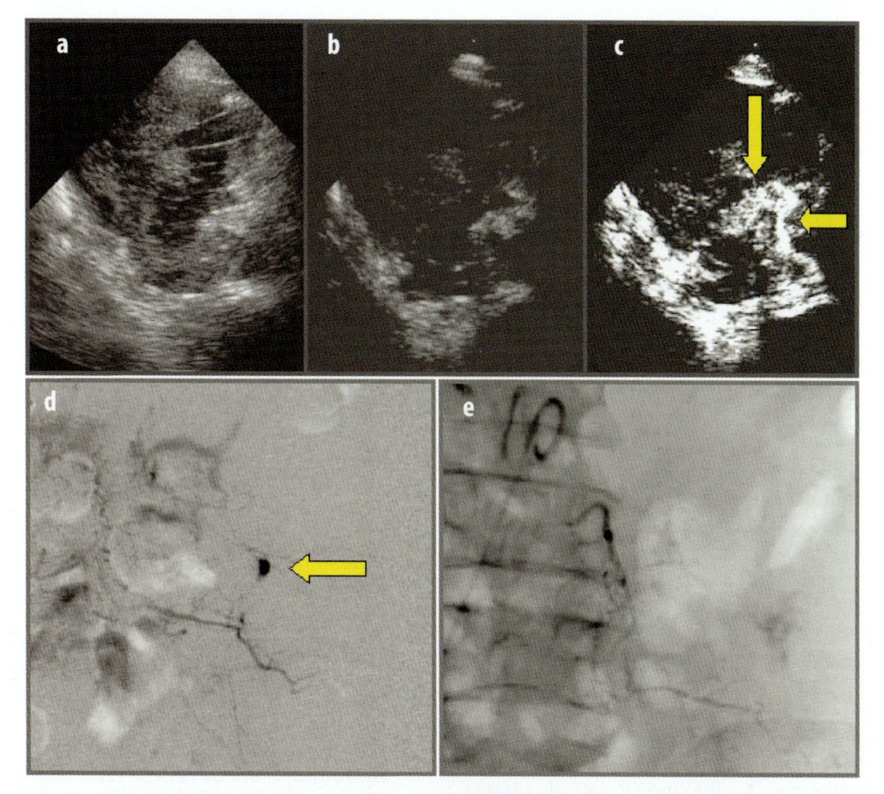

Fig. 22a-e. *Retroperitoneal perfused haematoma.* **a** Left hip transversal scan, B-mode. Expansive inhomogeneous echo-textured lesion with small anechoic internal areas: probable haematoma. **b, c** Left hip transversal scan, CEUS. Comparing to baseline CEUS scan (**b**), in which a complete cancellation of signal coming from steady tissue is obtained, 60 seconds after contrast administration (**c**) inside the haematoma an irregular and hyperechoic image (*yellow arrows*) becomes evident, corresponding to active bleeding. **d, e** DSA. The diagnostic angiography (**d**) shows a small nidus on contrast agent corresponding to active bleeding (*yellow arrow*). After embolisation (**e**), a vascular exclusion of the arterial branch afferent to the active bleeding area is demonstrated

Key Points

- Endoleak is defined as the presence of flow inside the residual peri-prosthesic aneurismatic sac.
- Contrast-enhanced ultrasound (CEUS) enables the demonstration of vascular prosthesis patency.
- The identification of ultrasound contrast agent is not dependent on blood flow velocity; even very slow flows are therefore depicted with CEUS.
- Ultrasound contrast agents are a useful tool for intraprocedural guidance for embolization of visceral aneurysms.

References

1. Taylor KJ, Holland S (1990) Doppler US. Part 1. Basic principles, instrumentation and pitfalls. Radiology 174:297-307
2. Winkler P, Hemke K, Mahl M (1990) Major pitfalls in Doppler investigations. Part II. Low flow velocities and colour Doppler applications. Pediatr Radiol 20:304-310
3. Wachsberg RH (2003) B-flow, a non Doppler technology for flow mapping: early experience in the abdomen. Ultrasound Q 19:114-122
4. Mattrey RF, Pelura TJ (1997) Perfluoro-carbon based ultrasound contrast agents. In: Goldeberg BB (ed) Ultrasound contrast agents. Martin Dunits, London, pp 83-87
5. Morel DR, Schwieger I, Hohn L et al (2000) Human pharmacokinetics and safety evaluation of Sono Vue, a new contrast agent for ultrasound imaging. Invest Radiol 35:80-85
6. Parent FN, Meier GH, Godziachvili V et al (2002) The incidence of type I and II endoleak: a 5-year follow-up assessment with color-duplex ultrasound scan . J Vasc Surg 35:474-481
7. Parodi JC, Palmaz JC, Barone HD (1991) Transfemoral intraluminal graft implantation for abdominal aortic aneurysms. Ann Vasc Surg 5:491-496
8. Parodi JC, Barone A, Piraino R et al (1997) Endovascular treatment of abdominal aortic aneurysms : lessons learned. J Endovasc Surg 4:102-110
9. White GU, Yu W, May J et al (1997) Endoleak as a complication of endoluminal grafting of abdominal aortic aneurysms. J Endovasc Surg 4:152-155
10. Thompson M, Boyle GR, Hartshorn T et al (1998) Comparison of computed thomography and duplex imaging in assessing aortic morphology following endovascular aneurysm repair. Br J Surg 85:340-350
11. Zannetti S, De Rango P, Parente B et al (2000) Role of duplex scan in endoleak detection after endoluminal abdominal aortic aneurysm repair. Eur J Vasc Endovasc Surg 19:531-535
12. Raman KG, Missig-Carroll N, Richardson T et al (2003) Color-flow duplex ultrasound scan versus computed tomographic scan in the surveillance on endovascular anerysm repair. J Vasc Surg 38:645-651
13. Lookstein RA, Goldman J, Pukin L et al (2004) Time-resolved magnetic resonance angiography as a noninvasive method to characterize endoleaks: initial results compared with conventional angiography. J Vasc Surg 39:27-33
14. McWilliams RG, Martin J, White D et al (1999) Use of contrast-enhanced ultrasound in follow up after endovascular aortic aneurysm repair. J Vasc Interv Radiol 10:1107-1114
15. Giannoni MF, Palombo G, Sbarigia E et al (2003) Contrast-enhanced ultrasound imaging for aortic stent-graft surveillance. J Endovasc Ther 10:208-217
16. Bendick PJ, Bove PG, Long GW (2003) Efficacy of ultrasound contrast agents in the non-invasive follow up of aortic stent grafts. J Vasc Surg 37:381-385
17. Golzarian J, Murgo S, Dussaussois L et al (2002) Evaluation of abdominal aortic aneurysm after endoluminal treatment: comparison of color-Doppler sonography with biphasic helical CT. AJR Am J Roentgenol 178:623-628
18. Napoli V, Bargellini I, Sardella SG et al (2004) Abdominal aortic aneurysm: contrast-enhanced US for missed endoleak after endoluminal repair. Radiology 233:217-225
19. Paulson EK, Kliewer MA, Hertzberg BS et al (1995) Color Doppler sonography of groin complications following femoral artery catheterization. AJR Am J Roentgenol 165:439-444
20. Liu JB, Merton DA, Goldberg BB et al (2002) Contrast-enhanced two and three-dimensional sonography for evaluation of intra-abdominal hemorrage. J Ultrasound Med 21:161-169
21. Goldberg BB, Merton DA, Liu JB et al (1998) Evaluation of bleeding site with a tissue-specific sonographic contrast agent: preliminary experiences in an animal model. J Ultrasound Med 17:609-616

Section IV

New Prospects in Clinical Application of Contrast Ultrasound

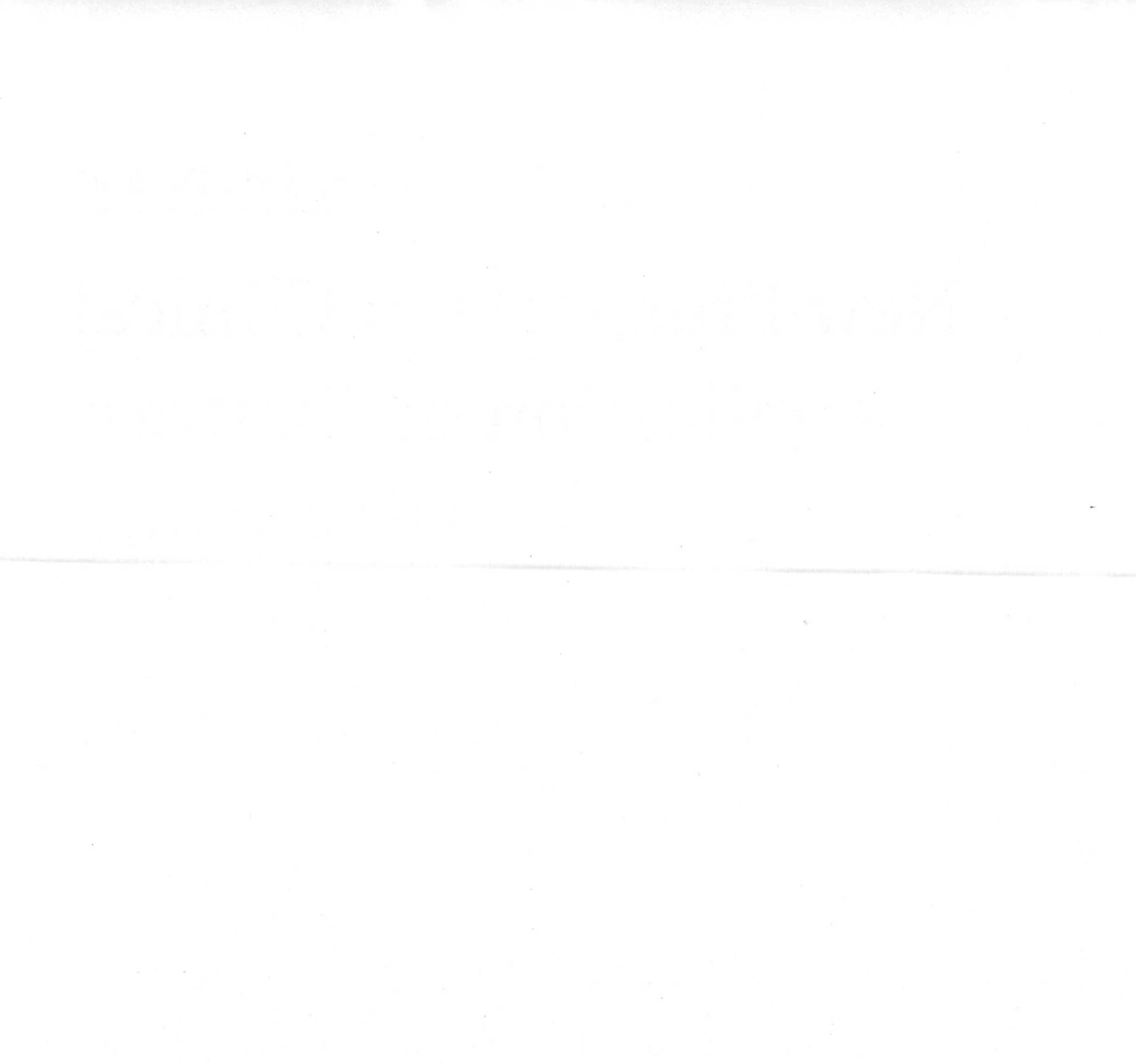

IV.1

Contrast-Enhanced Ultrasound of Focal Renal Lesions

Anders Nilsson

Introduction

Many small things have contributed to advances in diagnostic ultrasound brought about by contrast-enhanced ultrasound (CEUS). Among the most important are the development of contrast microbubbles that are stable enough for continuous scanning, at least at low mechanical index, and ultrasound machine software that enables us to produce images based on microbubble concentration rather than tissue echogenicity. This enables us to add a vast improvement in contrast resolution to the already excellent spatial and temporal resolution of ultrasound images. The image resolution of ultrasound can then be used to its full advantage also in patients where other modalities may not be possible, such as in impaired renal function or possible allergic reactions. Thus, techniques have been developed mainly for detection and characterisation of focal liver lesions [1-3]. As has been pointed out in previous chapters, the liver is particularly suited to CEUS, as the microbubbles get trapped and remain in the sinusoids but are washed out from tumour tissue.

However, applications are emerging for other tissues and organs as well. In the kidney, images based on contrast concentration can improve the detection of non-perfused focal lesions like cysts, abscesses, infarctions and post-radio-frequency ablation necroses. Normal renal parenchyma does not, of course, contain sinusoids, but preliminary work suggests that the perfusion differences between tissues with a normal capillary bed and the neovascularisation of tumours can be detected if the pattern of contrast-enhancement is followed over time, subjectively or with the aid of analysis programs, preferably built into the ultrasound machine itself [4].

Normal Kidney

The established phases of contrast-enhancement after a bolus injection that are seen in the liver are not seen in the kidneys due to differences in blood supply and vasculature. Similarly, however, different stages of renal enhancement exist and must be understood in order to avoid misdiagnosis. First the arteries enhance followed closely by a complete fill-in of the cortex. The pyramids then gradually enhance over the next 30-40 seconds to become isoechoic or almost isoechoic with the cortex. As there is no accumulation of contrast in the kidneys (as in the sinusoids of the liver), the enhancement decreases with the microbubble concentration in the general circulation. When this happens there may again appear a difference between the cortex and the pyramids, the latter becoming once more hypoechoic (Fig. 1).

Cysts

Ultrasound contrast agents are so-called blood pool agents, i.e., they do not, contrary to X-ray contrast media, leave the blood vessels. With the availability of ultrasound machine software that can detect the differences between an echo emanating from tissue and the signal sent out by a resonating contrast bubble, images can be formed based virtually only on the presence of microbubbles. As structures without perfusion will have no contrast uptake, they will have no brightness in the image, whether they are in the liver or elsewhere in the body, thus remaining dark with an excellent delineation against normal surrounding tissue. Simple cysts will then be dark even during the peak of a contrast bolus even if they contain

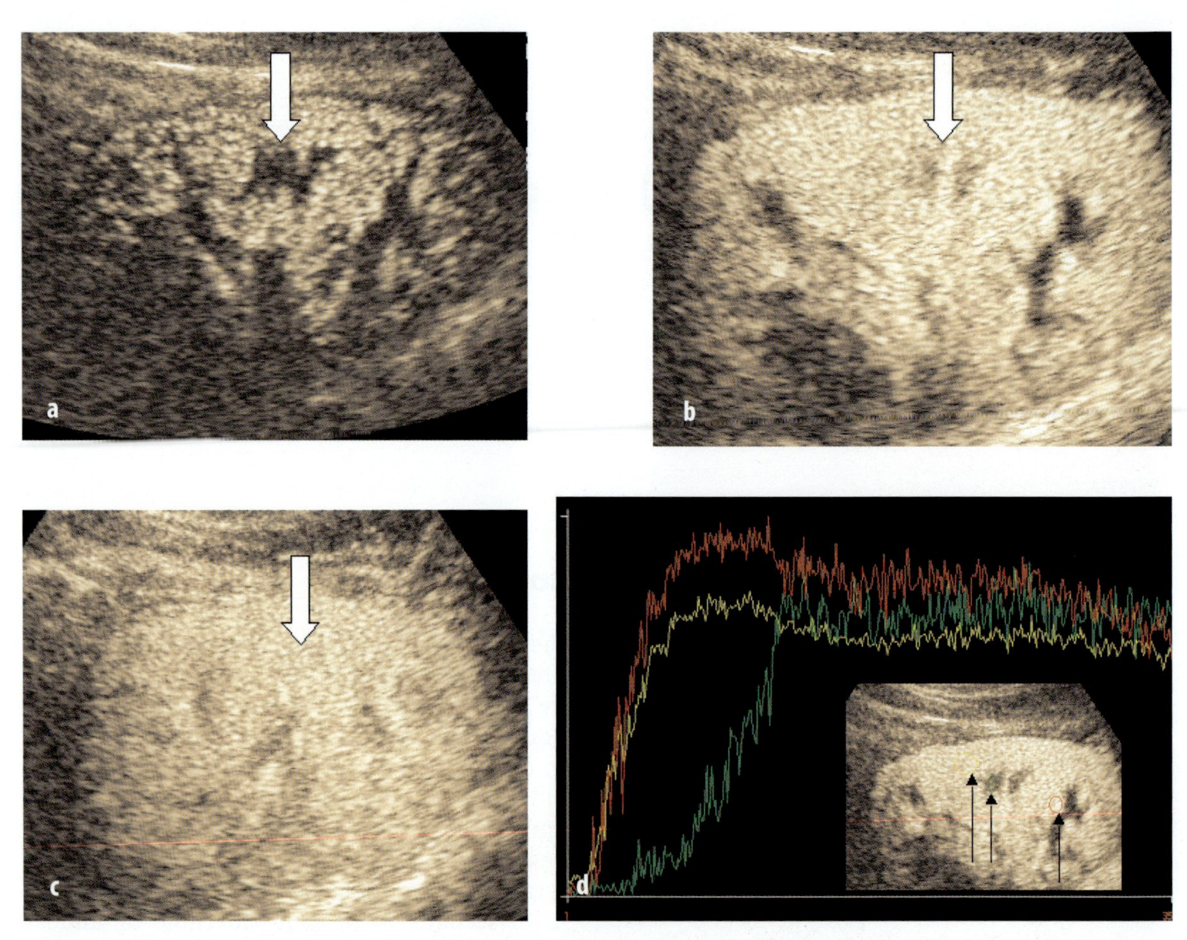

Fig. 1a-d. Normal renal enhancement after an iv bolus. Note the slower fill-in of the pyramids (*arrows*), also shown by the quantification graph, where a ROI has been placed in a segmental artery (*red*), cortex (*yellow*) and a pyramid (*green*)

echoes on native ultrasound. Thus smaller cysts can be detected. This may possibly be important in the early detection of conditions like polycystic kidney disease, but the main advantage is that the spatial resolution of ultrasound can be used for characterisation of indeterminate focal lesions detected on, for example, computed tomography (Fig. 2) [5]. As the sensitivity for detection of small amounts of contrast agent is improved in the newer software programs, possibilities open up also for detecting thin but perfused septae in the cysts, possibly indicative of malignancy rather than simple cysts.

Abscesses, Infarctions and Ruptures

It is important to remember that CEUS is an integral part of a complete ultrasound examination, not a separate entity. Whereas all things without contrast uptake will have the same brightness on CEUS, their appearance on native ultrasound will, of course, vary. Abscesses, especially when small, may derange normal renal anatomy but will otherwise contain an echogenicity that could make them difficult to detect. On CEUS they will, like cysts, remain dark. The sharp delineation against normal tissue will enable a detailed assessment of the lesions shape that may give clues to its nature; abscesses (like cysts) are often round. Infarctions and post-traumatic ruptures will, in the same fashion, appear dark, the spatial resolution of ultrasound helping in detecting even small lesions where a fissure can be seen as a narrow line and infarctions wedge-shaped near the kidney surface [6]. The case history will, of course, give more information and it could be said that the most important roles of CEUS are to detect the lesion and to ascertain that it is indeed non-enhancing (Figs. 3, 4).

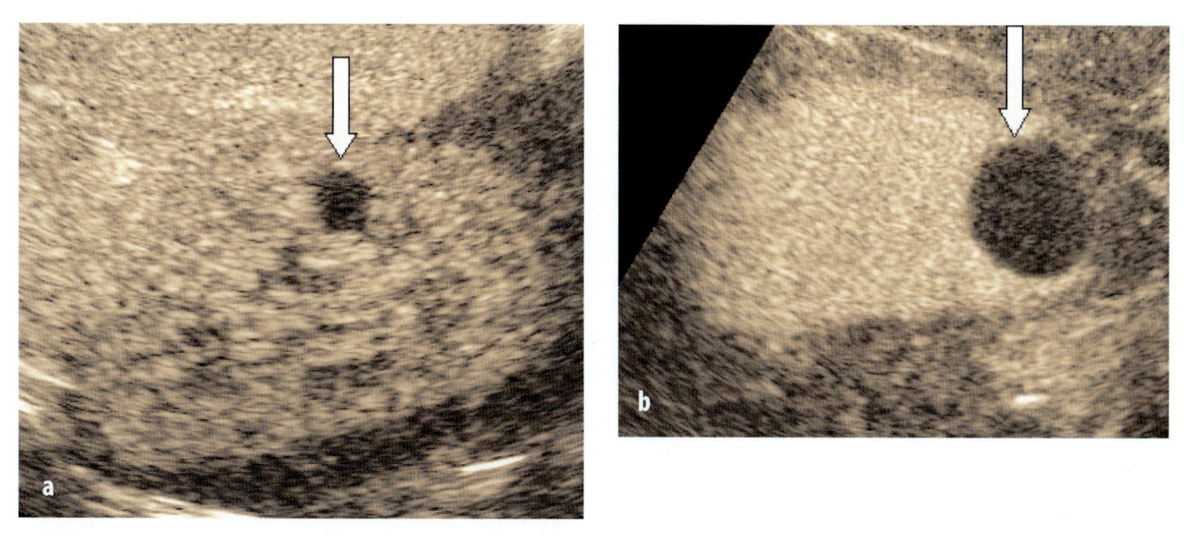

Fig. 2a, b. Cysts (*arrows*) show a clear demarcation and no contrast uptake, regardless of size

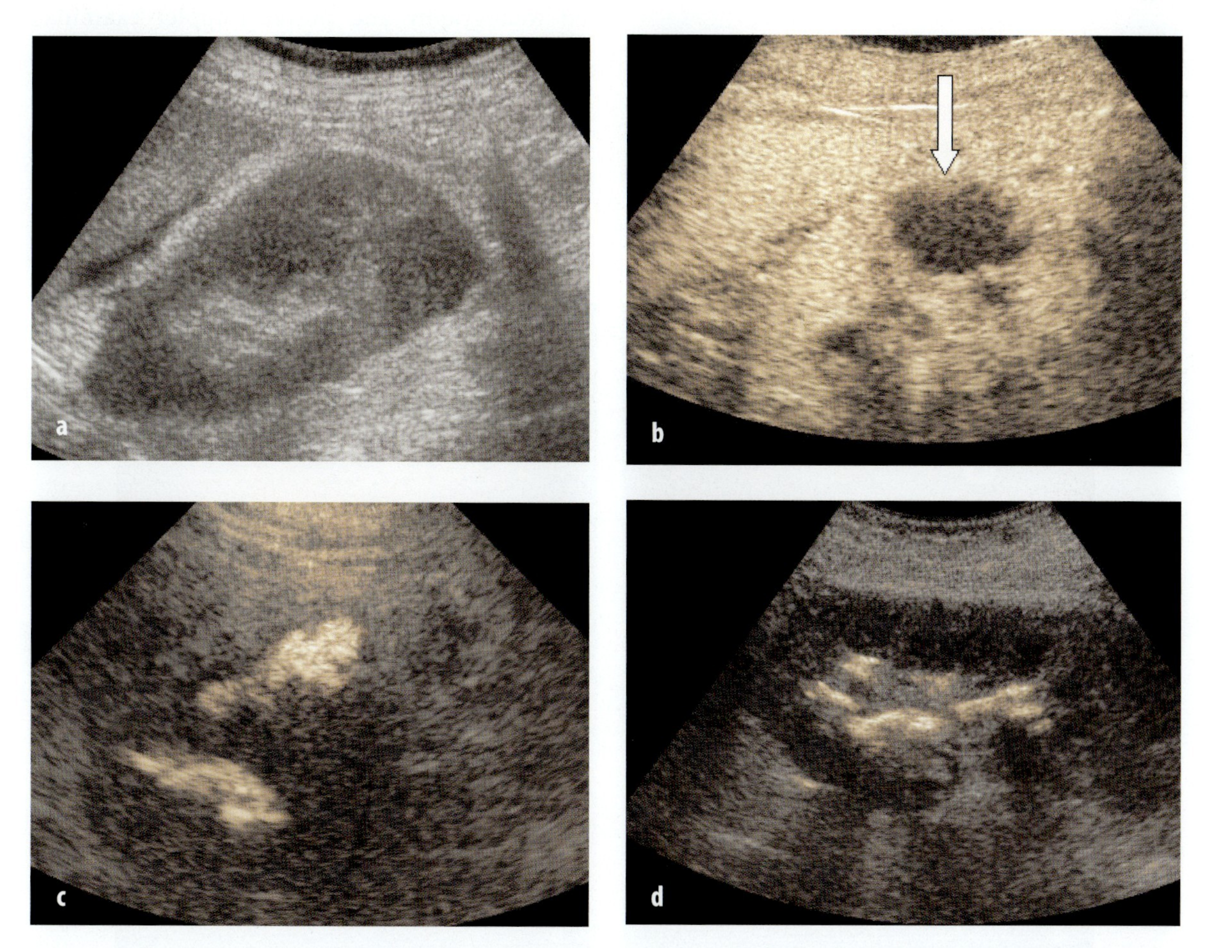

Fig. 3a-d. Renal abscess with minimal findings on B-mode, but with a clearly demarcated non-enhancing area on CEUS (*arrow*). After a CEUS-guided catheter drainage of the abscess, contrast has been injected through the catheter, delineating the abscess, but also showing the collecting system that fills up with contrast

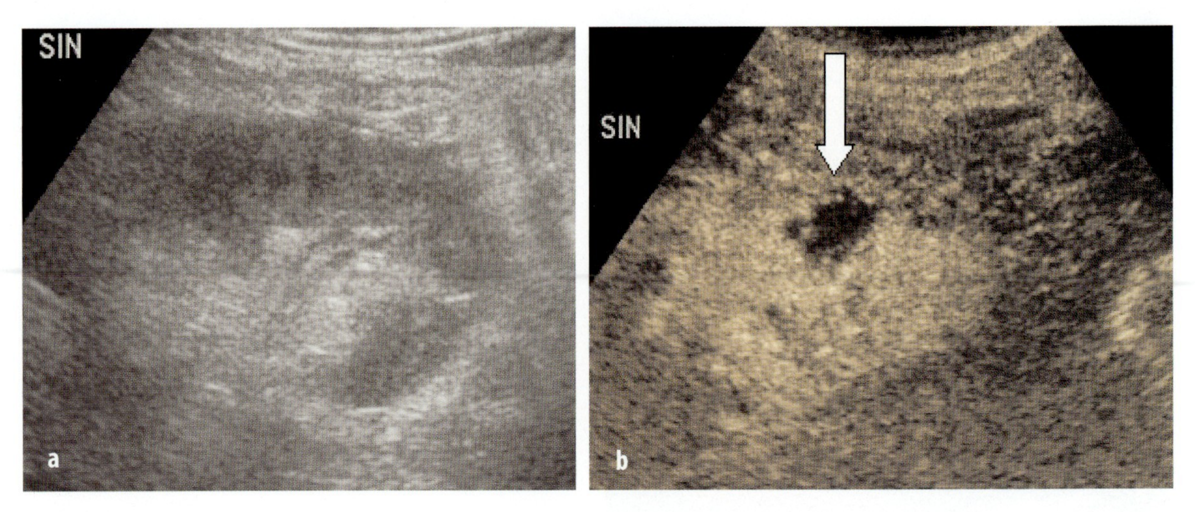

Fig. 4a, b. B-mode scan of a patient presenting with sudden severe left flank pain shows nothing, but CEUS depicts a non-enhancing, wedge-shaped area near the surface of the kidney, consistent with a small renal infarction

Infections

If the case history suggests a renal infection, it is important to be able to differentiate between an already formed abscess and a pyelonephritis. As described above, an abscess on CEUS will be dark, but early experiences indicate that the difference in perfusion caused by the parenchymal oedema around a pyelonephritis can also be detected, similar to contrast-enhanced computed tomography and power Doppler examinations [7, 8], appearing as an area with decreased brightness (Fig. 5). As this decrease is based on perfusion variations in tissues with the same blood vessel architecture otherwise, the differences are seen during all the phases of a CEUS examination, contrary to the differences seen with tumour vascularisation (see below).

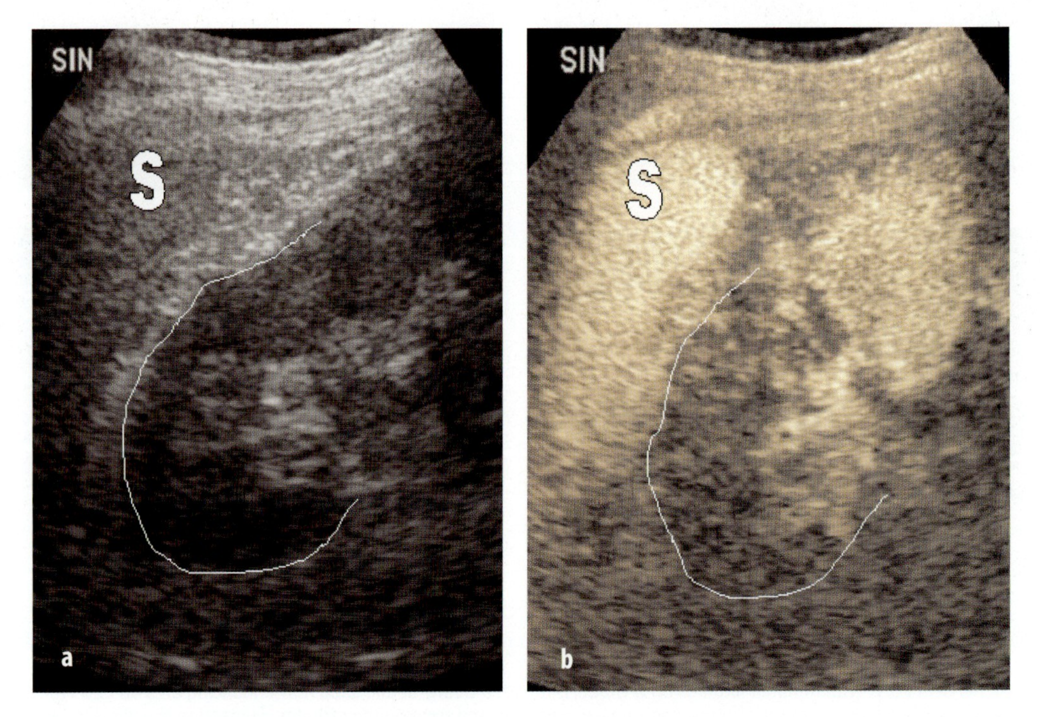

Fig. 5a, b. Scans through the left flank of a patient with flank pain and high fever. The kidney just caudal to the spleen (*S*) shows a normally enhancing lower pole but, by comparison, very sparse contrast uptake in the upper pole (*contour marked*)

Tumours

Many hypovascular tumours have very little enhancement on CT, not enough to make a confident diagnosis of a renal cell carcinoma. It is of value to be able to make this distinction rather than having to choose between additional, costly tests, a long follow-up or a mere assumption of a malignancy. CEUS, when performed with contrast-specific software, is very sensitive to microbubble presence, even in small quantities. Thus, intratumoural vasculature can be detected, possibly with the aid of quantification software that can detect an increase in image brightness even when a subjective assessment may leave doubts. In addition, small vessels may be depicted in mural nodules, septae or thickened cyst walls whereas the detection of such small vessels is difficult with Doppler (Fig. 6). Thus, CEUS may be used for the evaluation of CT/MR findings, atypical cysts or cyst-like lesions with echogenic contents, the existence of contrast within the suspected areas being equivalent to the existence of vessels, i.e. perfused viable tissue.

In the same manner, biopsies can be guided to non-necrotic areas of a suspected lesion, improving the diagnostic yield of the puncture [9].

Renal tumours seem to have a contrast pattern similar to the normal renal parenchyma, at least in the early stages of enhancement. There may be a rim enhancement in a pseudo-capsule [11] but, as there is no real accumulation of contrast in the kidneys, the detection rate of small tumours is unlikely to be as much improved by CEUS as is seen with focal liver lesions. However, malignant tumours do not have a proper capillary bed and early experiences indicate that contrast will remain in the capillaries even as it is

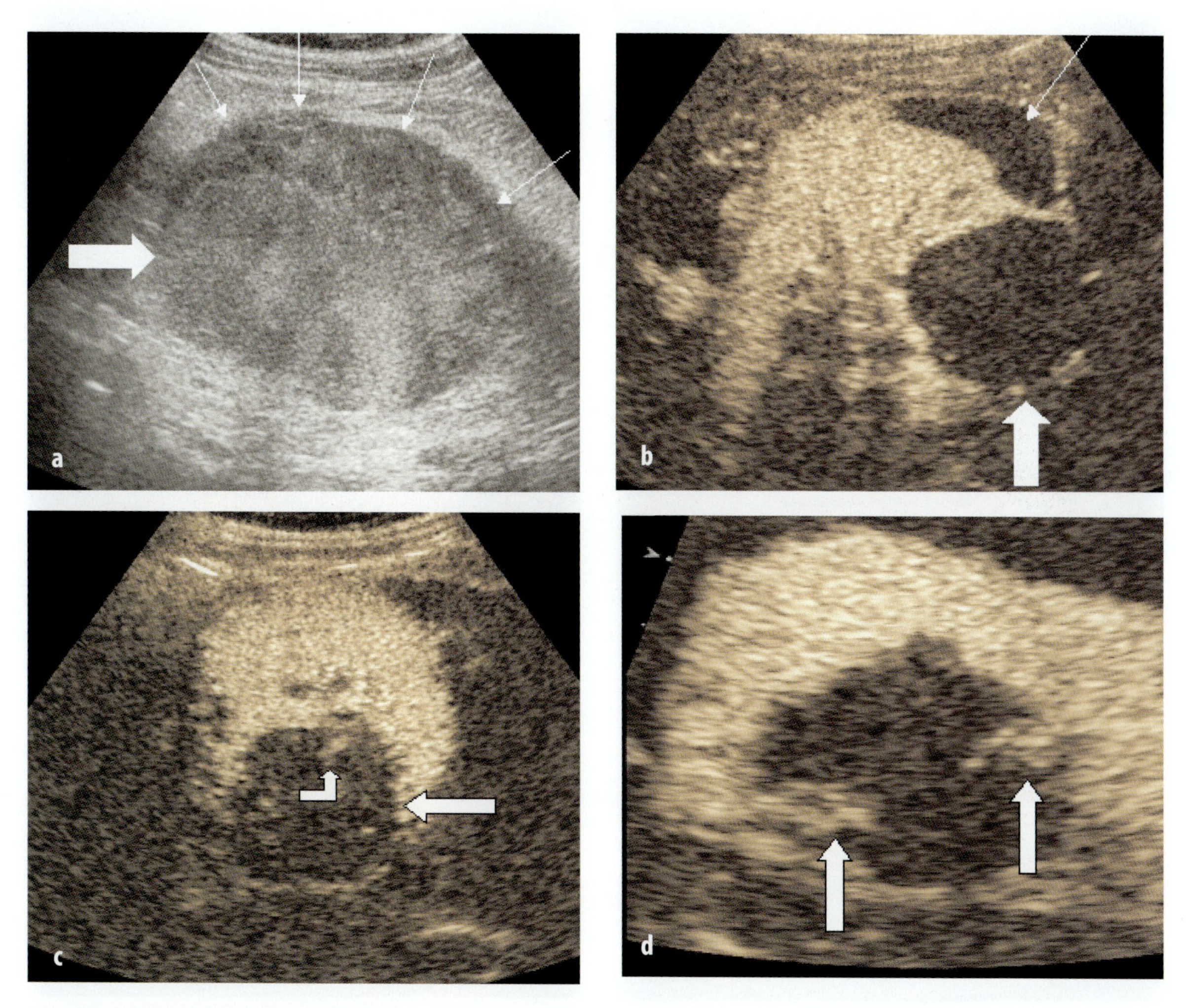

Fig. 6a-d. Patient with sudden flank pain. B-mode ultrasound shows the kidney (*fat arrow*) surrounded by a hematoma (**a**). On CEUS the hematoma is delineated (*thin arrow*) and a cyst is seen, possibly hemorrhagic, as it did not show up on B-mode (**b**). However, a careful CEUS scan also shows tiny perfused nodules within the cyst. A cystic renal cell carcinoma, probably the cause of the bleeding, was later removed (**c, d**)

washed out of the tumour neovasculature, creating a similar but weaker equivalent to the situation in the liver, possibly helping characterisation, if not detection [10]. Thus, malignant tumours tend to be slightly hypoechoic compared to normal parenchyma in the later phases. This could be helpful in evaluating normal variants, e.g., a prominent column of Bertin, and their differentiation from focal lesions suspected on basic ultrasound, especially under suboptimal imaging conditions. The area to be studied must then be followed to the later stages of the contrast-enhancement, at least for 1 minute. In most instances, a clear difference can be detected by analysis software at that stage and seen subjectively shortly thereafter, if not before (Figs. 7-9). A necrotic area in the tumour will, of course, remain dark, but as tumours with central necrosis tend to be large and thus easily detected and characterised on native ultrasound, this is likely to be of limited importance, except as guidance for biopsies.

There are, as yet, no scientific data proving an ability to help in the differentiation between benign and malignant focal lesions, but with improved knowledge of contrast-enhancement patterns this may only be a matter of time. Benign lesions like angiomyolipomas have been shown to enhance less than renal cell carcinomas in the arterial phase [12] and tend to retain the contrast better than a malignant tumour in the later phases, presumably due to vessel anatomy. However, knowledge about how a small, highly differentiated tumour would behave is limited, and the differentiation of benign from malignant in the individual patient remains difficult.

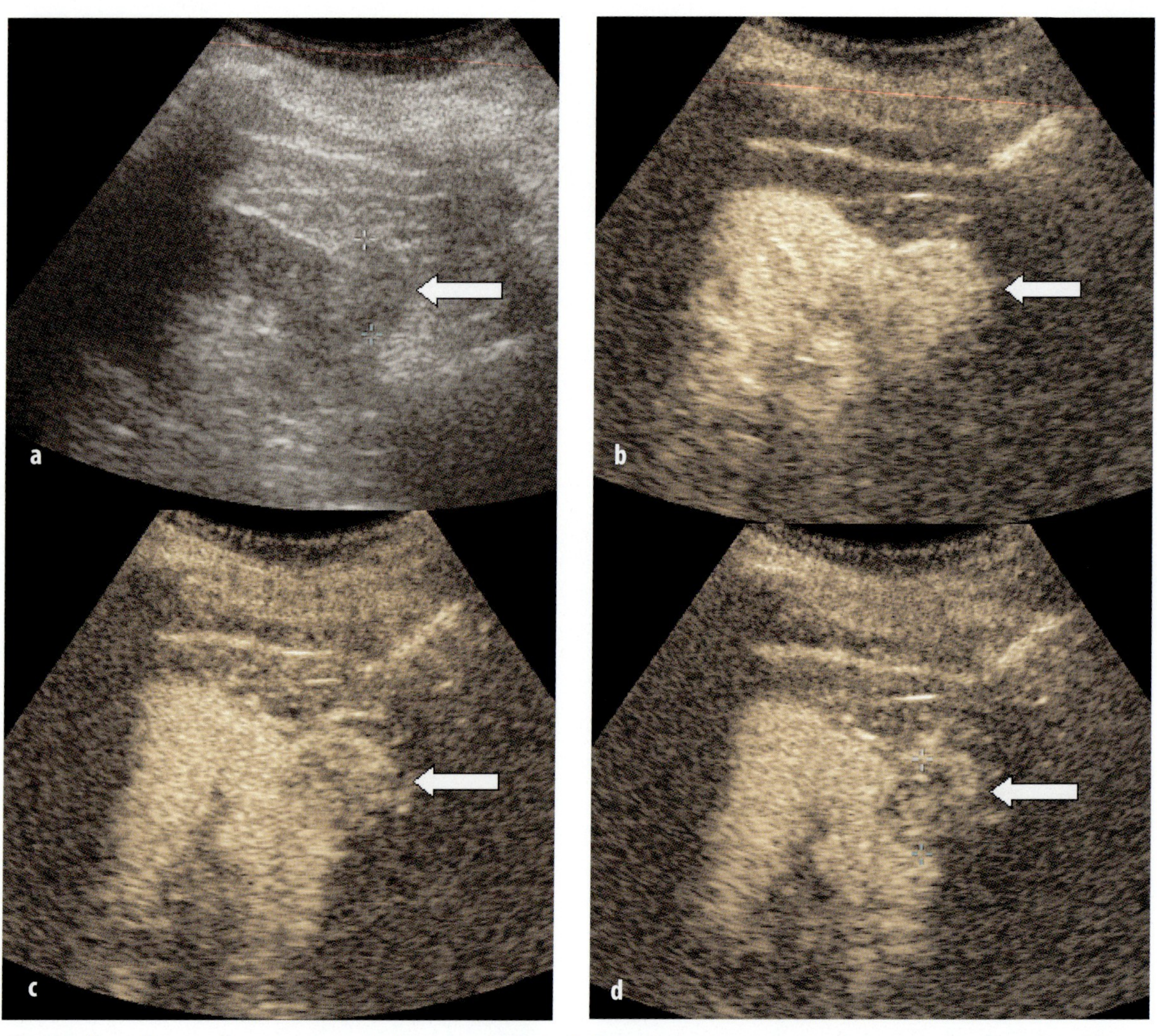

Fig. 7a-d. Small renal cell carcinoma seen both on B-mode (**a**) and CEUS with a typical contrast-enhancement, i.e., almost isoechoic with the normal parenchyma in the early stages (**b** = 15 sec) and then progressively hypoechoic (**c** = 30 sec, **d** = 60 sec)

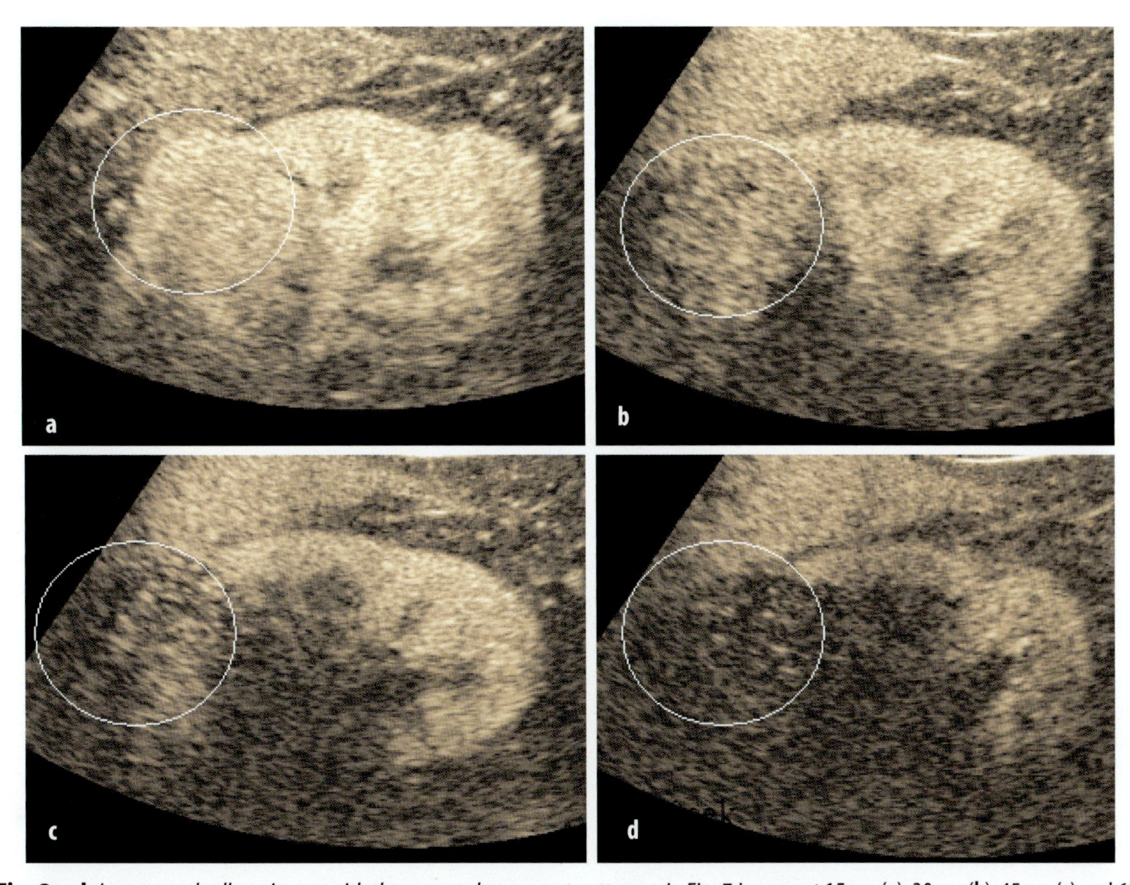

Fig. 8a-d. *Larger renal cell carcinoma with the same enhancement pattern as in Fig. 7.* Images at 15 sec (**a**), 30 sec (**b**), 45 sec (**c**) and 60 sec (**d**), by which time the tumour is virtually without enhancement, stressing the importance of following the enhancement patterns through all stages

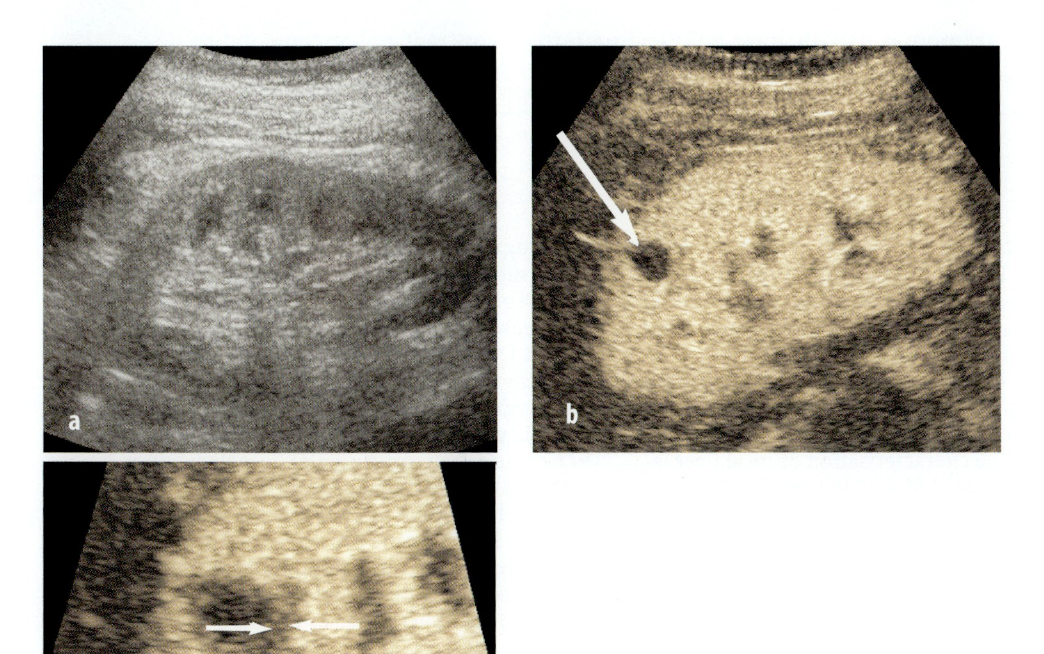

Fig. 9a-c. Patient referred for a high blood cell count. No lesion is seen on B-mode (**a**), but a cyst-like lesion appears in the early stages of CEUS (**b**). After 60 sec, however, contrast has left the previously normal-looking margin of the lesion, creating a hypoechoic rim around the non-enhancing portion (**c**). An erythropoietin-producing tumour was later removed

Conclusion

The intense enhancement of the normal kidney opens many possibilities for improved diagnosis and characterisation of renal lesions.

When CEUS is used with contrast-specific software, non-perfused areas are easily delineated and, conversely, minimal vascularisation can be detected. Possible uses include the detection of small cysts, parenchymal rifts, renal infarctions, abscesses or rifts/haematomas.

Local or focal differences in blood flow can be noted, offering an indication of diffuse renal disease or focal lesions impairing the blood flow to a portion of the kidney. Possible uses include the assessment of pyelonephritis, both in the detection of the lesion itself and the distinction against an abscess formation.

Small amounts of contrast can be seen because of the high detection sensitivity. This improves the ability to visualise tiny vessels, indicating a possible malignancy rather than a simple cyst. Possible uses include the characterisation of atypical cysts and indeterminate lesions.

Knowledge of a normal renal enhancement pattern may allow the differentiation of renal parenchyma with an abnormal shape from solid focal lesions. Possible uses include the characterisation of suspected focal lesions and, in the future, possibly the differentiation of benign from malignant lesions.

The arrival of both stable contrast agents and the development of dedicated contrast-specific software are fairly recent events. Much work is still to be done before the above described applications are properly explored and validated. It is important to remember that even though accumulated experience so far indicates that malignant tumours are hypoechoic in the later contrast stages, it cannot be inferred that a lesion that retains contrast is benign. Similarly, that a focal pyelonephritis can be seen as a hypoechoic lesion does not mean that an infection can, with some degree of certainty, be excluded because of a normal CEUS scan. To reach this stage a lot of research is necessary, but it is almost certain that the resulting improvement in diagnostic accuracy will be worth the effort.

Key Points

- CEUS of the kidneys can be used to get further information about the character of renal lesions.
- Renal cell carcinomas usually have a typical pattern of contrast-enhancement, but it is not yet possible to distinguish solid malignant lesions from benign ones.

References

1. Wilson SR, Burns PN, Muradali D et al (2000) Harmonic hepatic US with microbubble contrast agent: initial experience showing improved characterisation of haemangioma, hepatocellular carcinoma and metastasis. Radiology 215:153-161
2. Leen E, Becker D, Bolondi L et al (2003) Prospective open-label, multicentre study evaluating the accuracy of unenhanced versus SonoVue-enhanced ultrasonography in the characterisation of focal liver lesions. Ultrasound Med Biol 29 [Suppl 5]:S23
3. Albrecht T, Hoffmann CW, Schmitz SA et al (2001) Phase inversion sonography during the liver specific late phase of contrast-enhancement: improved detection of liver metastases. AJR 176:1191-1198
4. Cosgrove D, Eckersley R, Blomley M, Harvey C (2002) Quantification of blood flow. Ultrasound. ECR Categorical Course Syllabus. Springer, Berlin Heidelberg New York, pp 84-90
5. Correas JM, Claudon M, Tranquart F, Helenon O (2003) Contrast-enhanced ultrasonography; renal applications. J Radiol 84:2041-2054
6. Ascenti G, Zimbaro G, Mazziotti S et al (2001) Usefulness of power Doppler and contrast-enhanced sonography in the differentiation of hyperechoic renal masses. Abdom Imaging 26:654-660
7. Rosenfield AT, Siegel NJ (1981) Renal parenchymal disease. Histopathologic-sonographic correlation. AJR 137:793-798
8. Dacher JN, Pfister C, Monroe M (1996) Power Doppler sonographic pattern of acute pyelonephritis in children: comparison with CT. AJR 166:1451-1455
9. Krause J, Nilsson A (2003) Targeted tumor biopsy under contrast-enhanced ultrasound guidance. Eur Radiol 13 [Suppl 4]:L239-L240
10. Quaia E, Siracusano S, Bertolotto M et al (2003) Characterization of renal tumours with pulse inversion harmonic imaging by intermittent high mechanical index technique: initial results. Eur Radiol 13(6):1402-12
11. Ascenti G, Gaeta M, Magno C et al (2004) Contrast-enhanced second-harmonic sonography in the detection of pseudocapsule in renal cell carcinoma. AJR 182(6):1525-1530
12. Siracusano S, Quaia E, Bertolotto M et al (2004) The application of ultrasound contrast agents in the characterization of renal tumors. World J Uro 22(5):316-22

IV.2

Renal Transplant Follow-up

Thomas Fischer

Imaging of Kidney Transplants

Kidney transplant is the first method of choice for treating terminal renal failure. Only the timely transplant of a suitable donor kidney ensures optimal medical management and social rehabilitation of affected patients. There has been a steady increase in graft survival time through improved operative techniques in combination with better immunosuppressive medication [1, 2].

A kidney graft is susceptible to numerous post-operative complications and deleterious effects and therefore requires close post-operative follow-up. In the diagnostic management of kidney graft recipients, a number of imaging modalities such as ultrasound (US), magnetic resonance imaging (MRI), computed tomography (CT), and digital subtraction angiography (DSA) have a crucial role besides the clinical examination, paraclinical parameters, and the immunologic and histologic examination of graft biopsies. US is the most widely employed non-invasive modality for the post-operative assessment of kidney grafts. In particular, color duplex ultrasound (CDUS) is able to answer a number of diagnostic queries [2-11]. B-mode US provides morphologic information on the kidney graft and can be used to diagnose urinary retention, perirenal hematoma, lymphocele, or a tumor, while Doppler techniques such as CDUS or power Doppler (PD) mainly serve to evaluate perfusion of the anastomoses and kidney parenchyma. Other cross-sectional imaging modalities such as CT or MRI are rarely necessary [4, 9]. They are used for specific indications only, mostly prior to a surgical or urologic intervention, for instance, to identify active bleeding, to evaluate a hematoma prior to removal, or to exclude a malignant tumor [12]. The indication for invasive DSA is established on the basis of the CDUS findings [7, 13-14]. DSA simultaneously offers the option of treating renal artery stenoses by means of percutaneous angioplasty (PTA) or stenting.

Complications Affecting Kidney Grafts

Early and Late Nephrologic Complications

Hyperacute, accelerated, or acute rejection episodes can occur in the early phase after kidney transplant (in the first four weeks). Such rejection episodes must be differentiated from acute tubular necrosis (ATN) because the therapeutic management is different. Since a reliable differentiation is not possible on clinical grounds, histologic examination of graft biopsies is considered the diagnostic gold standard [1, 8, 15-17]. Despite the options of CDUS and PD, US may not yield a reliable diagnosis in individual graft recipients [18-19]. Nevertheless, close sonographic follow-up in the post-transplant phase is helpful in arriving at the correct diagnosis in conjunction with the clinical and paraclinical data and establishing the indication for biopsy [20]. Data in the literature varies widely with regard to the reported specificity of CDUS in diagnosing rejection, which is given as 25% [21] to 90% [22], with sensitivities ranging from 35% [23] to 94% [24].

In the late phase after kidney transplant, acute and chronic rejection, infection (primarily with cytomegalovirus [CMV]), cyclosporine toxicity, and recurrent or *de novo* glomerulonephritis become more important. In particular, various chronic kidney conditions share the features of interstitial sclerosis and glomerular obliteration in late disease, so their differential diagnosis by imaging is difficult. When there is chronic graft damage, angiography and 3D power Doppler show the typical 'leafless tree' appearance [25] (Fig. 1).

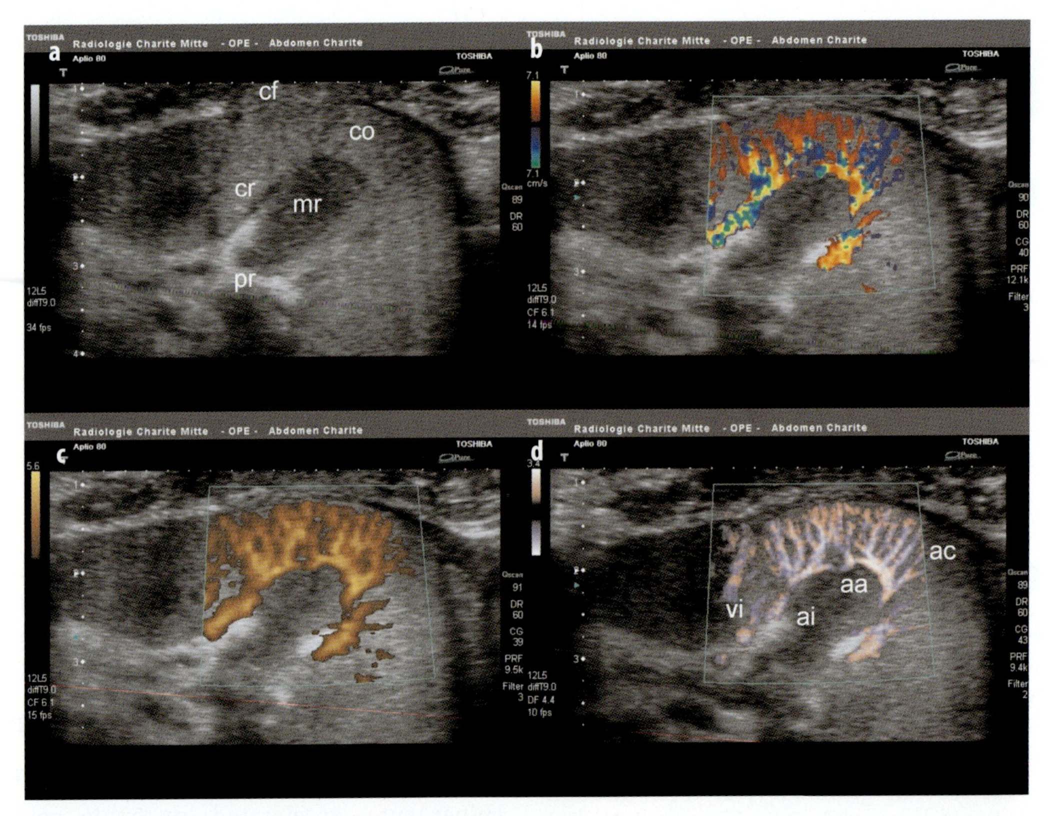

Fig. 1a-d. Normal appearance of the kidney on unenhanced B-mode ultrasound (**a**) with visualization of the fibrous capsule (*cf*), cortex (*co*), renal medulla (*mr*), renal columns (*cr*), and renal papillae (*pr*). High resolution ultrasound in a recipient with good graft function and superficial location of the kidney (technique: Aplio 80, Toshiba, 9 MHz, differential tissue harmonic imaging). CDUS (**b**) and power Doppler (**c**) reliably depict the vascular tree up to below the capsule. Wideband Doppler, Advanced Dynamic Flow, provides an artifact-free and detailed view of vascular anatomy (**d**) with reliable depiction of the interlobar artery and vein (*ai, vi*), the arcuate artery (*aa*), and the cortical arteries (*ac*)

Surgical Complications

The most common complication in kidney recipients is a perirenal fluid collection, which may indicate a hematoma, seroma, lymphocele, or urinoma [26]. Identification and volume measurement of such fluid collections are straightforward with B-mode US (Fig. 2). Fine-needle biopsy may occasionally be required to establish the differential diagnosis [27]. Possible compression of the renal vein by a fluid collection is evaluated by CDUS. As with native kidneys, B-mode scanning also allows differentiation of urinary obstruction with evaluation of the renal calices, ureter, and bladder. Correct positioning of a ureteral splint can also be evaluated.

Occlusion of the renal artery causes transplant ischemia, while thrombosis of the renal vein causes hemorrhagic infarction. Both conditions are rare complications, but must be taken into consideration in the early phase after kidney transplant [28]. CDUS reliably identifies a complete loss of perfusion of the main renal artery and is limited only in obese graft recipients and when the graft lies deep in the iliac fossa [29-31]. Renal vein thrombosis has an incidence of 1-4% [32]. Characteristic flow curves with peak systolic inflow and end-diastolic flow reversal, in combination with an increase in the graft volume, point to the differential diagnosis [33-34], but may be difficult to differentiate from the flow curves in ATN or rejection in individual cases (Fig. 3).

A typical late vascular complication is transplant renal artery stenosis (TRAS). Its incidence is 1.6-16% [35]. TRAS can eventually lead to transplant insufficiency and must be considered in kidney recipients with newly occurring hypertension. Most stenoses occur at the anastomotic site [36]. CDUS has a sensitivity of 67-100% and a specificity of 66-100% (Fig. 4) in diagnosing TRAS (Fig. 4). The diagnosis of TRAS by CDUS is examiner-dependent and correlates with the examiner's experience [37-39].

An arterio-venous (AV) fistula must be considered as a possible complication after renal core biopsy (Fig. 5). AV fistulas are typically detected incidentally as they have a high rate of spontaneous occlusion [40].

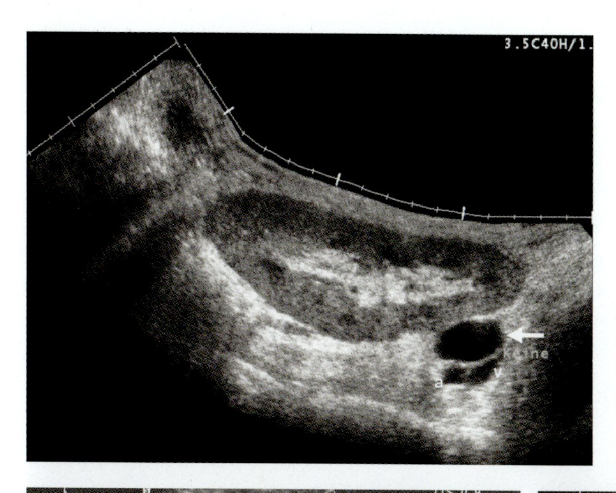

Fig. 2. Visualization of a transplant kidney throughout its length with SieScape panoramic imaging. A lymphocele measuring 2 cm (*white arrow*) is seen in the area of the pelvic axis (external iliac artery (*a*), external iliac vein (*v*)) immediately post-operatively (technique: Sonoline Elegra, Siemens, 3.5 MHz, SieScape)

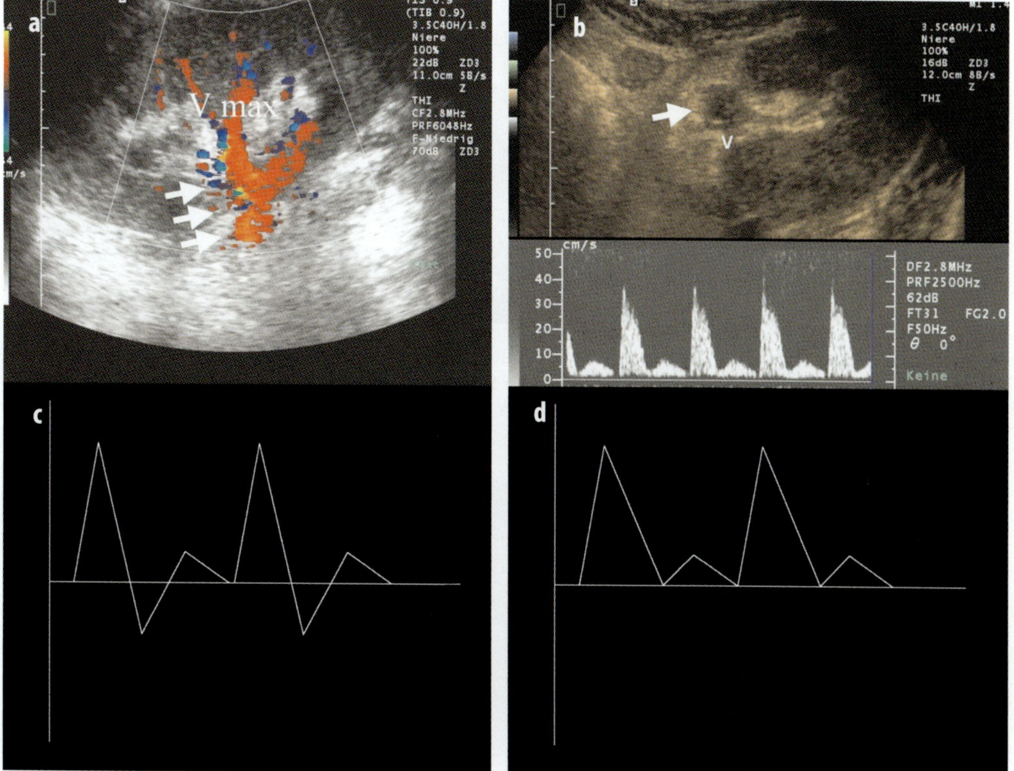

Fig. 3a-d. *Thrombotic occlusion of the renal vein (white arrows).* Normal appearance of the renal artery but nearly complete absence of venous flow on CDUS scan (**a, b**). Compression of the renal vein by a hematoma (*white arrow*) must be considered in the differential diagnosis as both venous thrombosis (**c**) and compression of the vein (**d**) have similar Doppler waveforms

Baseline Ultrasound

Color Duplex Ultrasound and Power Doppler

Features and Current Role in Clinical Practice

Determination of the resistance index (RI) and pulsatility index (PI) by means of color duplex ultrasound (CDUS) and of subcapsular perfusion by power Doppler (PD) are integral procedures in the diagnostic evaluation of suspected rejection [10, 11] but also serve to assess tumor vascularization, to evaluate recipients with suspected anastomotic stenosis, or to exclude venous thrombosis. The most important nephrologic complications in the early phase are ATN and acute rejection. These two conditions cannot be reliably differentiated using B-mode US alone [41-43]. An increase in graft volume or enlargement of the medullary cones with increasing loss of echogenicity are unspecific. Similar changes may also become prominent in infection. Although the advent of CDUS has improved the non-invasive diagnostic evaluation of kidney

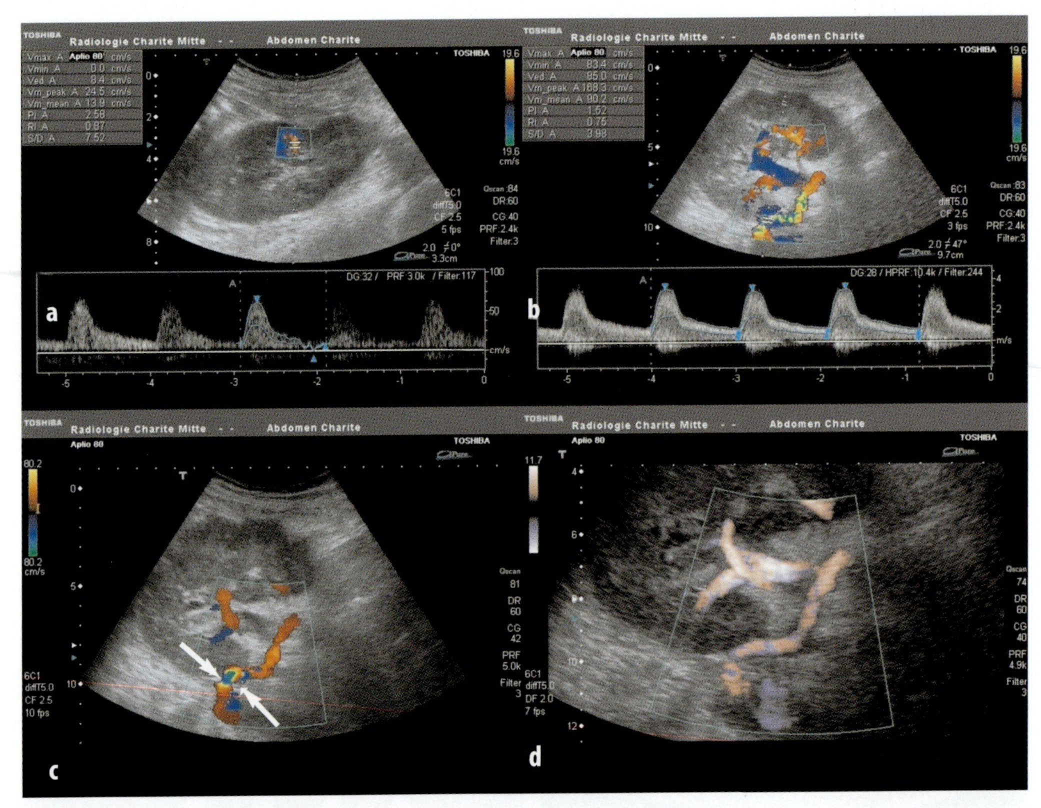

Fig. 4a-d. Increased resistance index (0.87) after long-standing untreated transplant renal artery stenosis (**a**). Markedly increased flow velocity (> 3 m/sec) and turbulent flow (**b**) with typical aliasing in the stenotic area **c**, (*white arrow*) on CDUS. Detailed visualization of the narrowing directly at the anastomosis in the Advanced Dynamic Flow mode (**d**)

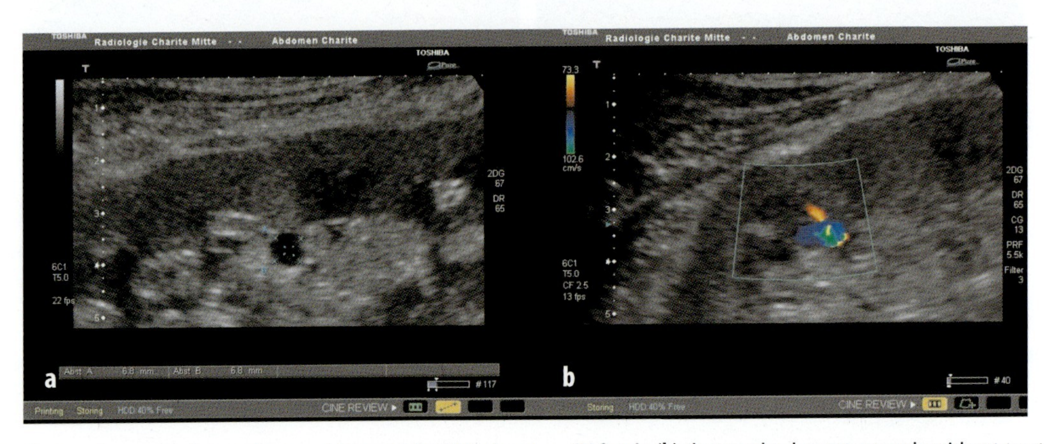

Fig. 5a, b. Anechoic cystic lesion after renal biopsy (**a**). CDUS shows an AV fistula (**b**) that resolved spontaneously without treatment. With the high PRF used, there is selective visualization of the AV fistula without other flow signals from the graft

grafts, differentiation of acute rejection and ATN appears almost impossible [44, 45]. Some authors claim that it is possible to differentiate acute rejection and ATN, on the one hand, from changes in the flow profile that are associated with cyclosporine toxicity, on the other [46]. Moreover, CDUS has the potential to evaluate the effects of rejection therapy and to estimate the prognosis in terms of transplant survival [10].

After initial evaluation of the kidney graft immediately after surgery for assessment of organ perfusion or documentation of surgical complications, duplex parameters like the RI and PI should be determined on the second postoperative day when an effect of initial edema at the anastomotic site can be largely excluded [47]. The RI and PI are calculated according to the formulas given in Table 1. Automated measurement is performed in the interlobar artery or the arcuate artery in the upper, lower, and mid-

Table 1. Calculation of the resistance index and pulsatility index

Index	Calculation	Normal range
Resistance index (RI)	Vmax – Vmin / Vmax	0.55-0.75
Pulsatility index (PI)	Vmax – Vmin / Vmean	1.12-1.26

dle third of the transplanted kidney [6, 37]. RI and PI are measures of peripheral resistance downstream of the site of measurement. They increase in the case of rejection after initial graft function. Together with the clinical and paraclinical findings, the RI and PI thus serve to differentiate rejection from a normal graft with good function [48]. Resistance increases because of edema formation in interstitial rejection or because of direct damage to the capillaries in vascular rejection [49]. Differentiation of rejection from ATN is crucial for initiation of adequate therapeutic measures, but is difficult. A steep increase in PI in conjunction with a pronounced increase in RI up to an RI of 1 are indicative of concomitant ATN and rejection. In individual cases with failure of graft function recovery, a graft biopsy may be necessary for definitive diagnosis [1, 8, 15]. Serial RI determination is desirable.

TRAS is the most important vascular complication in the late phase after kidney transplant. Criteria for diagnosis are a peak systolic velocity of 1.9 m/s [7] or 2.5 m/s [5] with a consecutive decrease in RI and PI below 0.6 and 0.5, respectively [50]. Again, it is important take into account the course of the RI decrease.

The color-coded information provided by CDUS is based on the analysis of the mean frequency shift, while PD processes the amplitude of the Doppler signal. Power Doppler US has a better signal-to-noise ratio compared with CDUS and can therefore be operated with a high gain and low pulse repetition rate (PRF), which enables sensitive detection of blood flow [51]. Histologically, chronic rejection is characterized by arteriopathy, intimal proliferation, necrosis, and medial thickening [52]. These changes are associated with reduced peripheral perfusion, which can be diagnosed by PD. The latter is thus a valid diagnostic modality for the detection of severe parenchymal damage in the late phase after kidney transplant [53]. The option of three-dimensional representation of the vascular tree [54] can be used for follow-up evaluation and standardization of the examination (Fig. 6). Chronic rejection, cyclosporine toxicity, and chronic CMV infection cannot be differentiated [55].

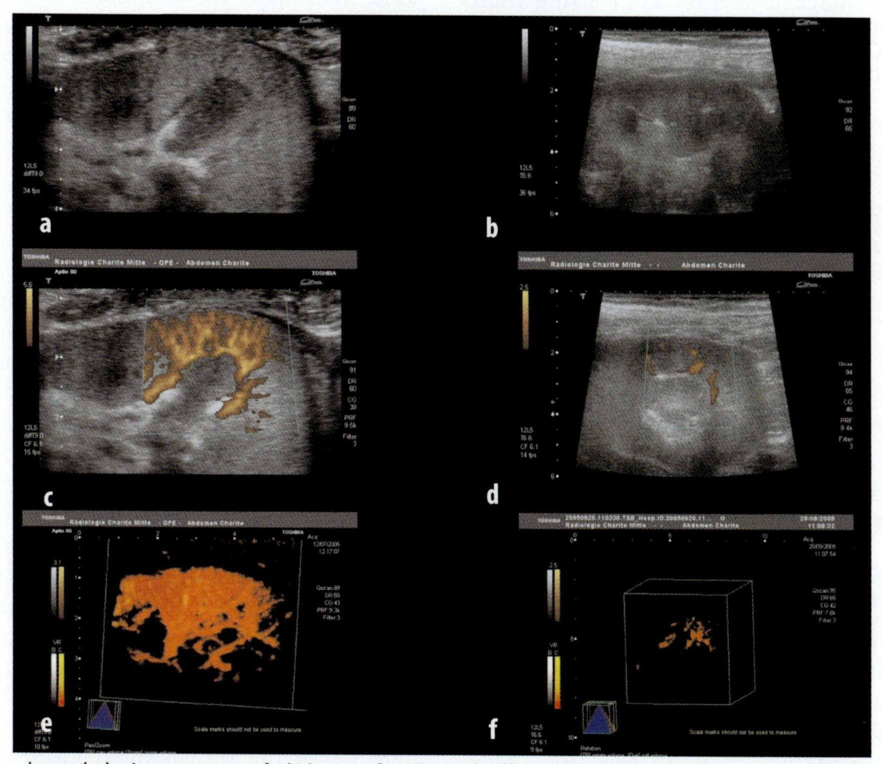

Fig. 6a-f. Normal morphologic appearance of a kidney graft with good differentiation of the medulla and cortex (**a**). Limited differentiation of the medulla and cortex (**b**) in a patient with chronic graft damage 24 years after transplant. Normal renal vascularization to below the capsule in the power Doppler mode (**c**). Rarefied vessels (**d**). Reconstructed 3D view of the patient with good transplant function (**e**) as compared with the patient with chronic transplant damage (**f**). So-called ' leafless tree' sign

Limitations

General limitations of the sonographic evaluation of a kidney graft are the known examiner dependence of US, as well as the restricted morphologic information obtained in obese graft recipients and when the kidney graft is located deep in the iliac fossa [29-31, 56]. These limitations can give rise to inadequate evaluation or misinterpretation. Other factors that may impair the assessment of transplant function are the site of measurement in the interlobar arteries, an increased intra-abdominal pressure, and an increased heart rate or arrhythmia [29-31]. Since each kidney graft represents an individual vascular bed, it is desirable to perform serial examinations, which provide more valid results than a single examination. Serial data is considered to be reproducible [22].

A number of individual factors, such as immunosuppressive therapy with cyclosporine, can affect the RI or PI [29, 55]. Although a kidney graft is not subject to the same laws as a native kidney due to denervation, systemic factors such as hypertension or atherosclerosis must be taken into account in interpreting the parameters determined by CDUS. Limitations of the scanning depth of CDUS in evaluating deeply located anastomoses have in part been overcome through the use of PD. PD assessment of chronic transplant damage is mainly done using high-frequency transducers [53]. This technique cannot be used in obese patients and does not allow evaluation of the entire graft.

Disorders occurring in the early phase after kidney transplant, such as acute rejection episodes or ATN cannot be reliably differentiated clinically or sonographically using CDUS or PD. The same holds true for chronic damage of the graft. Histology of a transplant biopsy continues to be the diagnostic gold standard [1, 8, 15-17].

Contrast Ultrasound

Fundamental Principles of Contrast Medium Administration in Kidney Transplants

Fundamental Principles and Potential Applications

The timely identification of early and late complications after kidney transplant poses a considerable challenge but is crucial for rapid initiation of adequate therapeutic measures. The clinical manifestation of early rejection, ATN, and drug-induced nephropathy is very heterogeneous and difficult to interpret reliably. Recent technological developments of ultrasound equipment [57-61] and the advent of ultrasound contrast media (USCM) have also widened the sonographic spectrum available for kidney graft evaluation [61-64]. USCM are very tiny gas bubbles (e.g., sulfur hexafluoride or air) stabilized with a coat of phospholipid (SonoVue, Bracco) or galactose (Levovist, Schering). The small size of the microbubbles of 1 to 5 μm on average allows them to enter the capillaries where they enhance the echoes in the scanning field, which is why they are also designated echo enhancers. The visualization of very small vessels down to the capillary level allows differentiation of cystic and malignant renal lesions by means of contrast-enhanced US [65].

The basic technique for evaluating renal vascularization is contrast medium imaging [66] with emission of very low amounts of sound energy to induce the individual microbubbles to reflect specific frequencies or emission of high energies, so-called stimulated acoustic emission (SAE), to produce a single high signal in the 'death struggle' of the microbubbles. Based on the emitted energy, two techniques of contrast-enhanced US for kidney graft evaluation can be differentiated as in the use of contrast-enhanced US for the characterization and detection of focal liver lesions. The emitted energy is described by the mechanical index (MI) and the corresponding techniques are designated as high MI technique (MI > 0.5) or low MI technique (MI < 0.3). High energies amplify the Doppler signal by about 30 dB, which was found to improve the visualization of TRAS in combination with administration of the echo-enhancer Levovist (intense signal at high sound energy with only little signal amplification at low sound energy). The technique used today is the so-called flash replenishment technique, in which single high ultrasound energy pulses are emitted [67] to destroy the microbubbles and the time to renewed accumulation of microbubbles is evaluated. With this technique, very minute perfusion signals in the renal capillary bed can be selectively depicted for characterization of renal blood flow in the different territories [68]. Low MI US is superior to the high MI technique in that it enables real-time scanning of a transplant kidney since the harmonic vibration of the microbubbles contributes to the signal and the bubbles are not destroyed. The sulfur hexafluoride-based microbubbles (SonoVue) provide good signal amplification at a very low sound energy [69] and enable straightforward real-time US of the transplanted kidney over some minutes. A low frame rate further increases the longevity of the microbubbles (< 10 fps). The low MI phase-inversion technique [70] uses the entire frequency spectrum for generation of the image and thus fully exploits the backscatter signal of the microbubbles, resulting in a further reduction of the transmit energy (MI < 0.1) with less destruction of the microbubbles as compared with harmonic imaging. Most second-generation ultrasound contrast agents (SonoVue, Sonazoid, Definity, Imavist) enable continuous scanning of renal blood flow (real-time perfusion imaging) [70-71)].

Conventional US techniques such as CDUS (determination of RI and PI) and PD for evaluation of subcapsular perfusion have been a component in the evaluation of kidney graft recipients for years [10], although their diagnostic yield is limited due to their low specificity [29-31]. The first improvement was achieved through enhancement of the color Doppler signal by means of the USCM Levovist (color Doppler imaging, CDI), which allowed reliable diagnosis of renal infarction and characterization of malignant tumors [72, 73]. This new technique did not evolve into a routine diagnostic procedure due to the fairly short time window after administration of the echo-enhancer, its inadequate pressure stability and the technical limitations of US equipment at that time. Initial results in the evaluation of kidney grafts by means of contrast-enhanced US [56, 62-65] using the low MI technique in combination with a second generation contrast medium (e.g., SonoVue) suggest that this is a promising candidate for a valid US technique that yields examiner-independent and reproducible results even under difficult anatomic conditions (obese patients) [56], though it has not yet established itself as a routine diagnostic procedure.

Specific Ultrasound Techniques

Various contrast-enhanced US methods have been used to evaluate renal vascularization or the vascularization of renal tumors. They rely on the phase or pulse-inversion technique (wideband harmonic imaging) that generates the image from the second harmonic echo response from the non-linear reflectors (microbubbles) after transmission of two sound pulses. The second pulse is inverted (180° out of phase) [74]. The aim is to scan the kidney transplant with a very low acoustic power (MI < 0.3). The MI (calculated as the peak negative sound pressure divided by the square root of the transmitted frequency) is the standard measure of the energy applied, though there is considerable variation depending on the ultrasound unit and the specific contrast-enhancement technique used. In addition, there is variation in the actual local pressure within the scanning field, e.g., through sound attenuation. Hence, MI values provide only a rough measure.

When USCM were first introduced, basically only abdominal 3.5 MHz probes had the capability of contrast-enhanced imaging, which is why the entire kidney graft was scanned after bolus administration or continuous infusion of the contrast medium [56, 65].

While renal vascularization or vascularization of a renal tumor can be evaluated visually as the inflow of the contrast medium into the kidney transplant (e.g., to identify a perfusion defect) [75], determination of renal perfusion requires quantitative procedures [69-71]. Various quantitative approaches for contrast-enhanced ultrasonography have been developed in recent years. A fairly simple and practical approach is the mathematical description of the time-intensity curve (TIC). The curve represents the temporal course of signal intensities after bolus administration of the echo enhancer in a region of interest (ROI) and can be generated using either the tools that are integrated in modern ultrasound units or external computer analysis [56]. The bolus kinetics are characterized by a wash-in and a wash-out phase. Typically, mean pixel brightness (intensity) is determined in a defined area (ROI) over time. Bolus kinetics follow the indicator dilution principle, with the height of the wash-out curve indicating the blood volume and the wash-out time, the blood flow. Measurement requires homogeneous distribution of the microbubbles in blood without extravasation. This requirement is fulfilled by second generation ultrasound contrast media, which are so-called blood pool agents. This is a technically feasible method, but the fact that the amount of contrast medium administered as a bolus is not exactly reproducible limits this method and makes it difficult to compare transplanted patients.

Together with evaluation of bolus kinetics, it is possible to simultaneously determine the transit time, i.e., the time needed for the USCM to flow through the graft. The first change in signal is determined in ROIs placed in the renal artery and the renal vein in the hilum. The transit time is the calculated difference in time between the two ROIs and serves as a measure for general kidney perfusion [56]. The significance of this parameter in evaluating kidney grafts is based on the assumption that the transit time is increased when transplant perfusion is globally increased (e.g., in chronic transplant nephropathy) and decreased in the presence of an arteriovenous shunt (acute rejection). A scanning protocol is summarized in Table 2.

Table 2. Suggested protocol for determining bolus kinetics in renal transplants

Technique	Parameter
High end US system	Aplio 80, Toshiba
Transducer	3.5 MHz wideband transducer
Low MI pulse-inversion technique	Contrast harmonic imaging
Mechanical index (MI)	MI < 0.1
Echo-enhancer	SonoVue, Bracco-Altana
Dosage	1.6 ml ,1 plus 5 ml NaCl as a bolus

Since the transplanted kidney is fixed in the iliac fossa and is subject to only a small amount of respiratory motion, the TIC and transit time can be determined from a fairly constant transducer position and with only few motion artifacts. Recent techniques such as ROI tracking contribute to the standardization of the method. When there is good transplant function, the TIC is characterized by a rapid increase in signal intensity to peak maximum and a relatively flat curve during wash-out of the contrast medium. Different mathematical parameters can be defined to describe the curve. For instance, the intensity level (mean pixel brightness) at the beginning of CM wash-in can be designated as the initial value (Ix), the time at which the first clear increase in signal is noted as t baseline and the corresponding intensity value as I baseline. The time at which maximum intensity (I peak) is reached is t. The decrease can be determined by the simple calculation of t decrease (tdecrease=tpeak+{tpeak-tbaseline}), which in turn defines I decrease [56-57]. Using these parameters, the increase and decrease of the time-intensity curve can be calculated in different vascular territories, such as the interlobar artery and the renal cortex.

$$\text{Increase} = \frac{(\text{I peak-I baseline})}{(\text{t peak-t baseline})}$$

$$\text{Decrease} = \frac{(\text{I peak-I decrease})}{\text{t decrease}}$$

For individual comparison within a graft that is independent of the patient's cardiocirculatory status, ratios of the slopes of the time-intensity curves in the interlobar artery and the renal cortex can be defined. This ratio has been designated as the perfusion quotient (PQ) in earlier studies.

$$\text{PQ} = \frac{\text{increase in the interlobar artery}}{\text{increase in the renal cortex}}$$

In addition, the difference in the time to peak between the two vascular territories can be determined from the TIC.

$$\Delta\text{t peak} = \text{t peak renal cortex - t peak interlobar artery}$$

With adequate settings, a further parameter can be calculated from the TIC, the arterio-venous time difference (transit time) between the renal artery and vein in the hilum. The problem of this approach is that it is difficult to achieve sufficiently constant ultrasound parameters (emitted energy, overall gain, size of ROI, distance of transducer from graft, time and site of bolus administration) for comparison of results in individual patients undergoing follow-up examinations (Fig. 7).

The longer and variable inflow time (so-called venous pooling) after intravenous (iv) bolus administration of the USCM poses a problem for analysis of bolus kinetics. Therefore, a second method for the complex mathematical description of blood flow in a vascular territory, so-called replenishment kinetics, has been described in a perfusion model of the kidney and compared with simple bolus kinetics [69-71]. This method measures the microbubble replenishment rate of a tissue area after destruction of microbubbles through a single high and short ultrasound pulse. Standardized scanning sequences with a destructive pulse followed by an ultrasound signal of low energy with repeated emission of the high-energy pulse can be defined. The resulting replenishment kinetics corresponds to an exponential curve and is described by a simple mathematical function that is now already implemented in some evaluation tools [69-71, 76, 77].

$$Y = s+A\,(1-e(-\text{beta}\ t))$$

A = blood volume

beta = speed of microbubble contrast replenishment

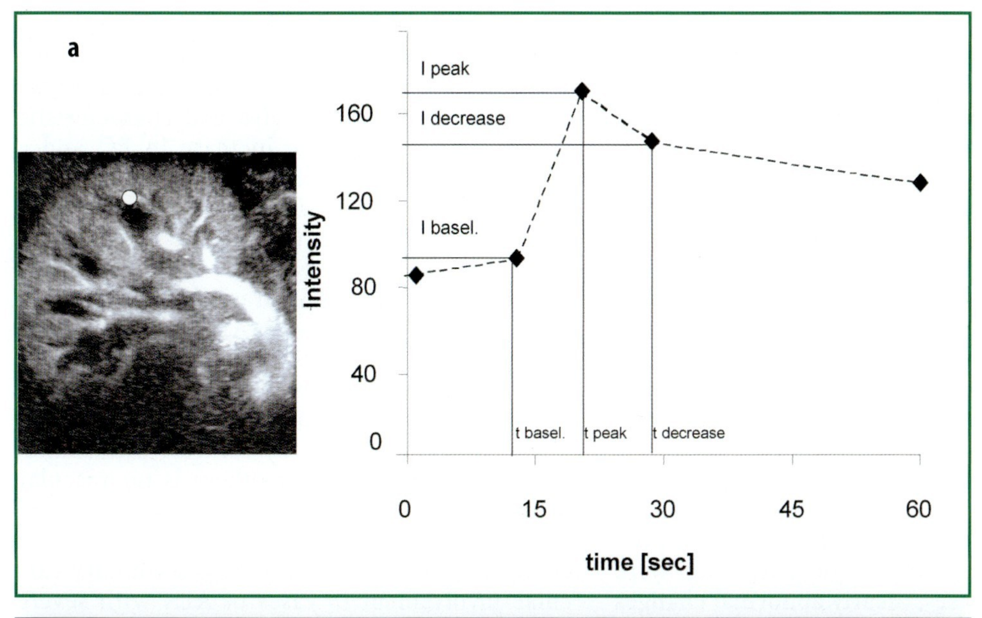

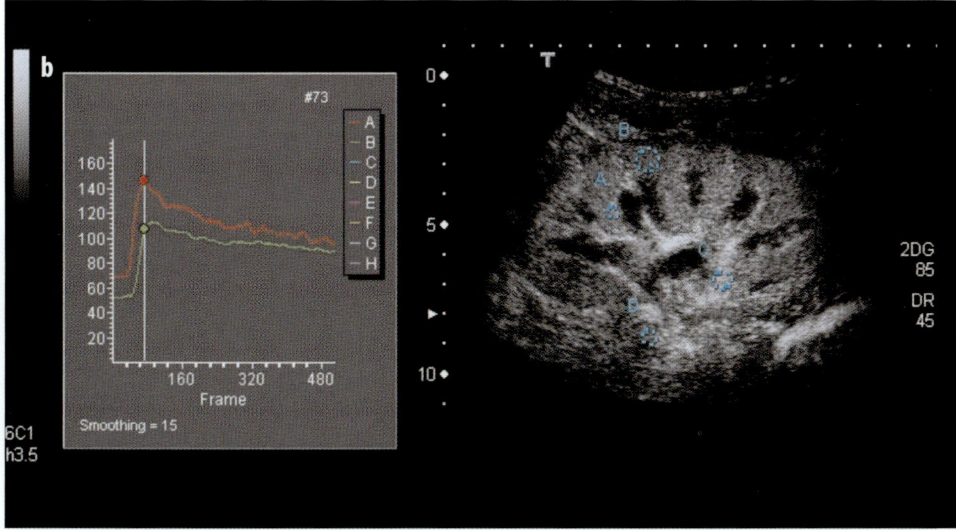

Fig. 7a, b. Depiction of the course of contrast-enhancement in the interlobar artery (**a**). The increase [(I peak – I baseline)/(t peak – t baseline)], decrease [(I decrease – I peak)/(t decrease – t peak)], and the time to peak intensity (t peak) were calculated from the time-intensity curves, defined ROIs in the interlobar artery and subcapsular parenchyma (**b**)

A constant level of contrast medium is achieved by continuous infusion. The replenishment model can be used to answer different questions and to quantify perfusion in different territories such as the kidney, myocardium, or cerebral parenchyma. Initial clinical results using this method are available for myocardial infarction [78], while most published results on renal perfusion have so far been obtained in animal experiments and flow models [69-71, 76, 77].

Role of Contrast Ultrasound in Clinical Practice

Detection of Nephrologic Complications in the Early and Late Phase after Transplant Using Ultrasound Contrast Medium

In the first four weeks after kidney transplant, it is crucial to differentiate acute rejection from ATN because these two conditions require different treatment approaches. A basic distinction is made between vascular and interstitial rejection and different stages are distinguished histologically. Borderline rejection may also be interpreted as a cover term for different disorders such as ATN. The histologic findings in turn need to be interpreted in conjunction with the imaging results and the clinical and paraclinical parameters.

Initial clinical studies in 22 [56] and 50 kidney graft recipients [79] found contrast ultrasound to be superior to B-mode graft volume evaluation and RI determination. Changes in the inflow and outflow patterns of the USCM correlate very well with the histological changes. While volume measurement or RI determination did not allow diagnosis of definitive pathology, contrast ultrasound showed suspicious flow phenomena for which histologic correlates were identified in all cases. Clearly abnormal changes were seen in the rejection group with vascular involvement (Banff II). These and all other patients included in the study underwent ultrasound assessment with administration of an echo-enhancer (1.6 ml SonoVue) on day 5 to 7 after kidney transplant. Arterial inflow and the parenchymal phase were digitally stored over 60 seconds at a frame rate of 10 fps, followed by quantification of perfusion using the ultrasound unit's integrated TIC software. ROIs were placed in the main renal artery, the interlobar artery, the subcapsular renal cortex, and the renal vein. The ROIs were adjusted in size to the respective vessel diameters and were smaller than the largest vessel diameter in order to eliminate slight motion artifacts. The zoom function was used for maximum visualization of the kidney graft, which also served to reduce possible motion artifacts. The ROIs were then checked by watching the entire digital clip and their positions corrected in case of deviation. Intensity was defined as the mean pixel brightness in the ROI. Contrast medium kinetics were then evaluated in the interlobar artery and the renal cortex using the integrated TIC software. A perfusion quotient (PQ) was calculated as the ratio of the upslopes of the TIC (PQ = increase in the interlobar artery/increase in the renal cortex). In addition, the difference in the time to peak between both vascular territories was determined (Dt = time to peak renal cortex - time to peak interlobar artery).

Kidney graft recipients assigned to the normal group in the study had a PQ of 1, as the upslopes in the interlobar artery and the renal cortex did not differ much. In contrast, the PQ was twice as high in patients with vascular rejection. Patients with ATN also had characteristic curves with a moderate increase in PQ and a longer time difference. The patients with Banff II rejection received anti-rejection therapy with 500 mg methylprednisolone (Urbason) on three successive days. All patients showed marked improvement and their transplants recovered function. The patients with ATN did not receive anti-rejection therapy. They showed spontaneous functional improvement in the further course. Banff I rejection (interstitial rejection) could not be identified by contrast ultrasound, which is not surprising as there is no vascular involvement and contrast US is a vessel-oriented diagnostic modality. However, there may be changes in contrast US if there is secondary vascular involvement in cases of ATN with severe interstitial edema (Fig. 8). Preliminary follow-up results in patients with Banff I rejection showed that the time-intensity curves became abnormal only in the second week after transplant or when there was histologic deterioration of the diagnosis. A definitive analysis of the changes in this patient group is not yet available. The suspicious flow phenomena depicted by contrast US in vascular rejection were interpreted as early indications of rejection-related changes. This was an important clue for the clinician that allowed early initiation of further histologic diagnosis and early initiation of anti-rejection therapy. Since contrast ultrasound has no side-effects, we consider it desirable to follow-up patients in whom anti-rejection therapy has been initiated, so that treatment may be adjusted if the contrast US findings show no improvement.

Only case reports are available on the use of contrast US in patients with chronic graft changes. Also, PD and 3D PD are excellent tools for the characterization of peripheral vessel rarefaction. The appearance resembles a 'leafless tree'. The potential benefit of contrast US remains to be defined, especially since different conditions occurring in the late phase after kidney transplant share the same features at their terminal stage. The identification of segmental perfusion defects and transplant evaluation in obese patients might further contribute to the standardization of the US examination. Moreover, it might be possible to not only differentiate rejection, but also perform interventions in a single session.

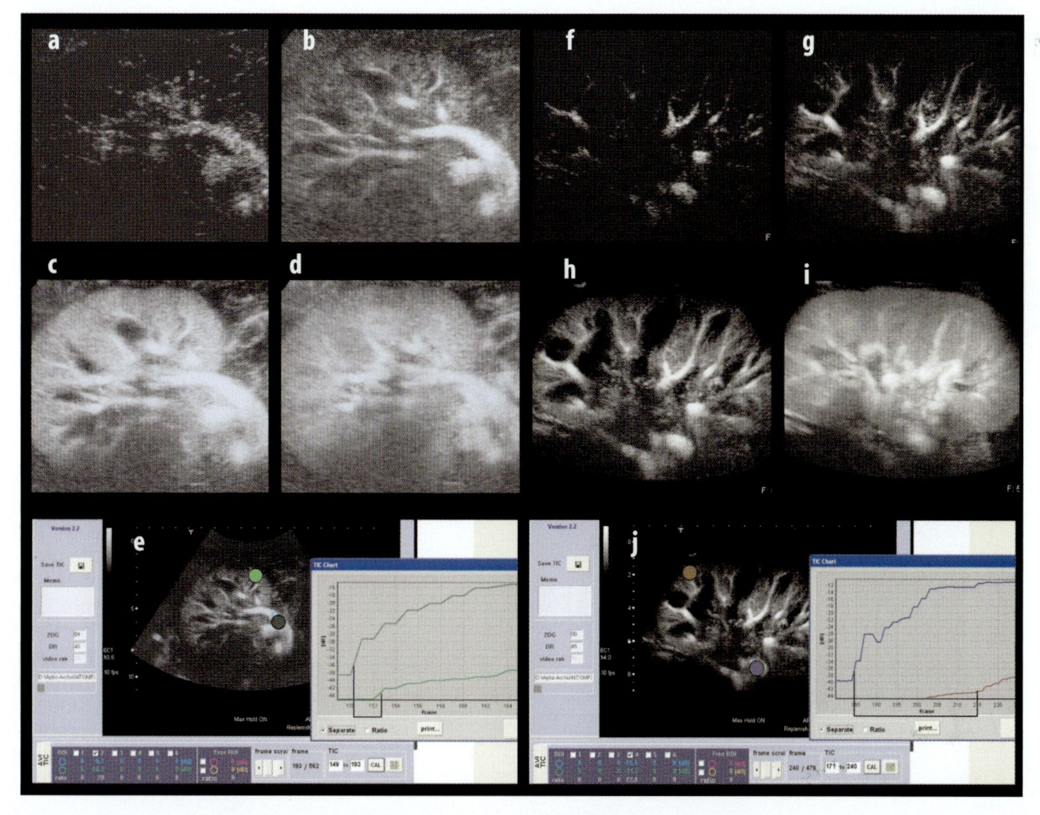

Fig. 8a-j. Temporal course of CM inflow after bolus administration of 1.6 ml of SonoVue via the left cubital vein. Patient with good graft function shown at 0 sec (**a**), 2 sec (**b**), 5 sec (**c**), and 10 sec (**d**). Analysis shows that signal intensity in the cortex increases as early as 0.2 sec after the increase in the main renal artery (**e**). Delayed inflow in the renal cortex in a patient with histologically proven borderline rejection and signs of acute tubular necrosis. Again, arterial inflow of the USCM is shown after 0 sec (**f**), 2 sec (**g**), 5 sec (**h**), and 10 sec (**i**). Analysis shows that the signal intensity in the cortex increases as late as 2 sec after the increase in the main renal artery (**j**)

Detection of Surgical Complications by Contrast Ultrasound

Common surgical complications in the immediate post-operative phase are hematoma, seroma, lymphocele, and urinoma [26]. Detection of a fluid collection and determination of its volume are straightforward by B-mode ultrasound, while delineation of a perirenal or subcapsular hematoma may be more difficult. Initial results suggest that contrast US is superior to B-mode US in detecting a perirenal or subcapsular hematoma. This superiority is based on the fact that hematomas may be isoechoic with the kidney parenchyma on conventional US, while contrast US differentiates them from the perfused parenchyma as non-perfused lesions (Fig. 9). In this study, a combined US examination was performed in which the perfusion parameters were determined first, and then, after homogeneous opacification, the entire graft and its immediate surroundings were scanned. Perirenal hematoma was shown to compromise subcapsular perfusion [56, 79]. A hematoma must be considered in the differential diagnosis of rejection in interpreting bolus kinetics. At the same time, the US examination can serve to establish the indication for removal of a hematoma prior to repeat surgical intervention.

Rare early complications of kidney transplant are occlusion of the renal artery with subsequent graft ischemia and thrombosis of the renal vein with hemorrhagic infarction [28]. In general, both events can be diagnosed by CDUS, but the method is limited in obese recipients and when the graft is located deep in the iliac fossa [29-31]. Another possible indication is exclusion of a perfusion defect in recipients with difficult anastomosis of pole vessels (Fig. 10). Partial ischemia seen as a perfusion defect results if, for technical reasons, a polar artery is not connected to the circulation. Compared to PD, contrast US identifies such defects without problems and allows exact measurement of its area. If there are additional complications, such as rejection, a reliable histologic diagnosis is possible only if the graft biopsy is not obtained from the area of the perfusion defect, which cannot be reliably delineated in the B-mode or by PD.

Transplant renal artery stenosis (TRAS) is a typical late vascular complication [35] that the clinician should think of in kidney recipients

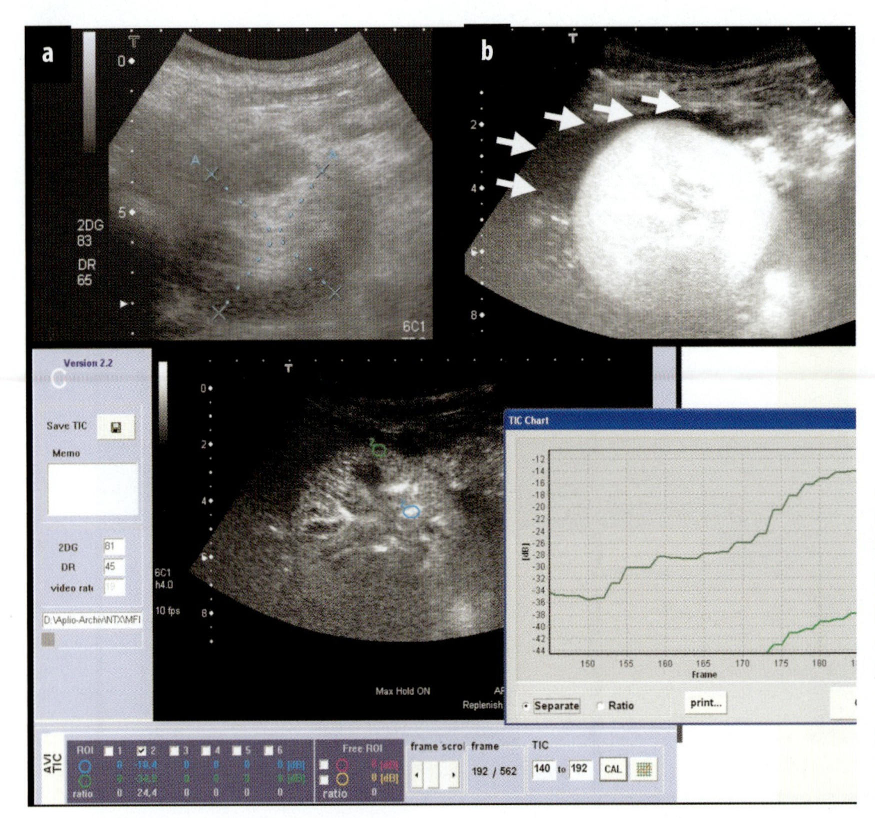

Fig. 9a, b. Transverse view of a transplant kidney obtained in the unenhanced B-mode (**a**). Normal appearance of the graft with a hematoma almost isoechoic with the renal parenchyma. Contrast ultrasound clearly demonstrates a non-enhancing perirenal hematoma (*white arrows*) (**b**). TIC analysis shows a delayed increase in signal intensity in the cortex (**c**). This curve must be differentiated from the curve in acute rejection

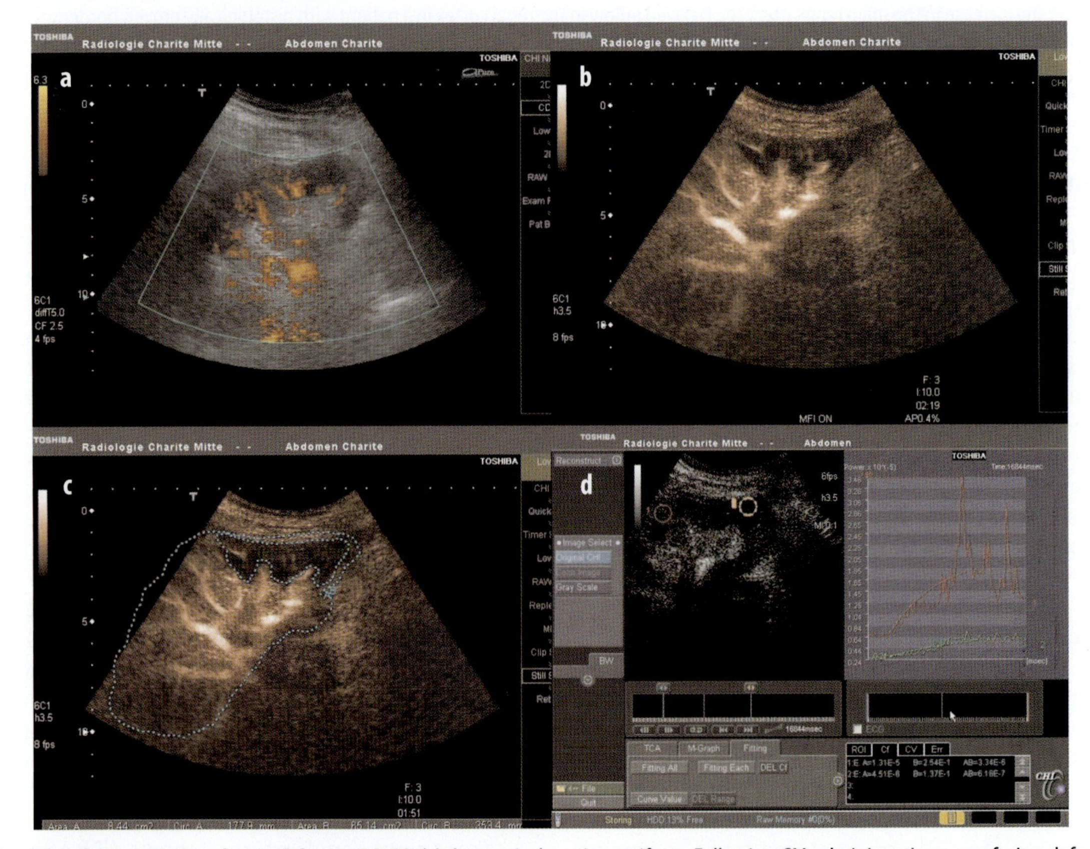

Fig. 10a-d. No typical perfusion defect on 3D-PD (**a**), but typical motion artifacts. Following CM administration, a perfusion defect is depicted in the polar area (**b**) covering about 10% (**c**). Raw data analysis identifies slight perfusion in the area of the defect with flattening of the curve and reduced signal intensity (**d**)

with newly occurring hypertension. A stenosis typically occurs at the anastomotic site [36], where it can be identified by contrast US even in difficult anatomic situations. Nevertheless, the potential benefit of contrast US is controversial [80-82]. CDUS already has a sensitivity and specificity in diagnosing TRAS of 66-100%, but is examiner-dependent [37-39]. Contrast US has advantages in assessing therapeutic outcome, since parameters of renal perfusion provide clues as to the prognosis of treatment of TRAS (stent, PTA). Systematic studies addressing this aspect are not yet available (Fig. 11).

In the long-term follow-up of kidney graft recipients, the identification and differentiation of cystic and solid tumors becomes important. Contrast US allows differentiation of benign and malignant tumors [72, 83], as has already been reported in the literature for native kidneys. In the aftercare of kidney graft recipients, this becomes even more of an issue as early diagnosis may enable tumor enucleation and thus spare the patient a transplant nephrectomy and return to hemodialysis. Clinically, it is important to differentiate a hemorrhagic cyst [84] from renal cell carcinoma (Fig. 12). Following administration of an echo-enhancer, a hemorrhagic cyst retains its low echogenicity and, similar to a perfusion defect, is delineated from the enhancing surrounding renal parenchyma. Renal cell carcinoma is characterized by an abnormal vascular supply and wash-out of the echo-enhancer in the parenchymal phase. Simple subjective evaluation of CM inflow into the kidney tumor can be supplemented by additional perfusion analysis using the bolus kinetics or replenishment model [77]. It has not yet been investigated whether it is possible, for instance, to reliably differentiate an angiomyolipoma (Fig. 13) from a renal cell carcinoma. This is probably due to the fact that MRI enables reliable identification of an angiomyolipoma on the basis of its fatty content. When the renal parenchyma is normal, subjective analysis alone enables reliable differentiation of the medulla and cortex on the basis of the temporal course of contrast medium inflow (Fig. 14). It should be emphasized again, however, that contrast US enables nearly complete evaluation of renal perfusion down to the level of very small capsular vessels in a standardized manner [56, 79].

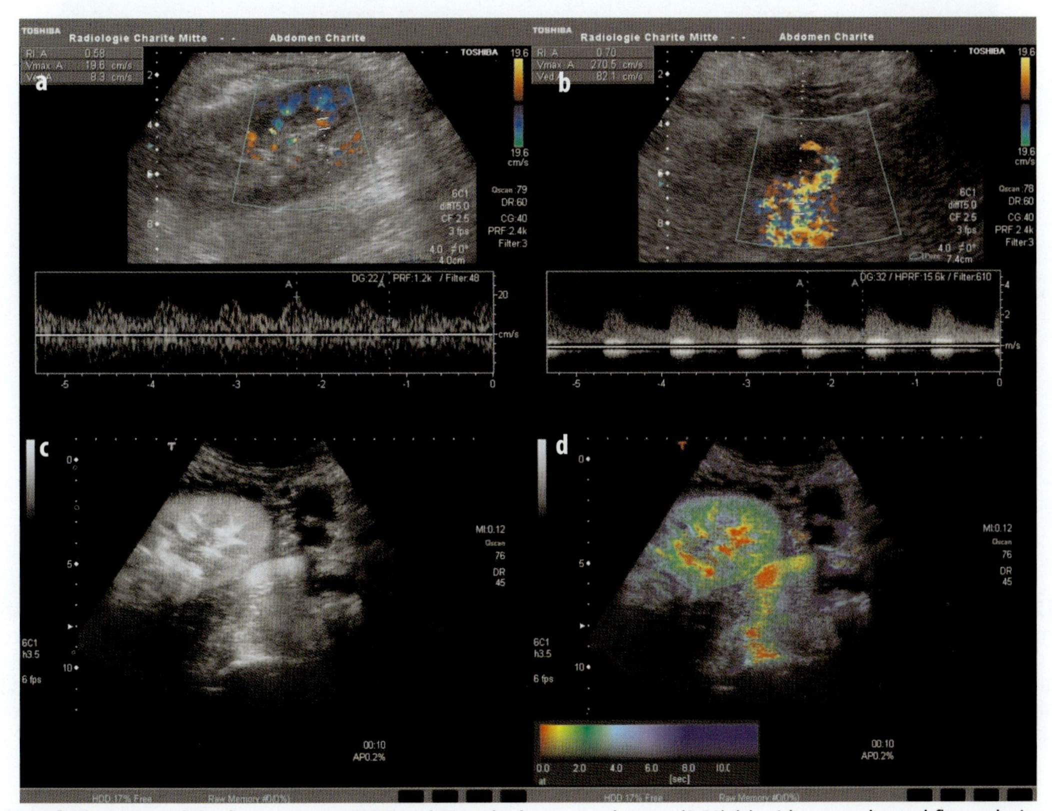

Fig. 11a-d. Flattening of the flow curve on CDUS and RI in the low normal range (0.58) (**a**) with an accelerated flow velocity of 270 cm/sec at the site of anastomosis and turbulent flow (**b**). Perfusion image obtained 10 sec after USCM administration (**c**). Generation of the parametric image from the time-intensity curve depicting the course over the first 10 sec after the first increase in the renal artery (**d**). Delayed inflow into the renal cortex (*blue margin*)

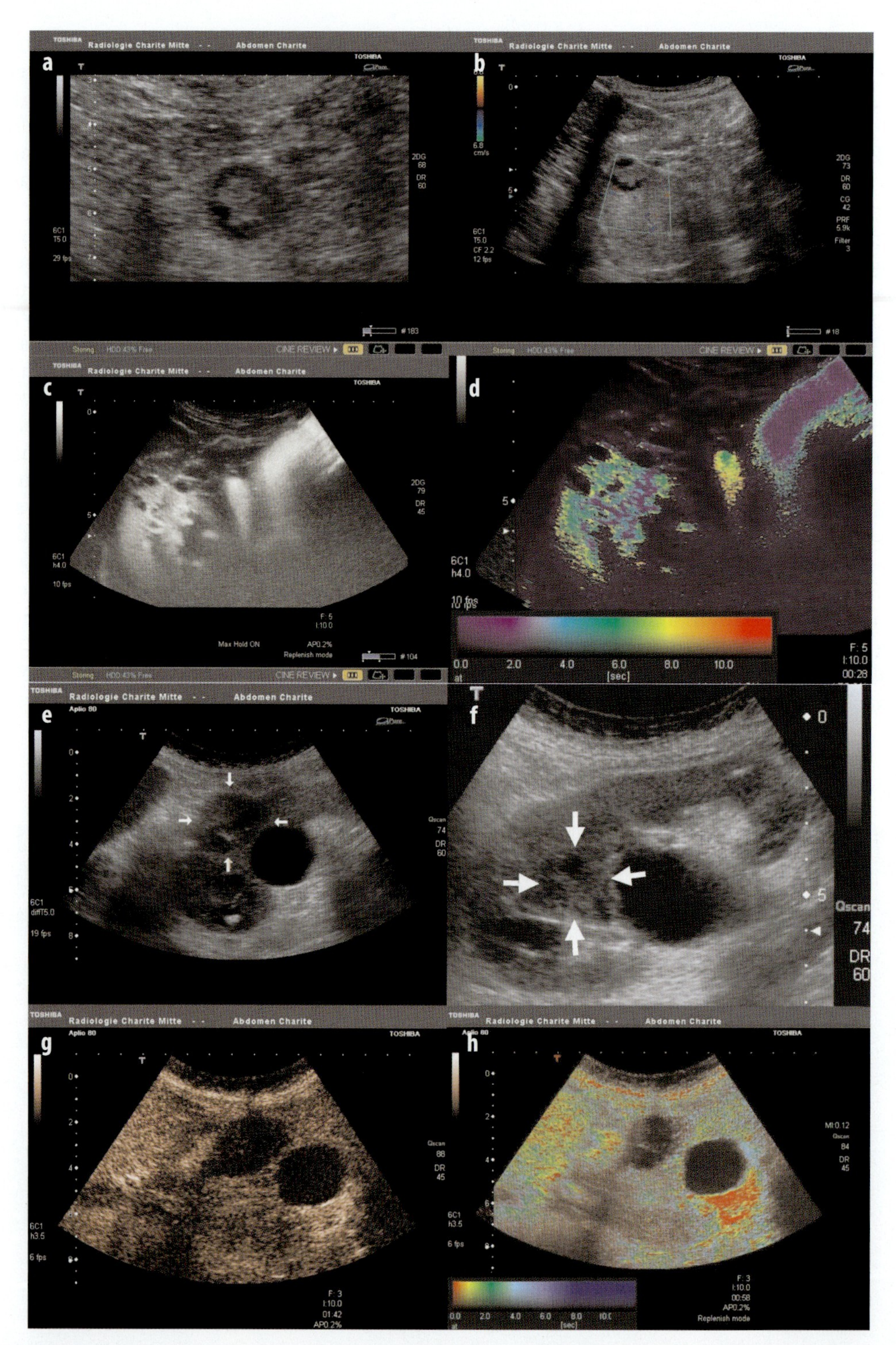

Fig. 12a-h. Lesion with complex echo pattern indicating solid and cystic portions (**a**). CDUS showed only negligible vascularization of the tumor (**b**). A hemorrhagic cyst was diagnosed by unenhanced CT. Contrast US demonstrated tumor vascularization with enhancement of the central tumor portions (**c**). The parametric image shows that maximum intensity in the central tumor portions is reached at the same time as in the renal cortex (**d**). Nearly isoechoic circular lesion (white arrows) adjacent to an uncomplicated cyst shown on transverse view (**e**) and longitudinal view (**f**). No enhancement of the lesion after USCM administration (**g**). There is likewise no enhancement of the lesion over time in the parametric image (**h**). MRI confirmed the diagnosis of a hemorrhagic cyst

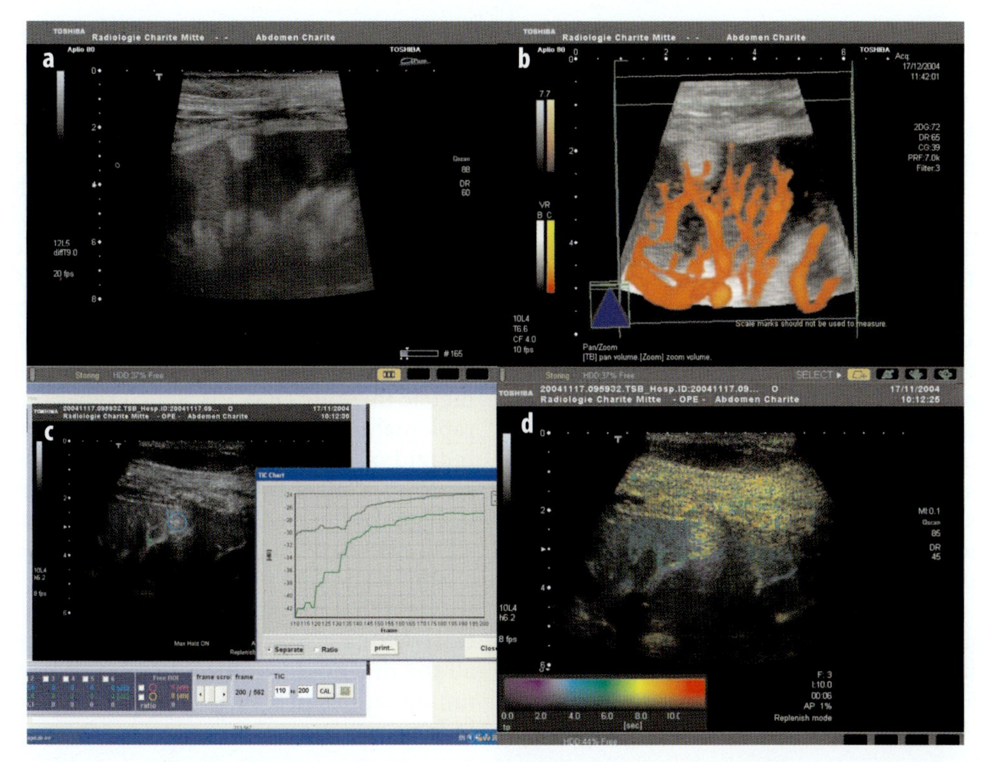

Fig. 13a-d. Depiction of a homogeneously hyperintense and sharply delineated tumor in the middle parenchymal third of the transplanted kidney (**a**). The reconstructed 3D view shows rather moderate tumor vascularization with otherwise normal appearance of the vascular tree (**b**). Delayed and protracted enhancement of the lesion as compared with the interlobar artery (**c**). Good depiction of the tumor also in the parametric image of USCM arrival time (**d**)

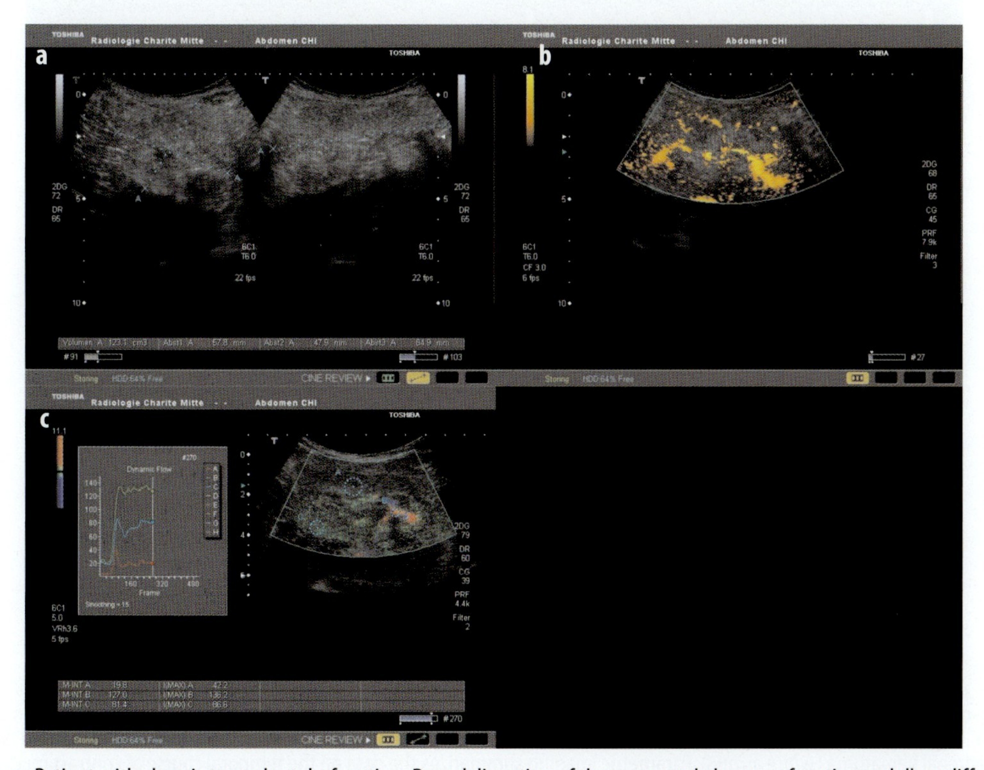

Fig. 14a-c. Patient with chronic transplant dysfunction. Poor delineation of the organ and absence of corticomedullary differentiation in the B-mode (**a**). Power Doppler shows pronounced rarefaction of vessels in the periphery (**b**). Inhomogeneous enhancement of the kidney on vascular recognition imaging with depiction of the blood flow direction in the renal artery (red) and of the stationary bubbles (green) in the renal parenchyma. Interestingly, the curves from the areas with different enhancement show identical times to peak, but different signal intensities as an indication of reduced vascular density in the periphery (**c**)

Finally, contrast US has the potential to be used to monitor the outcome of ablation therapy of renal cell carcinoma as it may serve to guide the minimally invasive intervention and document the ablation defect in a single session [85].

Potential, Prospects, and Limitations of the Method

Studies on the use of contrast ultrasound are limited by the fact that only a fairly small number of patients have been investigated so far. Future studies should therefore aim to enrol large numbers of patients and to evaluate the examiner-dependence of the method. Various options such as the low MI pulse-inversion technique, models for the description of renal perfusion (bolus kinetics and flash replenishment), and the already known applications of contrast US provide a large enough basis for the wide clinical use of this new modality in the routine setting. However, as a 'vessel-oriented modality', contrast US is not able to diagnose Banff I rejection as there is no vascular involvement.

New applications of contrast US will arise from the further technical development of the ultrasound equipment. The rapid technical advances seen in recent years are followed by the introduction of new software tools for the analysis of the raw datasets or the improved visualization of microbubbles at very low energy, for instance by means of techniques that sum and depict the signals from the microbubbles over time (Micro Flow Imaging, Toshiba). This new technique in turn is the basis for so-called parametric imaging (Fig. 15), which relies on bolus or replenishment kinetics and is able to analyze individual curve parameters, such as the time to peak on a pixel-by-pixel basis. The information is displayed in a color-coded image that presents all the US data in a standardized manner. This is a simple and fast technique with a high diagnostic yield that may improve the acceptance of contrast US as a routine diagnostic tool providing all the diagnostic information on contrast medium dynamics in a single image of the transplant kidney.

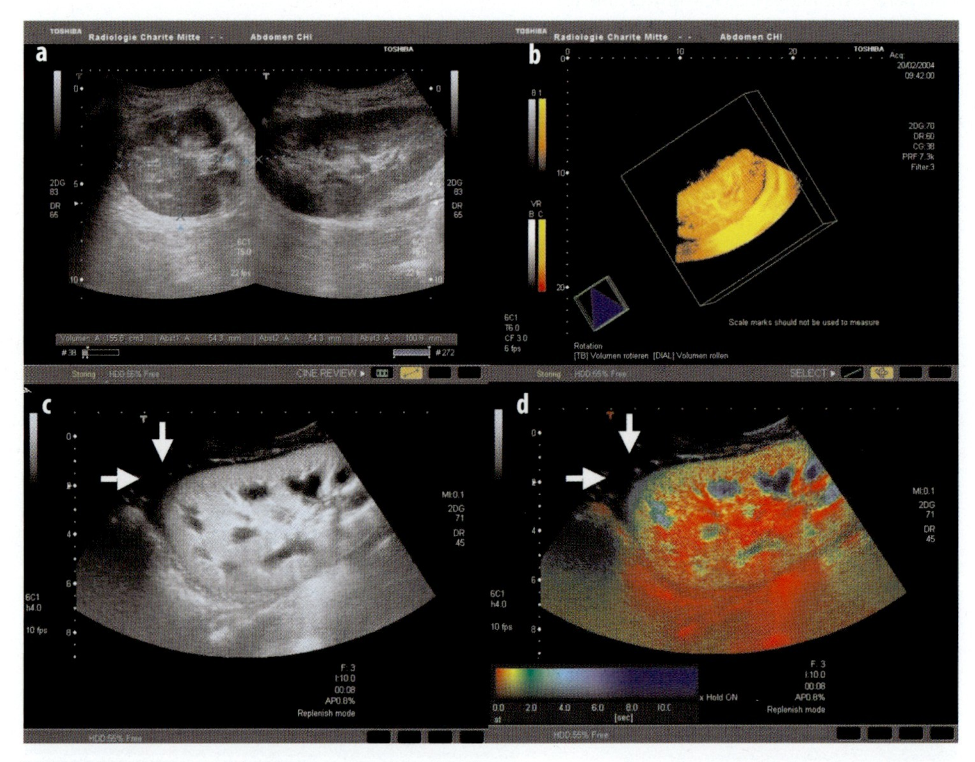

Fig. 15a-d. Normal B-mode scan after kidney transplant (**a**). Homogeneous and good vascularization of the kidney on 3D power Doppler (**b**). Rapid and homogeneous enhancement of the kidney without perfusion defects after CM administration (**c**) and delineation of small perirenal hematoma (*white arrows*). Parametric imaging summarizes the data on the temporal course of contrast medium arrival in a single image. The curve shows rapid enhancement of the renal cortex with a delay only in the area of the hematoma (**d**)

Key Points

- Contrast ultrasound is a promising and straightforward method that is superior to established sonographic techniques such as conventional B-mode scanning (volume measurement, demonstration of hematoma) and color Doppler (rejection, perfusion defects, vascularization) for the diagnostic evaluation of kidney grafts.
- Moreover, contrast US has the potential for tumor characterization in transplanted kidneys. A single examination by contrast ultrasound can answer a variety of questions in the early post-operative phase (rejection) and long-term follow-up (chronic damage).
- Initial studies show that efficient and early diagnosis of rejection or ATN is possible as these conditions have characteristic bolus kinetics curves. Surgical complications, such as perfusion defects secondary to thrombosis of a polar artery or post-operative hematoma, are also identified.
- Perfusion effects of a hematoma can also be assessed.

References

1. Diethelm AG, Deierhoi MH, Hudson SL et al (1995) Progress in renal transplantation. A single center study of 3359 patients over 25 years. Ann Surg 221:446-458
2. Lee HM, Posner MP, King AL et al (1993) Status of long-term (25 years) survival of kidney transplant patients. Transplant Proc 25:1336-1337
3. Alvarez G, Gonzalez-Molina M, Cabello M et al (1991) Pulsed and continuous Doppler evaluation of renal dysfunction after kidney transplantation. Eur J Radiol 12:108-112
4. Arima M, Ogino T, Hosokawa S et al (1989) Functional image diagnosis of kidney transplants using ultrasonic Doppler flowmetry and magnetic resonance imaging. Transplant Proc 21:1907-1911
5. De-Gaetano AM, Boldrini G, Nanni G et al (1989) Noninvasive surveillance of allografted kidneys by ultrasonic duplex scanning. Angiology 40:705-715
6. Flückner F, Steiner H, Horn S et al (1990) Farbkodierte Duplexsonographie and Widerstandsindex bei Nierentransplantaten mit Dysfunction. RoFo 153:692-697
7. Grenier N, Douws C, Morel D et al (1991) Detection of vascular complications in renal allografts with color Doppler flow imaging. Radiology 178:217-223
8. Hollenbeck M (1994) New diagnostic techniques in clinical nephrology. Colour coded duplex sonography of renal transplants – tool or toy for the nephrologist? Nephrol Dial Transplant 9:1822-1828
9. Steinberg HV, Nelson RC, Murphy FB et al (1987) Renal allograft rejection: evaluation by Doppler US and MR Imaging. Radiology 162:337-342
10. Radermacher J, Mengel M, Ellis S et al. (2003) The renal arterial resistance index and renal allograft survival. N Engl J Med 349:182-184
11. Restrepo-Schafer IK, Schwerk WB, Muller TF et al (1999) Intrarenal doppler flow analysis in patients with kidney transplantation and stable transplant function. Ultraschall Med 20:87-92
12. Letourneau JG, Day DL, Feinberg SB (1987) Ultrasound and computed tomographic evaluation of renal transplantation. Radiol Clin North Am 25:267-79
13. Dodd GD, Tublin ME, Shah A et al (1991) Imaging of vascular complications associated with renal transplants. AJR Am J Roentgenol 157:449-59
14. Hollenbeck M, Kutkuhn B, Grabensee B (1994) Colour Doppler ultrasound in the diagnosis of transplant renal artery stenosis. Bildgebung 61:248-54
15. Townsend RR, Tomlanowich SJ, Goldstein RB et al (1990) Combined Doppler and morphologic sonographic evaluation of renal transplant rejection. J Ultrasound Med 9: 199-206
16. Weskott HP (1995) Power US: Phantom measurement of slow flow. Radiology 197:337
17. Waiser J, Schreiber M, Budde K et al (2000) Prognostic value of the Banff classification. Transpl Int 13:106-111
18. Bude RO, Rubin JM, Adler ED (1994) Power versus conventionel color Doppler sonography: comparison in the depiction of normal intrarenal vasculature. Radiology 192:777-780
19. Genkins SM, Sanfilippo FP, Caroll BA (1989) Duplex Doppler sonography of renal transplants: Lack of sensitivity and specificity in establishing pathologic diagnosis. AJR Am J Roentgenol 152:535-539
20. Hollenbeck M, Hilbert N, Meusel F et al (1994) Increasing sensitivity and specificity of Doppler sonographic detection of renal transplant rejection with serial investigation technique. Clin Investig 72:609-615
21. Phillips AO, Deane C, O´Donnell P et al (1994) Evaluation of Doppler ultrasound in primary non-function of renal transplants. Clin Transplant 8:83-86
22. Rigsby CM, Burns PM, Weltin GG et al (1987) Doppler signal quantitation in renal allografts: comparison in normal and rejecting transplants, with pathologic correlation. Radiology 162:39-42

23. Mallek R, Mostbeck G, Kain R et al (1990) Vaskuläre Nierentransplantatabstoßung – Ist eine duplexsonographische Diagnose möglich? RoFo 152:283
24. Hollenbeck M, Stuhrmann M, Trapp R et al (1994) Farbkodierte Dopplersonographie zur Früherkennung von Abstoßungsreaktionen nach allogener Nierentransplantation. Dtsch med Wochenschr 116:921-927
25. Kuo P, Monaco AP (1993) Chronic rejection and suboptimal immunosuppression. Transplant Proc 25:2082
26. Pozniak MA, Dodd GD, Kelcz F (1992) Ultrasonographic evaluation of renal transplantation. Radiol Clin North Am 30:1053-66
27. Fahlenkamp D, Schönberger B, Lindeke A et al (1993) Laparaskopische Lymphozelendrainage nach Nierentransplantation. Z Urologie 2:55-56
28. Benoit G, Bensadoun H, Jardin A (1993) Surgical complications of kidney transplantation. European Urology Update Series 2:178-183
29. Martinoli C, Bertolotto M, Crespi G et al (1998) Duplex Doppler analysis of interlobular arteries in transplanted kidneys. Eur Radiol 8:765-769
30. Takano R, Ando Y, Taniguchi N et al (2001) Power Doppler sonography of the kidney: effect of Valsalva's maneuver. J Clin Ultrasound 29:384-390
31. Schwerk WB, Restrepo IK, Prinz H (1993) Semiquantitative analysis of intrarenal arterial Doppler flow spectra in healthy adults. Ultraschall Med 14:117-122
32. Delbeke D, Sacks GA, Sandler MP (1989) Diagnosis of allograft renal vein thrombosis. Clin Nucl Med 14:415-420
33. Duckett T, Bretan PN, Cochran ST (1991) Noninvasive radiological diagnosis of renal vein thrombosis in renal transplantation. J Urol 46:403-406
34. Laplante S, Patriquin HB, Robitaille P et al (1993) Renal vein thrombosis in children: evidence of early flow recovery with Doppler US. Radiology 189:37-42
35. Birkeland SA, Rohr N, Elbirk A et al (1995) Chronic rejection in kidney transplant patients receiving cytomegalovirus prophylaxis with acyclovir. Transplant Proc 27: 2040-2041
36. Jordan ML, Cook GT, Cardelle CJ (1982) Ten years of experience with vascular complications in renal transplants. J Urol 128:689-692
37. Baxter GM, Ireland H, Moss JG et al (1995) Colour Doppler ultrasound in renal transplant artery stenosis: which Doppler index? Clin Radiol 50:618-622
38. Maia CR, Bittar AE, Goldani JC et al (1992) Doppler ultrasonography for the detection of renal artery stenosis in transplanted kidneys. Hypertension 19:207-209
39. Snider JF, Hunter DW, Moradian GP et al (1989) Transplant renal artery stenosis: evaluation with duplex sonography. Radiology 172:1027-1030
40. Deane C, Cowan N, Giles J et al (1992) Arteriovenous fistulas in renal transplants: color Doppler ultrasound observations. Urol Radiol 13:211-217
41. Griffin JF, McNicholas MM (1992) Morphological appearance of renal allografts in transplant failure. J Clin Ultrasound 20:529-537
42. Jansen O, Rob PM, Schmidtke V et al (1992) Follow-up study of renal transplants by duplex Doppler and grey scaleultrasound. Eur J Radiol 15:26-31
43. Renowden SA, Blethyn J, Cochlin DL (1992) Renal transplant sonography: correlation of Doppler and biopsy results in cellular rejection. Clin Radiol 46:265-269
44. Blane CE, Gagnadoux MF, Brunelle F et al (1993) Doppler ultrasonography in the early postoperative evaluation of renal transplants in children. Can Assoc Radiol J 44:176-178
45. Saarinen O (1991) Diagnostic value of resistive index of renal transplants in the early postoperative period. Acta Radiol 32:166-169
46. Di Palo FQ, Rivolta R, Elli A et al (1993) Effect of cyclosporin A on renal cortical resistances measured by color doppler flowmetry on renal grafts. Nephron 65:240-244
47. Stevens PE, Gwyther SJ, Hanson ME et al (1993) Interpretation of duplex Doppler ultrasound in renal transplants in the early postoperative period. Nephrol Dial Transplant 8:255-258
48. Hollenbeck M, Hetzel GR, Hilbert N et al (1995) Dopplersonographische Beurteilung der Effektivität einer Abstoßungstherapie nach Nierentransplantation. Dtsch med Wschr 120:277-282
49. Häyry P, Yilmaz S (1994) Chronic allograft rejection: An update. Transplant Proc 26:3159-3160
50. Saarinen O, Salmela K, Edgren J (1994) Doppler ultrasound in the diagnosis of renal transplant artery stenosis-value of resistive index. Acta Radiol 35:586-589
51. Rubin JM, Bude RO, Carson PL et al (1994) Power Doppler US: potentially useful alternative to mean frequency-based color Doppler US. Radiology 190:853-856
52. Mihatsch MJ, Ryffel B, Gudat F (1993) Morphological criteria of chronic rejection: differential diagnosis, including cyclosporine nephropathy. Transplant Proc 25:2031-2037
53. Bude RO, Rubin JM, Adler RD (1994) Power versus conventional color Doppler sonography: comparison in the depiction of normal intrarenal vasculature. Radiology 192:777-780
54. Mutze S, Overhoff M, Filimonow S et al (1996) Ultraschalldiagnostik der Transplantatniere. Radiologe 36:31-37
55. Pallardó LM, Sánchez J, Puig N et al (1995) Chronic rejection in 500 kidney transplant patients treated with cyclosporine: incidence and risk factors. Transplant Proc 27:2215-2216
56. Fischer T, Mühler M, Kröncke TJ et al (2004) Early Postoperative Ultrasound of Kidney Transplants: Evaluation of Contrast Medium Dynamics Using Time-intensity Curves. RoFo 176:472-477
57. Pudszuhn A, Marx C, Malich A et al (2003) Prospective Analysis of Quantification of Contrast Media Enhanced Power Doppler Sonography of Equivocal Breast Lesions. RoFo 175:495-501
58. Dietrich CF (2002) 3D real time contrast-enhanced ultrasonography, a new technique. RoFo 174:160-163
59. Hohmann J, Skrok J, Puls R et al (2003) Characterization of focal liver lesions with contrast-enhanced low MI real time ultrasound and SonoVue. RoFo 175:835-843
60. Quaia E, Bertolotto M, Calderan L et al (2003) US characterization of focal hepatic lesions with intermittent high-acoustic-power mode and contrast material. Acad Radiol 10:739-750

61. Basilico R, Blomley MJ, Harvey CJ et al (2002) Which continuous US scanning mode is optimal for the detection of vascularity in liver lesions when enhanced with a second generation contrast agent? Eur J Radiol. 41:184-191
62. Schlosser T, Pohl C, Veltmann C (2001) Feasibility of the flash-replenishment concept in renal tissue: which parameters affect the assessment of the contrast replenishment? Ultrasound Med Biol 27:937-944
63. Wei K, Le E, Bin JP et al (2001) Quantification of renal blood flow with contrast-enhanced ultrasound. J Am Coll Cardiol 37:1135-1140
64. Girard MS, Mattrey RF, Baker KG et al (2000) Comparison of Standard and Second Harmonic B-mode Sonography in the Detection of Segmental Renal Infarction with SonographicContrast in a Rabbit Model. J Ultrasound Med 19:185-192
65. Nilsson A (2004) Contrast-enhanced ultrasound of the kidneys. Eur Radiol 8:104-109
66. Bokor D, Chambers JB, Rees PJ et al (2001) Clinical safety of SonoVue, a new contrast agent for ultrasound imaging, in healthy volunteers and in patients with chronic obstructive pulmonary disease. Invest Radiol 36:104-109
67. Correas JM, Claudon M, Tranquart F et al (2003) Contrast-enhanced ultrasonography: renal applications. J Radiol 84:2041-2054
68. Lucidarme O, Franchi-Abella S, Correas JM et al (2003) Blood flow quantification with contrast-enhanced US: "entrance in the section" phenomenon-phantom and rabbit study. Radiology 228:298-299
69. Nahar T, Li P, Kuersten B et al (2003) Detection of resting myocardial perfusion defects by SonoVue myocardial contrast echocardiography. Echocardiography 20:511-517
70. Schlosser T, Veltmann C, Lohmaier S et al (2004) Determination of the renal blood flow in macro- and microcirculation by means of pulse inversion imaging. RoFo 176:724-730
71. Bouakaz A, Krenning BJ, Vletter WB et al (2003) Contrast superharmonic imaging: a feasibility study. Ultrasound Med Biol. 29:547-553
72. Siracusano S, Quaia E, Bertolotto M et al (2004) The application of ultrasound contrast agents in the charcterization of renal tumors. World J Urol 22:316-322
73. Lacourciere Y, Levesque J, Onrot JM et al (2002) Impact of Levovist ultrasonographic contrast agent on the diagnosis and management of hypertensive patients with suspected renal artery stenosis: a Canadian multicentre pilot study. Can Assoc Radiol J 53:219-227
74. Lefevre F, Correas JM, Briancon S et al (2002) Contrast-enhanced sonography of the renal transplant using triggered pulse-inversion imaging: preliminary results. Ultrasound Med Biol 28:303-314
75. Robbin ML, Lockhart ME, Barr RG (2003) Renal imaging with ultrasound contrast: current status. Radiol Clin North Am 41:963-978
76. Krix M, Kauczor HU, Delorme S (2003) Quantification of tissue perfusion with novel ultrasound methods. Radiologe 43:823-830
77. Pollard RE, Sadlowski AR, Bloch SH et al (2002) Contrast-assisted destruction-replenishment ultrasound for the assessment of tumor microvasculature in a rat model Technol Cancer Res Treat 1:459-470
78. Wei K, Jayaweera AR, Firoozan S et al (1998) Quantification of myocardial blood flow with ultrasound -induced destruction of microbubbles administered as aconstant venous infusion. Circulation 97:473-483
79. Fischer T, Ebeling V, Giessing M (2006) A new method for standardized diagnosis following renal transplantation: ultrasound loith contrast-enhancement. Urologe A 45(1):38-45
80. Argalia G, Cacciamani L, Fazi R et al (2004) Contrast-enhanced sonography in the diagnosis of renal artery stenosis: comparison with MR-angiography. Radiol Med 107:208-217
81. Blebea J, Zickler R, Volteas N et al (2003) Duplex imaging of the renal arteries with contrast-enhancement. Vasc Endovascular Surg 37:429-436
82. Teixeira OU, Bortolotto LA, Silva HB (2004) The contrast-enhanced Doppler ultrasound with perfluorocarbon exposed sonicated albumin does not improve the diagnosis of renal artery stenosis compared with angiography. J Negat Results Biomed 3:3
83. Ascenti G, Gaeta M, Magno C et al (2004) Contrast-enhanced second -harmonic sonography in the detection of pseudocapsule in renal cell carcinoma. AJR Am J Roentgenol. 182:1525-1530
84. Kreft B, Schild HH (2003) Cystic renal lesions. RoFo 175:892-903
85. Veltri A, De Fazio G, Malfitana V et al (2004) Percutaneous US-guided RF thermal ablation for malignant renal tumors: preliminary results in 13 patients. Eur Radiol 14:2303-2310

IV.3

Contrast-Enhanced Ultrasound in Low-Energy Blunt Abdominal Trauma

Lars Thorelius

Introduction

Emergency clinics in general are confronted with a wide variety of trauma cases involving the abdomen. High-energy trauma often causes major damage to the parenchymal organs as well as to large vessels, resulting in life-threatening intra-abdominal bleeding. Sometimes the patient requires immediate surgical attention in order to survive, leaving no time for medical imaging to detect the source of the haemorrhage. Contrast-enhanced computed tomography (CT) is the modality of choice when the patient is stable enough that the time of imaging can be tolerated. With modern multi-slice CT scanners, a high-resolution exam of the entire thorax and abdomen is acquired in a minute or less. Multi-format 3D volumes are available almost immediately after the exam. With decreasing trauma energy there is less likelihood of life-threatening or disabling injuries. However, patients appearing at the emergency clinic after minor abdominal trauma may also be affected by abdominal injuries and haemorrhage. Sports injuries, playground falls and horse riding accidents are a few examples of common causes of low-energy trauma that occasionally cause parenchymal damage, with the potential risk of further haemorrhage. Fortunately, a substantial number of these patients are unharmed. Any abdominal injury is often limited and generally involves the spleen, liver or kidneys. Other organs are only rarely involved. Hence, medical imaging is indicated following low-energy trauma as a precautionary measure rather than as a necessity. To date, contrast-enhanced CT is the only relevant modality for excluding parenchymal injuries. With access to faster CT scanners the number of such precautionary exams is likely to increase in the future. Considering the high incidence of low-energy trauma with negative CT exams, and the usually conservative treatment when an injury is discovered, the drawbacks of radiation exposure and high doses of iodine contrast cannot be ignored. The fact that many of the patients are otherwise young and healthy individuals even further emphasises the gravity of exposing them to radiation through CT exams.

Baseline Ultrasound

Today ultrasound (US) has an established role in many emergency centres in cases of multi-trauma as a quick and readily available first-line imaging modality for the detection of free fluid. Focused Assessment with Sonography in Trauma (FAST) is a fast selective approach for the assessment of fluid in the peri-cardium and the abdomen. A significant amount of free fluid is an indication of substantial haemorrhage requiring immediate surgical attention. In other cases, FAST can guide the clinician to further exams with angiography or CT. Severe trauma may cause injuries to any abdominal structure, and US is not sufficient for extensive abdominal trauma screening for a number of reasons, of which poor access due to gas and bone are important limiting factors. CT is mandatory in such cases. The lack of free abdominal fluid is by no means a guarantee for intact parenchymal organs. According to one report, up to 40% of trauma patients without free fluid have parenchymal damage. Despite much research and many efforts, US unfortunately remains ineffective for accurate visualisation of parenchymal injuries and haematomas. This inefficiency means that US is not recommended for use in stable trauma patients.

The spleen, liver and kidneys are usually readily accessible with US in suitable patients. Unfortunately, even large parenchymal lacerations and subcapsular haematomas are often isoechoic with the adjacent parenchyma. The structural difference to the parenchyma is often not obvious. When the laceration can be seen with US the size of the damage is usually very difficult to determine. The extent of the injury is frequently underestimated. Consequently, there is no proper place for US in the assessment of parenchymal damage. Hence, US should not be used to try to rule out parenchymal damage in low-energy trauma. Contrast-enhanced CT has to date been the only relevant modality for this purpose.

Contrast Ultrasound Features

With the introduction of Ultrasound Contrast Agents (UCA) that sustain continuous exposure to US with low mechanical index (MI), Contrast-Enhanced UltraSound (CEUS) may have the potential to become an efficient and welcome alternative to CT for the visualisation of parenchymal lacerations and haematomas.

We use Siemens Acuson Sequoia machines equipped with CPS, which is a special UCA option. This option can colour-code fundamental frequency US reflections that are unique to microbubbles, making CEUS truly contrast-specific. With this technique the contrast sensitivity is greatly increased over harmonic imaging at the expense of a slight reduction of spatial resolution and a moderate reduction of frame rate. In practice, different brands of US machines perform differently with regard to CEUS. The suggestions presented here may not apply entirely to other machines. Also, different UCAs may perform differently. We have used SonoVue (Bracco, Italy) for our studies. Our experiences may not apply directly if another UCA is used.

A brief elaboration on the dynamics behind imaging of vascular focal lesions is relevant in order to clarify the principles behind CEUS detection of traumatic parenchymal damage.

Obviously, contrast agent imaging modalities like CEUS, CT and magnetic resonance imaging (MRI) can depict the concentration of their contrast agents. After a bolus injection of contrast, the human eye is not very efficient at determining the absolute quantity of the enhancement of a parenchyma, but it can visualise enhancement differences between a focal lesion and the adjacent organ parenchyma quite well. The difference in bolus enhancement dynamics between the focal lesion and the surrounding organ parenchyma adds a dynamic component to the morphological pattern of structures, with the normal parenchymal parts of the pattern acting as a known reference. Although the enhancement difference between the lesion and the parenchyma may be small, and the duration of the pathology-specific moment may be short, the method of comparing the enhancement differences between the lesion and the parenchyma with the naked eye over time is considered to be quite reliable for characterisation of focal lesions with the different modalities. When there is a certain degree of sustained enhancement difference in the late vascular phase, the visual detection of focal lesions is also generally accepted. There is scientific support for the fact that the bolus characteristics of different focal lesions in the liver are equal or very similar when comparing CEUS with CT and MRI. Studies have also supported the observation that CEUS is not less sensitive than CT or MRI at detecting liver metastases. Although not yet scientifically proven, the parenchyma of the spleen also seems very similar when compared on the different modalities. However, there is a big difference between CEUS when compared to CT and MRI regarding the renal parenchyma, since microbubbles are a pure blood pool agent which lack a urine excretory phase, as opposed to contrast media for CT and MRI.

The similarities between CEUS and CT discussed above are very important when considering new CEUS applications where CT is well established, such as traumatic parenchymal injuries. In our experience, using proper software, US is extremely sensitive to the presence of minute concentrations of microbubbles. In fact, we find that the sensitivity to the difference between the presence and absence of small concentrations of contrast is generally considerably greater with CEUS than with CT. In other words, we think that the absence of contrast signal in a structure is of higher predictive value for the tissue being truly avascular when examined with CEUS rather than with CT, provided that there is a strong detectable contrast signal in the adjacent structures. Our experience is based on exams of known avascular structures, mainly simple cysts in the liver and kidneys and necrotic parts of tumours that have been examined with contrast-enhanced CT and referred to the US department for biopsy. With the CPS contrast-specific software, the cysts are completely black against the brightly enhancing and software-coloured parenchymal enhancement that surrounds it. In tumours there is sometimes a diffuse gradual decrease of CT contrast towards necrotic areas, which makes it difficult to exactly pinpoint the margins of remaining vascularity. With CEUS, the enhancement of the margins is usually delineated from the necrosis with a sharp edge. Sometimes CEUS detects minimal strands of vascular tissue containing slowly moving contrast-enhancing dots in the necrotic margins. These strands often have no evident counterparts in the CT exam. By the appearance of the dots in the least enhancing structures it seems that the CPS software is sensitive to small conglomerates of microbubbles, or maybe even to single microbubbles, that are grossly exaggerated in size by the software and thus visible on the screen as dots of light. Sometimes these dots clearly move with the circulation. These dots seem to constitute the smallest possible quanta of contrast signal. By appearance the next step down would be total absence of microbubbles. The corresponding minute concentration of iodine contrast is probably not detectable with CT (Fig. 1.)

Our experience of CEUS for parenchymal injuries began in 2002, and to date we have regularly performed exams on parenchymal damage. Although this series includes one pancreatic contusion, the spleen, liver and kidneys (in that order) have been most commonly observed both with regard to suspected injuries and positive results. Several cases have been multi-trauma cases where CEUS was performed because of unclear CT findings or unexpected symptoms. Such cases are beyond the scope of this article, but of course they contribute to our overall experience of parenchymal injuries.

Our hypothesis is that CEUS is well suited for the detection and mapping of traumatic parenchymal injuries considering the conspicuous nature of avascular areas in enhanced parenchyma. Blunt parenchymal trauma may cause a variety of injuries including lacerations, contusions, haematomas, capsule ruptures and vessel tears of different severity. In low-energy blunt abdominal trauma there is often no parenchymal damage at all, and in cases of injuries, these are mild to moderate and treated conservatively in the vast majority of cases. Regardless of injury type and severity they all share a common denominator, which is hypovascular contusions or avascular haematomas in lacerations or outside the parenchyma and the capsule of the organ. After the immediate haemorrhage has stopped there is no connection between the blood stream and haematomas, rendering them avascular structures. Parenchymal contusion areas have various degrees of decreased perfusion because of crushing rather than tearing of the parenchyma. Presumably, the less intact the perfusion, the worse and more vulnerable is the contusion injury. Some contusion areas are vaguely visible, maybe representing only an oedema and not true tissue disruption. When being presented to a trauma patient we know in advance that we will concentrate our CEUS exam on finding or ruling out avascular haematomas or hypovascular injuries. We do not have to take any dynamic vascular patterns of the injuries into account.

Normally the liver circulation is divided into the arterial phase, the portal phase and the late phase. In the search for fissures and other haemorrhagic injuries of blunt trauma, a different and simpler bolus phase description can be used to explain how to administer the UCA. In our experience, for this purpose the bolus circulation can be divided according to the visual appearance of homogeneity in the parenchyma. When disregarding identifiable vessels and studying a homogeneous part of any normal organ parenchyma with CEUS including the liver, there are three phases to consider. The first phase begins when the first small arterial vessels appear, and ends when the last parenchymal enhancement variations disappear. At this point the second phase begins, lasting until the appearance of the first

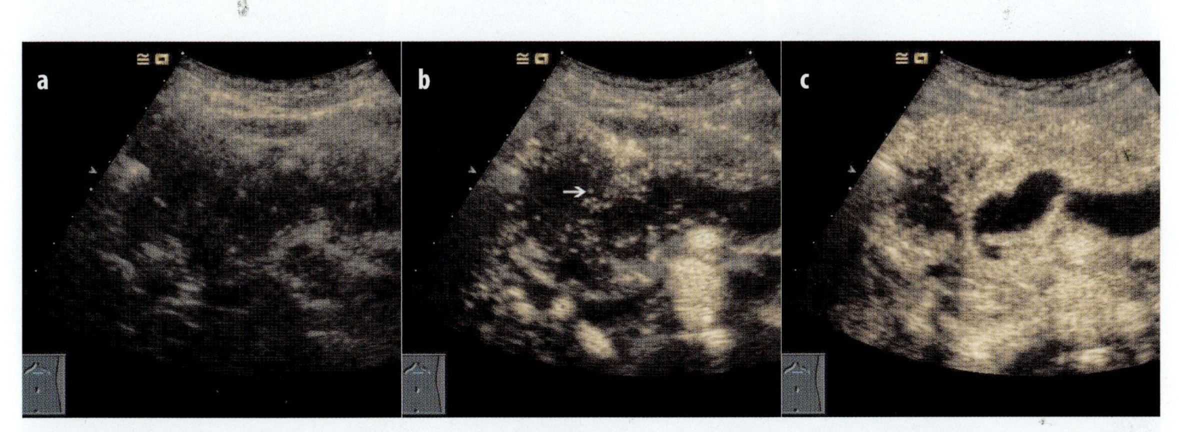

Fig. 1a-c. The arterial phase of a necrotic pancreas cancer. **a** Before arterial phase. **b** Early arterial phase showing the first individual "dots" of enhancement. **c** Later arterial phase with homogeneous enhancement

visible signs of microbubble destruction with diffuse irregular strands or patches of inhomogeneous enhancement, or until wash-out of the UCA begins to reveal a disturbing image of small contrast dots. Thus, the third phase begins with the first visible sign of irregular enhancement and continues until the absence UCA.

During all three phases, traumatic injuries lack or have very little enhancement and are potentially detectable. Although many fresh injuries are visible already in phase one, the second phase provides the optimal conditions for the detection of the thinnest lacerations and haematomas due to the homogeneity of the parenchymal background enhancement. In phase three the conditions deteriorate rather quickly. Phase two is the truly efficient injury detection phase, and I choose to call this phase 'the homogeneous phase' since it describes the mechanism behind its efficiency. Again, observe that these phases are not analogous with the traditional arterial, portal and late phases that are relevant for vascular parenchymal lesions. To our knowledge, the homogeneous phase is useful only for the detection of structures with no or very little vascularisation (Fig. 2). We have observed a minute contrast-enhancement in some cases of otherwise very sharply delineated and quite wide lacerations, whereas others have been totally void of any enhancement. To our knowledge, this slight enhancement within some sharply margined presumed rifts has not been clearly demonstrated with other modalities that lack the extreme contrast sensitivity of CEUS. These cases of slight enhancement are difficult to explain, but evidently they point to a complexity of parenchymal damage mechanisms with the existence of previously unrecognised tear-like contusions (Fig. 3).

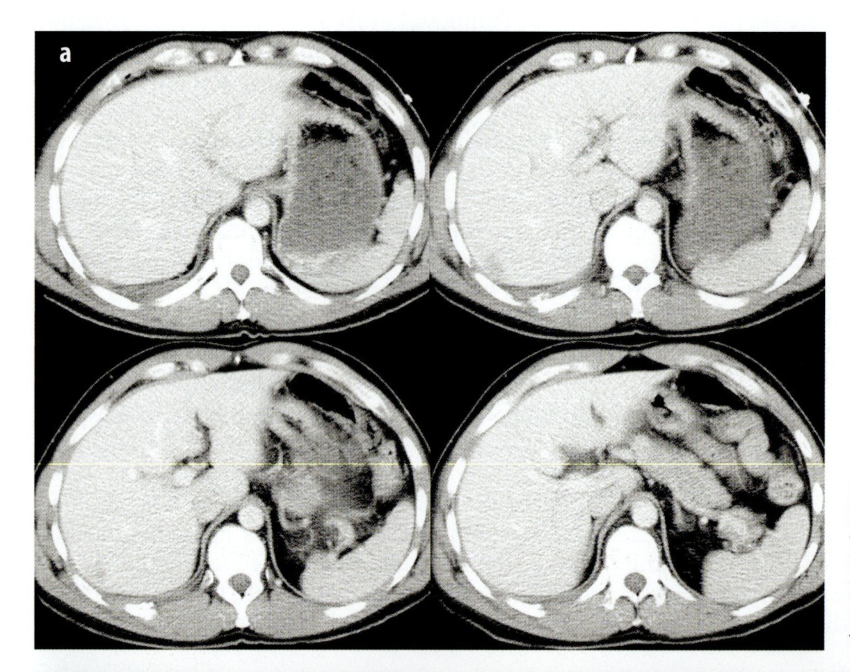

Fig. 2a, b. a CT of small trauma injury in the liver surface. **b** First image is US with trauma findings. Second to fifth images are CEUS in the early phase going to the homogeneous phase. The laceration is hidden among irregularities before the homogeneous phase

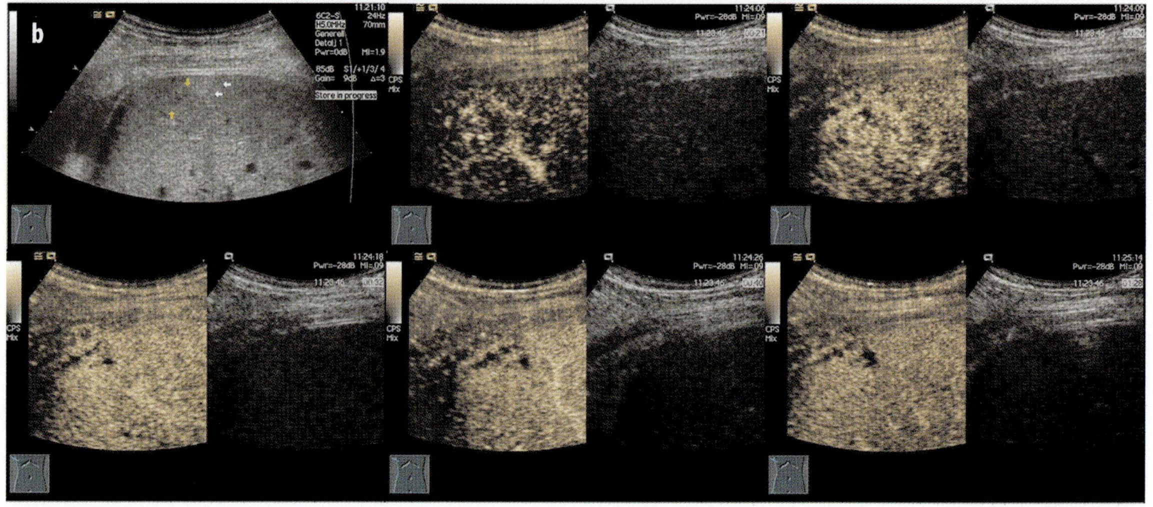

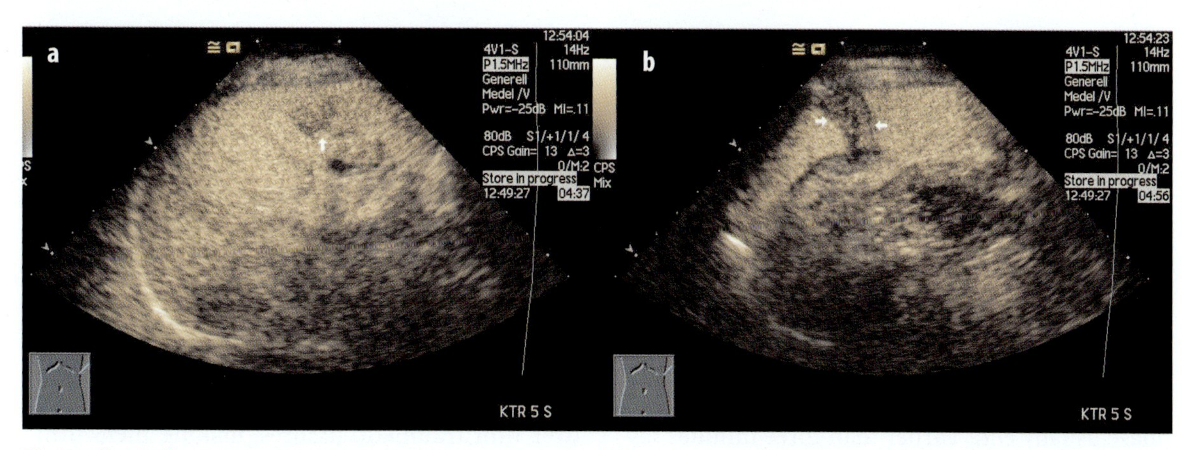

Fig. 3a, b. a Well vascularised contusion or oedema in splenic injury. **b** Sharply demarcated laceration with small amount of remaining circulation

The spleen enhances very brightly and has a first enhancement phase with an initial image of diffuse irregular patches, also well known from CT. Phase two may not begin until close to one minute from the injection. The accumulation of UCA in the parenchyma seems quite robust and usually allows the injury detection phase to last until about five minutes after injection. This is usually more than enough to cover the spleen to satisfaction. One disturbing factor that is not correlated with the three enhancement phases described is a common, quite rapid decrease of UCA concentration in the parenchymal splenic veins. About two to three minutes following the injection the veins turn dark, and are subsequently virtually black. This is probably due to an effective filtration of microbubbles from the circulation by the spleen. We have observed a clear reduction of the UCA concentration in the splenic vein compared to the superior mesentery vein in late phases of portal vein studies. This observation probably supports the filtration theory. In the beginning this phenomenon was somewhat confusing, as the veins could be mistaken for lacerations, but with the problem in mind it is not difficult to separate the two phenomena. If in doubt, a few enhancing dots can always be seen passing the vein. With the combination of grey-scale and colour-coded contrast it is often still easier to separate the black veins from the usually grey lacerations. A re-injection is another efficient solution to the problem. With proper video documentation, a re-run of loops will almost always disclose the fact that a thin laceration is extended beyond the shape of a tubular structure. Far from the hilum this problem does not exist in practice (Fig. 4). The liver has the fastest practical onset of the homogeneous phase, beginning about 40 seconds after injection, or slightly earlier. The homogeneous phase lasts until about four minutes after injection. For some reason, some individuals have a fast decrease of enhancement in the parenchymal

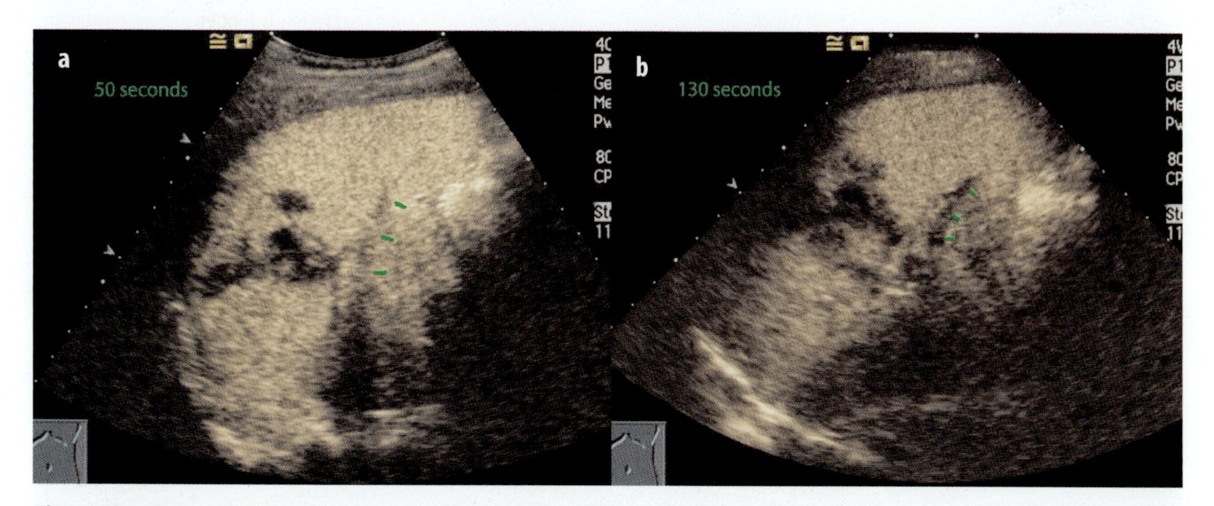

Fig. 4a, b. a Quite wide laceration in the spleen following blunt left flank trauma. Injuries of this size are clearly seen in all contrast phases, here 50 seconds after bolus. Large vein marked green. **b** After 130 seconds the vein is very dark with a few dots of UCA passing. Laceration is still conspicuous

veins, similar to that of the spleen. This reduction has never been observed to be as complete as in the spleen so there is little practical risk of confusion with lacerations. However, livers that do not display the early vein darkening are less disturbing to examine. In this majority of cases, exclusion of tiny injuries may be slightly more efficient.

The kidneys have the most complex bolus enhancement pattern and the fastest third phase. Initially there is strong enhancement of the cortex, followed by gradual filling of the pyramids from the periphery. The pyramids are filled about 30-40 seconds after injection. The homogeneous phase usually ends earlier than three minutes following injection. Usually there is enough time to cover one kidney satisfactorily, but the two kidneys require separate injections. With a proper dose of UCA, the enhancement of the pyramids is visually slightly weaker than that of the cortex because of their substantially lower perfusion. In the relatively few cases of renal injury that we have seen, this has not caused any diagnostic problems. The enhancement of the pyramids is still an efficient background for traumatic lesions, proven by the conspicuous blackness of small simple renal cysts that are frequently encountered in cases of renal CEUS. The third phase of the kidneys is caused more by wash-out than by UCA deterioration. We have not observed darkening of the renal veins. There is quite a dense flow of contrast dots in the veins even very late in the third phase.

For the special purpose of injury detection, a long homogeneous phase is desirable. Since practically no enhancement occurs in the injuries, the second phase can be prolonged by additional injections of UCA until the organ is sufficiently covered. Usually the homogeneous phase provides plenty of time for a full organ exam, but the liver sometimes requires an additional injection of half the original bolus about four minutes after the first injection. A continuous infusion would probably be ideal, but we have no experience of infusion in trauma patients.

Generally speaking, regardless of different organ characteristics, UCA doses in trauma should be kept lower than for most other applications. An injection of too much UCA seems to result in a thin, diffuse zone of 'bleeding' of the contrast echo into structures immediately adjacent to enhanced parenchyma. This artefact sometimes has a negative effect by casting a 'glare' over thin traumatic fissures, making them difficult to detect. Such fissures are sometimes only a few millimetres wide, although they may extend from side to side of the organs. Another disadvantage of an enhancement that is too intense is that it masks the decrease in perfusion caused by oedema surrounding a laceration or in a contusion. In CT, such diffuse oedemas in the parenchyma are very clear and may have a tendency to exaggerate the size of non-viable injuries in the parenchyma. Opposed to this, usually CEUS displays the viability of the entire parenchyma very distinctly, but if too much UCA has been injected the enhancement decrease of mild contusions cannot be appreciated visually. In our experience, this artefact can be avoided by continuous examination of the parenchyma as the microbubble concentration decreases, but it is better to try to avoid the artefact by injecting less UCA than normally recommended for other indications. Oedematous contusion areas with remaining circulation are especially easy to see in the early homogeneous phase with a apropriately low initial dose. A slow injection of the UCA and the subsequent saline also decreases the intensity of the initial arterial enhancement peak (Fig. 5).

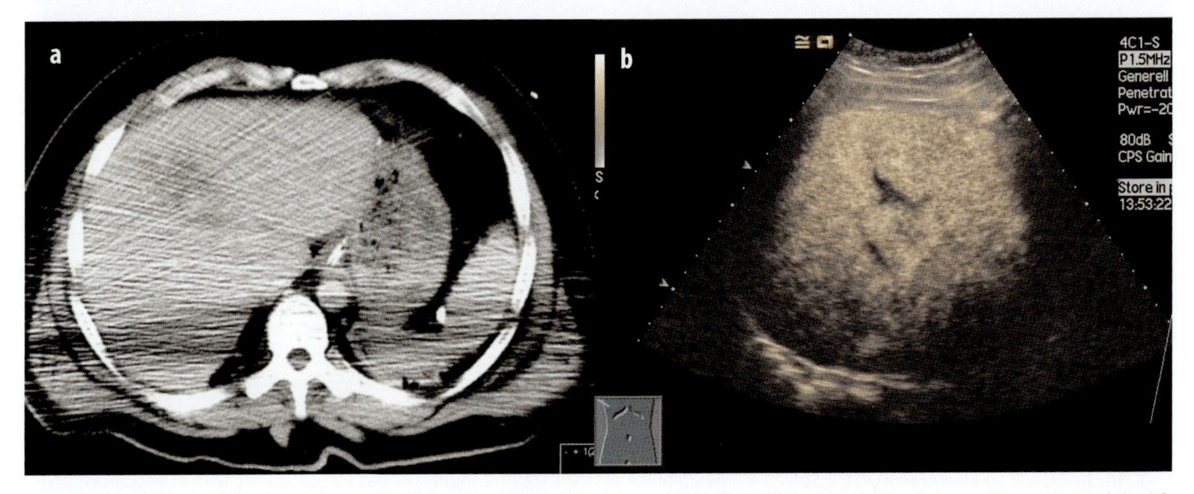

Fig. 5a, b. a Motorcycle trauma. CT with artefacts shows diffuse dark area in liver. **b** CEUS depicts sharp margins of laceration, while diffuse margin on CT is believed to be viable parenchyma with oedema

Dose Recommendations

Generally speaking, patient size and shape are obviously important determinants when deciding the optimal contrast dose for different organs and indications. In trauma there are two kinds of pathology mainly responsible for determining the optimal dose. In our practice, CEUS is performed on about 20% of all our patients, annually about 1400 CEUS patients. Some of our patients are children, on whom we also perform CEUS for an accurate result in individual cases, if necessary. On some indications paediatric use of CEUS is essential for an accurate outcome, and parenchymal traumatic injury is a very clear indication for CEUS since US inefficiently assesses parenchymal damage. To date, we have given SonoVue about 120 times to children, ranging in age from newborn to 17 years-old, in doses from 0.05 ml to 4.8 ml. We have never encountered any adverse effects of SonoVue in any of our 4000 patients, including the children. The single most frequent indication in children has been blunt abdominal trauma. So far SonoVue has an exceptional tolerance level among our patients. SonoVue doses have not been officially established for use in children, but in our experience so far a dose roughly calculated by the following formula has given good imaging results:

Dose (millilitres) = Patient age (years)/10 for the liver, and half that dose for the spleen and kidneys, not below 0.1 ml.

Using the regular 1.5 MHz CPS transducer with the lowest possible MI, a 0.1 ml bolus followed by injection in the foot of 1 ml of saline using a thin needle was very useful for the diagnosis of a renal infarction in a full-term newborn baby with haematuria. The injection provided the enhancement of the retroperitoneal fat necessary to prove the blackness of the kidney. Initially, a bolus of 0.05 ml was tried, but was not sufficient. Such a small dose is technically difficult to handle without dilution. Peritoneal and retroperitoneal fat enhancement is normally clearly seen also in adults following normal contrast doses.

There are many factors involved in determining the optimal dose for children, and we do not claim to be in control of all parameters. The most important observation is the absence of adverse effects in combination with good imaging results. On that basis, we propose the formula above as a starting point for further fine-tuning of the recommendations. Meanwhile, we are quite convinced that our suggested doses will provide good imaging results in clinical cases where CEUS can be expected to deliver valuable medical information. We also believe that this procedure is safe for the children.

Of course, our experience of contrast administration in adults is considerably larger. In parenchymal trauma in non-obese adults it is advisable to use about 1.2-1.6 ml for the liver and 0.6 ml for the spleen and kidneys. If too much UCA is given, the parenchymal accumulation of contrast becomes so dense that the US energy is attenuated in the shallow areas, making the deeper parts of the organ difficult to access.

In all patients, including children, we use the CPS-optimized 1.5-2.5 MHz sector transducer for CEUS, with 1.5 MHz as the default. The 1.5-2.5 MHz CPS-optimised vector transducer with smaller footprint is used, when necessary, for proper access, but this slightly reduces the spatial resolution. There is also a 2-3 MHz CPS-optimised sector transducer with excellent resolution, but in our opinion it is generally not contrast-sensitive enough to replace the other transducers in most trauma applications, with the exception of small children or very thin adults. With the default transducers, the resolution of the image can also be increased by choosing the higher frequencies, but this is at the expense of a signal intensity. Generally speaking, the highest sensitivity to thin fissures is obtained by the high signal intensity of the default setting. This setting also provides the best penetration. It is essential to maintain a high frame rate, preferably above 15 fps. Using the zoom box to carefully zoom in on the organ is an efficient way to increase frame rate and noticeably optimize overall image quality, but MI must then be lowered to compensate for the increase of frame rate and scan line density in order not to disrupt the microbubbles. If in doubt, I advise a small sacrifice of sharpness to reach a sufficient frame rate, since thin fissures are easily overlooked if the frame rate is too low.

Ultrasound in Clinical Practice

In our practice, CEUS is increasingly used as the first modality for patients with low-energy blunt abdominal trauma, preferably to one side, if a senior sonologist is on duty. In the absence of a qualified sonologist, no trauma patients are examined with US or CEUS, and CT is performed instead. We discourage any use of US alone for these patients. On the other hand, CT referrals are increasingly being converted to CEUS in suitable trauma cases in the presence of an experienced sonologist, especially in young patients. If we determine that the patient is not able to cooperate well enough for accurate results, or if the essential organs are inaccessible with US, the patient is transferred to CT. The optimal CEUS procedures for trauma are of course subject to discussion and may very well be altered by ourselves or others. Today, with reference to our other CEUS experience, we have decided to work as described in the effort to build up a structured knowledge base for further improvements. In the following text the descriptions of UCA doses are limited to adults. Children are presently given doses in accordance with the formula discussed earlier.

For our CEUS procedures in general we depend to great extent on our dedicated US workstations and organ specific 5-10 second-long standardised scans mixed with free scanning. Parenchymal trauma is no exception. Of course, much of the diagnostic work is done bedside, but as for all CEUS procedures, storage of full frame rate dynamic clips is required for softcopy reading of details. With some experience, this method is quick and efficient. At the workstation we quite often find additional valuable information that was overlooked bedside. The re-evaluation procedure has often spared the time of another injection and examination.

We begin by assessing free fluid according to the FAST protocol. We always perform US and CEUS on the side of obvious discomfort and, depending on the case, also on the other side. During US, the optimal patient positions, breath positions and the accessibility of the organ are assessed for planning of CEUS. For the liver subcostal, access is mandatory for full coverage and cannot be replaced by intercostal scans. If the left decubitus position does not give subcostal access, the patient is transferred to CT. The different enhancement characteristics of the organs mean that they require different examination approaches. For left side trauma, a bolus of 0.6 ml is given. The left kidney is examined immediately and continuously, until the end of the homogeneous phase. It is often stunning how much easier it is to sharply delineate the kidney with CEUS than with US. The standardised scans should be slow and steady, covering the kidney in 5-7 seconds in the longitudinal plane, and about 10 seconds in the transverse plane. It is an advantage if the transducer can be held in the plane of the long axis of the kidney, but a slight tilt to avoid ribs does not seem to decrease the detectability of lacerations. The same applies to the transverse scans. The complexity of the kidneys means that it is important to use at least two roughly perpendicular scan planes, and if possible to alternate between two intercostal spaces when the ribs cannot be avoided. An alteration in position and breath levels is also an advantage. One has to pay special attention to the medial parts of the parenchyma adjacent to the hilum: for reasons not yet understood these areas sometimes look dark, with a lack of information. This can usually be overcome by an increase in MI. Some attenuation of energy may be seen in cases where an excessively large dose has been given, but it decreases with the rapid wash-out of microbubbles (Fig. 6).

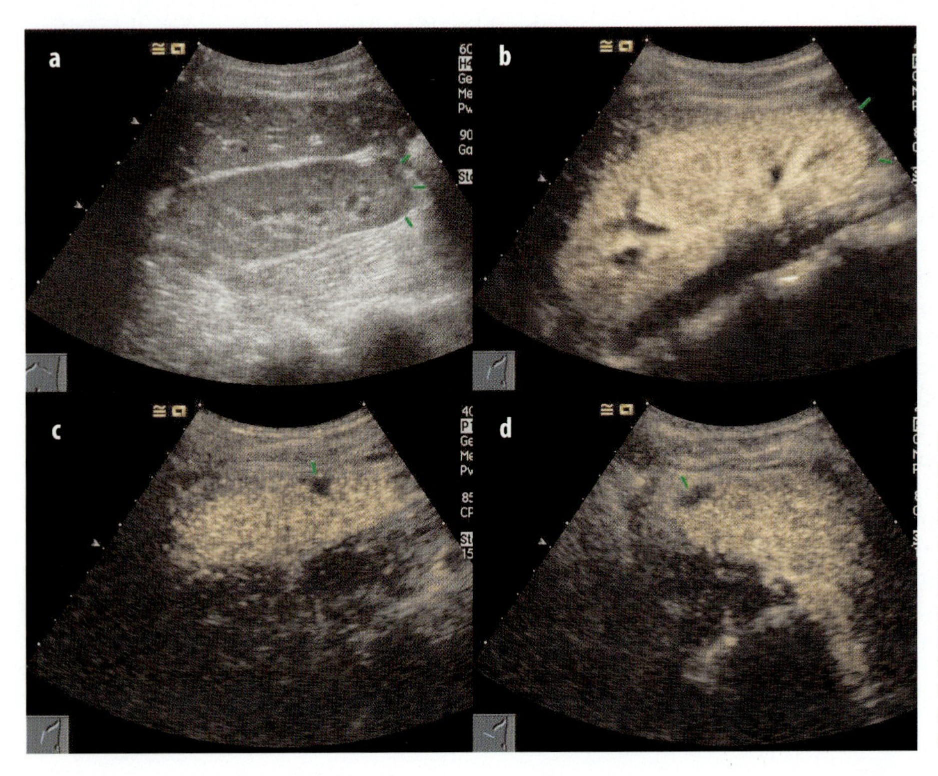

Fig. 6a-d. Adult with minor right flank trauma and light haematuria. **a** Small haematoma by caudal pole revealed by US, but no parenchymal injuries. **b** CEUS beginning of homogeneous phase with same small haematoma. **c** A small superficial laceration in the lateral renal surface is seen clearly. **d** Same laceration in perpendicular view

When the homogeneous phase of the kidney ends, the transducer is moved for scanning of the spleen, which is now in its homogeneous phase. For best resolution, it is first scanned intercostally level-by-level with the sector transducer, followed by the vector transducer for the perpendicular plane. Some people have a very small spleen located far from the thoracic wall. Such spleens are sometimes difficult to see, but by a combination of breath position and different approaches the problem is often solved. As stated before, the contrast accumulation of the spleen is very stable, allowing plenty of time for extensive scanning. The dorsocaudal margin of the spleen is usually easily viewed in great detail by finding the right intercostal space just below the margin. It is more difficult to reach the ventrocranial aspect of the spleen because of the lung, but with breathing movements and change in angles, it can also be properly covered in most cases. The energy attenuation effect caused by too much contrast is extreme in the spleen. If the ordinary liver dose of 2.4 ml is mistakenly injected, the depth of penetration into the spleen is usually reduced to a few centimetres, while the deeper structures are blocked from access for many minutes. Through experience, I know that the unprepared examiner can be quite confused by this phenomenon the first time it is encountered; a spleen that should be easily examined with US is replaced after injection by an impenetrable bright tissue wall just inside the intercostal space, hiding the other regions of the spleen. If this happens, the solution is to destroy all microbubbles in the spleen by scanning it through using normal MI colour Doppler and let it refill with the microbubbles in circulation. Normally, the enhancement will be properly balanced at this stage, but on a few occasions two bubble destructions have been required to bring the enhancement down to a homogeneous level. Mild attenuation can occur even with the recommended dose. It may not be obvious, but it is easy to see when it comes to mind so that penetration can be increased for better detectability. If in doubt, a new exam with 0.3 ml of UCA is recommended after bubble destruction (Fig. 7).

For right side trauma, 0.6 ml of contrast is injected following US. The kidney is examined as described earlier, after which another 1.2 ml is injected. The liver is already in its homogeneous phase from the first injection and can be examined immediately, but optimal enhancement will arrive within 40 seconds of the second injection. It may be preferable to divide the second dose into two boluses given 1-2 minutes apart. In flank trauma, the right lobe is most likely to be injured, so when examining the liver for trauma we make an exception from our liver standard and begin with the right lobe, with inclusion of the segment four area, preferably using the left decubitus position for the best subcostal access. The scanning protocol will not be discussed at length, but basically it consists of alternating longitudinal and transverse scans covering the different parts of the liver, and one or two intercostal scans. The rib-covered lateral and ventral surface parts of the right lobe are most easily overlooked, but with the breathing cooperation of the patient, it is usually not difficult to achieve good access. We have found that the deepest breath often is not optimal, since it pushes the transducer away. An intermediate inhalation is often the best position. After covering these parts of the liver, the patient turns to the supine position and the left lobe is

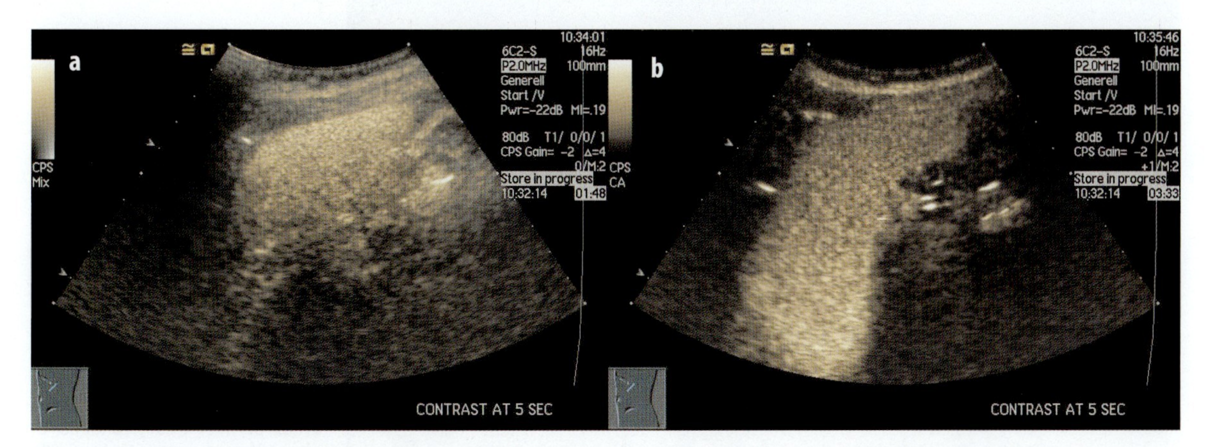

Fig. 7a, b. a Much too dense attenuetion in the spleen due too a large bolus coveres the medial part of the spleen. **b** Soon after bubble destruction the medial part of the spleen is visible

covered in a similar way. The caudate lobe seems to be the area outside the right lobe that is most susceptible to being overlooked, due mainly to shadowing from the falciform ligament. Often it is quite easy to find access around the ligament from a different angle or position of inhalation. We have not seen attenuation by too dense contrast in the liver (Fig. 8).

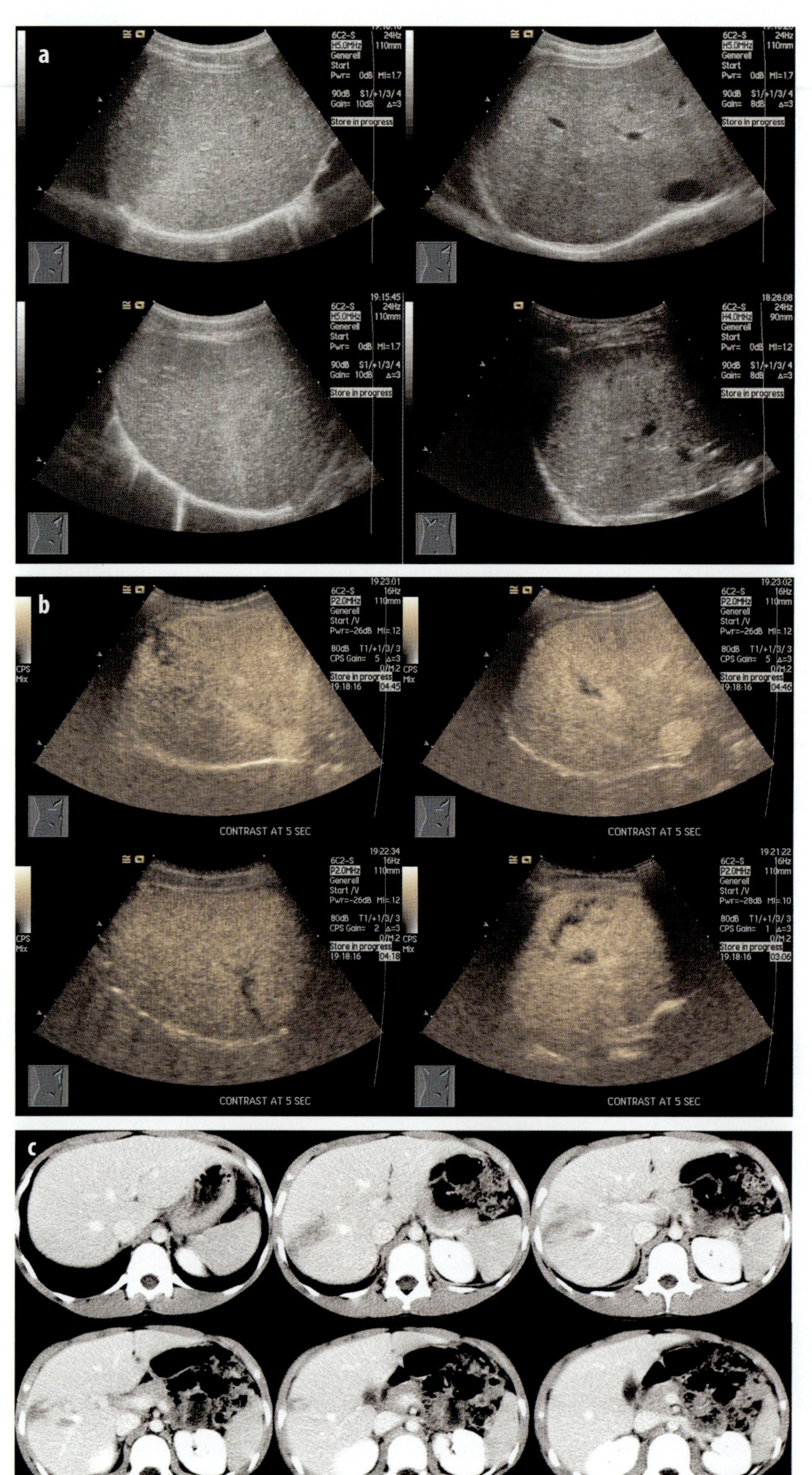

Fig. 8a-c. Images of 10 year old who fell in playground. **a** US in four positions sees low- and high-echo areas of liver injury. **b** CEUS in about the same positions as US. shows exact extent of lacerations. **c** CT less than one hour later is very similar to CEUS

From our experience of injuries examined with both CT and CEUS, we know that mapping of parenchymal lacerations is possible. With the difference in scan planes between the modalities it is sometimes difficult to transfer the exact position of a rift from one modality to the other. This is probably of minor importance since follow-ups are generally done only with standardised CEUS exams. We have had no significant problems assessing the lacerations' depth from the organ surface or hilum. The existence of an efficient high frame rate, wide-angle 4D solution would be an elegant method for overcoming the positioning dissimilarities if there is ever need for exact comparison. It is our definite impression that CEUS in practice finds more of the very thin lacerations than CT. Larger injuries found by CT have usually been easy to find with CEUS, but often, additional small rifts have been evident with CEUS. Subcapsular haematomas have similar appearance in the three organs. They are sharply delineated conspicuously dark or black structures on the surface of the enhancing parenchyma. The enhancement of surrounding fat further emphasises these haematomas. Among our positive cases many had no signs of free abdominal fluid or subcapsular haematoma.

With experience, we rely increasingly on CEUS in combination with FAST to rule out lacerations in the spleen, liver and kidneys. In recent cases, with findings of parenchymal damage, CT has not usually been performed, since mapping of the lacerations and haematomas for comparison with subsequent exams is possible with standardized scanning protocols. CEUS and FAST are not sufficient for the evaluation of abdominal trauma in all individual cases. Poor patient cooperation and obesity are probably the most frequent limiting factors, although obesity does not always prevent successful exams. Other limitations are obstruction by gas or bone and unfavourable organ locations where parts of the organs cannot be accessed. Of course, we add CT if, after CEUS, we determine that for some reason the organs have not been properly accessed or penetrated. We also take the patient's present symptoms into account when deciding whether CT is preferable. It is important to communicate with the patient to find out any additional information not expressed in the referral. Sometimes there is not a clear correlation between the trauma history and the symptoms. If the patient complains of epigastrial pain or the symptoms in other ways give reason to suspect injuries other than to the liver, spleen or renal injuries, we are naturally very liberal in adding CT. So far, our experience of CEUS in parenchymal trauma is encouraging, but we remain careful, since our negative and positive trauma cases are few in comparison to all our CEUS patients. This is especially true for the kidneys. However, as long as our clinical results continue in the same positive direction we must aim for wider trauma use by other CEUS-experienced sonologists and for properly designed further studies. The alternative is acceptance of unnecessary radiation exposure to a large and increasing number of otherwise healthy young individuals.

Key Points

- Low-energy blunt abdominal trauma rarely causes major parenchymal injury.
- Precautionary contrast-enhanced CT is often negative, but exposes an often young population to ionising radiation.
- US has a low sensitivity to parenchymal injuries.
- Under proper conditions, CEUS is very promising for detecting and excluding parenchymal injuries, even small ones.
- Provided scientific proof of efficacy, CEUS may replace CT in a vast number of future trauma cases.

Suggested Readings

Amoroso T (1999) Evaluation of the patient with blunt abdominal trauma: An evidence-based approach. In: Emergency medicine clinics of North America 17. Saunders, Philadelphia, pp 63-75

Blaivas M, DeBehnke D, Sierzenski PR, Phelan MB (2002) Tissue harmonic imaging improves organ visualization in trauma ultrasound when compared with standard ultrasound mode. Acad Emerg Med 9:48-53

Brooks A (2001) The role of ultrasound in trauma. J R Army Med Corps 147:268-273

Brown MA, Casola G, Sirlin CB, Hoyt DB (2001) Importance of evaluating organ parenchyma during screening abdominal ultrasonography after blunt trauma. J Ultrasound Med 20:577-583

Catalano O, Lobianco R, Mattace Raso M, Siani A (2005) Blunt hepatic trauma: Evaluation with contrast-enhanced sonography. J Ultrasound Med 24: 299-310

Catalano O, Lobianco R, Sandomenico F, Siani A (2003) Splenic trauma: evaluation with contrast-specific sonography and a second-generation contrast medium. J Ultrasound Med 22:467-477

Miller MT, Pasquale MD, Bromberg WJ, Wasser TE, Cox J (2003) Not so fast. J Trauma 1:52-60

Murphy R, Ghosh A, Mackway-Jones K (2002) Ultrasound or computed tomography in paediatric blunt abdominal trauma. Emerg Med J 19:554-556

Nilsson A, Loren I, Nirhov N, Lindhagen T, Nilsson P (1999) Power Doppler ultrasonography: alternative to computed tomography in abdominal trauma patients. J Ultrasound Med 18:669-672

Poletti P, Platon A, Becker C, Mentha G, Vermeulen B, Buhler L, Terrier F (2004) Blunt abdominal trauma: Does the use of a second-generation sonographic contrast agent help to detect solid organ injuries?. AJR 183: 1293-1301

Stengel D, Bauwens K, Sehouli J, Nantke J, Ekkernkamp A (2001) Discriminatory power of 3.5 MHz convex and 7.5 MHz linear ultrasound probes for the imaging of traumatic splenic lesions: a feasibility study. J Trauma 51:37-43

Stengel D, Bauwens K, Sehouli J, Porzsolt F, Rademacher G, Mutze S, Ekkernkamp A (2001) Systematic review and meta-analysis of emergency ultrasonography for blunt abdominal trauma. Br J Surg 88:901-912

IV.4

Prostate Carcinoma

Ferdinand Frauscher

Introduction

Prostate carcinoma is the most common non-skin cancer affecting men in Europe and the United States, and is second only to lung cancer as a cause of cancer deaths in men. In the United States, an estimated 230 000 men were diagnosed with prostate cancer in 2004, and nearly 30 000 will die of the disease [1]. Nevertheless, the fact that the vast majority of tumors are now detected either localized to the prostate or regionally spread, while only a small percentage are detected at the metastatic stage [1], has highlighted the importance of earlier detection and diagnosis of the disease. The use of prostate-specific antigen (PSA) testing has allowed physicians to detect tumors at much earlier stages of disease, and the recognition of finer points of disease pathology has enabled physicians to establish more comprehensive and detailed staging criteria [2, 3].

Current research in the areas of detection and diagnosis are primarily focusing on two main areas: identification of risk factors for disease in the general public that warrant regular screening; identification of imaging strategies for early detection of disease and disease progression, and use of these imaging strategies in predicting outcomes in different patient populations. The imaging techniques used include US, magnetic resonance imaging (MRI), and positron emission tomography (PET) [4].

Prior to the widespread use of PSA screening in asymptomatic men, prostate cancer was detected via digital rectal examination (DRE), and only 25% of newly diagnosed prostate cancers were clinically organ-confined [5, 6]. Since the advent of PSA testing, the percentage of newly diagnosed organ-confined and locally advanced disease has increased to more than 80% [1]. Currently, clinical practice guidelines recommend the use of both PSA and DRE in asymptomatic men [7, 8]. Although PSA testing can detect tumors at a far earlier stage than DRE, DRE as part of a comprehensive physical exam can help physicians better assess the extent of the disease and its effect on surrounding organs. Of note, the positive predictive value (PPV) of DRE increases with higher PSA levels, and the addition of DRE can more than double the predictive value in patients with a PSA level of more than 4 ng/mL [9]. The use of PSA as a screening tool can be challenging. Although its name suggests that it is produced and secreted solely by the prostate gland, PSA is produced by other tissues as well, including the peri-urethral glands, parotid gland, and adrenal and renal cell tumors, albeit at very low concentrations [10]. Transient or persistent elevations in serum PSA concentrations can also reflect changes in the prostate gland due to chronic or recurrent inflammation, trauma, ejaculation, urinary retention, and benign proliferation or enlargement [11-13]. Certain medications, including herbal supplements, can also cause changes in serum PSA [12-14]. A careful history and repeat PSA measurements can help distinguish between transient PSA rises due to these conditions and persistent rises due to prostate cancer, potentially minimizing unnecessary biopsy of non-cancerous tissue. Of these, elevated PSA measurements due to benign conditions, particularly benign prostatic hyperplasia (BPH), most directly underscores the difficulty in making a decision about the need for biopsy in asymptomatic men, even though cancerous prostate tissue releases up to 30 times more PSA into the serum than hyperplastic tissue [10,16]. BPH remains the most common cause of elevated serum PSA concentration [12]. However, while PSA testing has high sensitivity, it lacks specificity.

The standard care in patients with an elevated PSA and or an abnormal DRE is transrectal US-guided (TRUS) systematic biopsy of the prostate [17]. Since gray-scale US has a low sensitivity and specificity for prostate cancer detection, with the chance of detecting a hypoechoic lesion - which is the most common appearance of prostate cancer on gray-scale US - varying between 3% and 51%. Specifically, TRUS is limited by the inability to detect isoechoic tumors (Fig. 1) and by the often heterogeneous appearance of the prostate. Therefore Hodge et al. [18] introduced the 'sextant biopsy approach' in 1989, which is still a standard technique worldwide. However, numerous studies have shown that the sextant technique misses up to 35% of clinically relevant cancers [19]. This has resulted in studies using new biopsy strategies with more laterally directed cores and a higher number of cores overall (i.e., saturation biopsies with up to 45 cores). Analyzing the results, several studies have reported no significant improvement when performing a higher number of cores [20].

In order to improve the detection of prostate cancer, additional three-dimensional/four-dimensional (3D/4D) (Fig. 2) color and power Doppler US have been used. Color Doppler US has been applied to evaluate vascularity within the prostate and the surrounding structures [29-34]. The motivation behind the application of color Doppler US is to detect tumor neovascularity. Cancerous tissue generally grows more rapidly than normal tissue, and demonstrates increased blood flow, as compared to normal tissue and benign lesions. Color Doppler US may demonstrate an increased number of visualized vessels, as well as an increase in flow rate, size and irregularity of vessels within prostate cancer. Three different flow patterns may be associated with prostate cancer: diffuse flow, focal flow and surrounding flow [21]. The most frequently identified flow pattern is diffuse flow within the lesion. Early results have suggested that up to 85% of men with prostate cancers greater than 5 mm in size have visibly increased flow in the area of tumor involvement. In addition, hypervascularity may be seen in patients with more difficult to identify isoechoic and hyperechoic lesions (Fig. 3).

In a recent study Halpern et al. [35] assessed the value of gray-scale, color and power Doppler

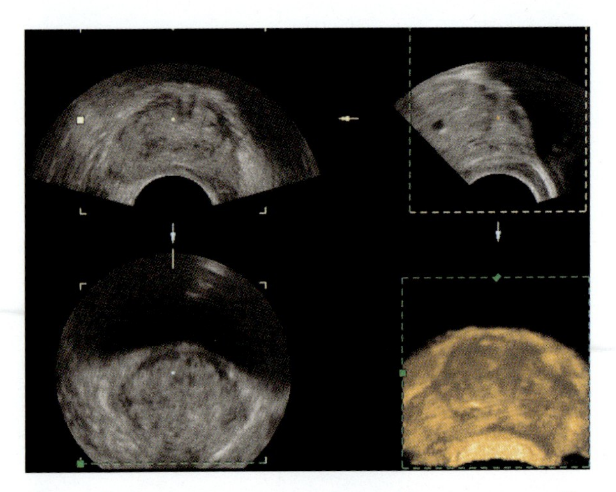

Fig. 2. 4D ultrasound image in a patient with prostate cancer. No focal abnormality is seen. The cancer was detected by systematic biopsy at the right base (Reprinted with permission from [17a])

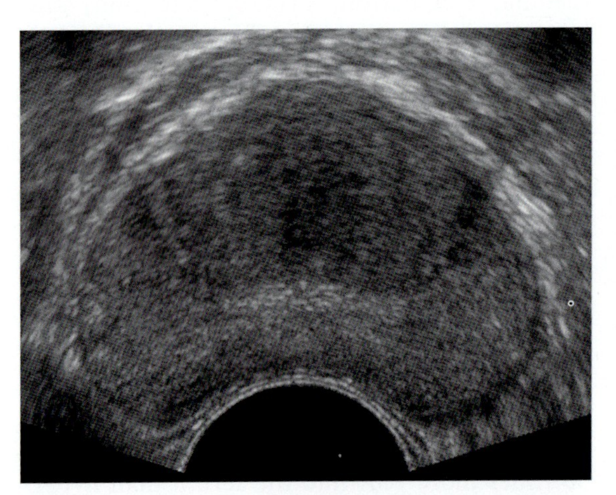

Fig. 1. Transrectal gray-scale ultrasound of the prostate. The transverse ultrasound scan shows no focal abnormality. The isoechoic cancer was located at the left side (Reprinted with permission from [17a])

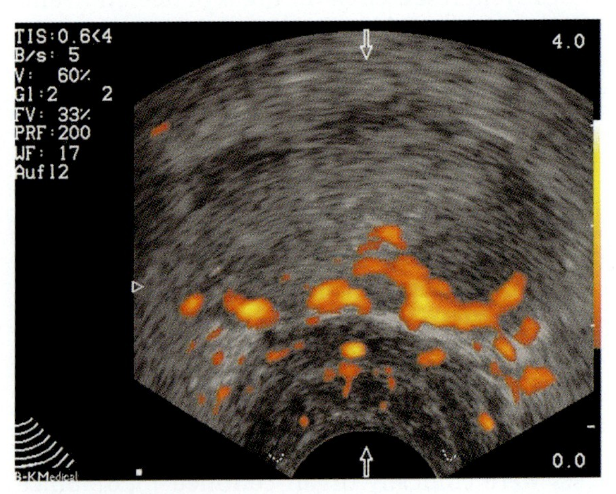

Fig. 3. Power Doppler ultrasound of the prostate. A hypoechoic hypervascular lesion is seen on the left side representing prostate cancer (Reprinted with permission from [17a])

US for the detection of prostatic cancer. They investigated 251 patients prior to biopsy. Each biopsy site was prospectively scored for gray-scale abnormalities and Doppler flow. Cancer was detected in 211 biopsy sites from 85 patients. Overall agreement between sonographic findings and biopsy results as measured with thc kappa statistic was minimally superior to chance (kappa = 0.12 for gray-scale, kappa = 0.11 for color Doppler, kappa = 0.09 for power Doppler). Among patients with at least one positive biopsy for cancer, foci of increased power Doppler flow were 4.7 times more likely to contain cancer than adjacent tissues without flow. They concluded that power Doppler may be useful for targeted biopsies when the number of biopsy passes must be limited, but that there is no substantial advantage of power Doppler over color Doppler. Other investigators suggest that although Doppler flow patterns may correlate with microvascular density, Doppler imaging does not provide sufficient sensitivity to preclude biopsy.

Clinical Application

Contrast-Enhanced Ultrasound

Color/Power Doppler Ultrasound

Recently developed US contrast agents can improve the detection of low-volume blood flow by increasing the signal-to-noise ratio [36-39]. Intravascular contrast agents allow a more complete delineation of the neovascular anatomy, by enhancing the signal strength from small vessels. Furthermore, these agents may be used to time the transit of an injected bolus. Unlike radiographic contrast media, which diffuse into the tissue and may obscure smaller vessels, microbubble echo-enhancing agents are confined to the vascular lumen, where they persist until they dissolve. Contrast agents are made of gas bubbles small enough to cross through capillary beds. They have two important acoustic properties. First, they are many times more reflective than blood, thus improving flow detection. Second, their vibrations generate higher harmonics to a much greater degree than surrounding tissues. The half-life of contrast agents is dependent on bubble construction. Bubbles can be free or encapsuled in soft or hard shells. The duration of enhancement after injection may lasts from a few seconds to many minutes, depending on the bubble type.

Radge et al. [40] performed TRUS microbubble contrast angiography of the prostate in 1996 in 15 patients with PSA elevations. Fourteen had a negative prior biopsy (1-3 x). Prostate cancer was detected in five patients. Microvascular patterns were judged abnormal in eight patients, two of which proved malignant, two of which were benign, and one of which was diagnosed with prostatitis. False-negative results were observed in three patients, whose positive biopsy sites were from the prostate apex. The authors concluded that following contrast agent administration, prostate blood vessel image enhancement was noted in all patients, and there were no adverse reactions during or after EchoGen administration with the dose employed. Watanabe [41] reported the use of a microbubble contrast agents (SH/TH508) in nine cases with prostate cancer. Blood flow images were enhanced in all these cases. Even in cases of localized cancer, blood flow images were visualized clearly in the cancer lesion.

In a previous study at our institution, we examined the use of contrast-enhanced color Doppler US in 72 patients identified by PSA screening. Using a quantitative scale to characterize the degree of vascularity, the technique had a sensitivity of 53%, specificity of 72%, and a PPV of 70% in distinguishing prostate cancer from benign lesions [42].

Bree at al. [43] reported the potential use of contrast-enhanced color Doppler to increase the diagnostic yield in a group of 17 patients with normal gray-scale TRUS and elevated PSA values. Correlation of biopsy sites with color Doppler US abnormalities revealed a sensitivity of 54%, a specificity of 78%, a PPV of 61%, and a negative predictive value (NPV) of 72% for the detection of prostate cancer. Three of the cases with a positive contrast-enhanced biopsy site had negative TRUS random biopsy within the previous year [31].

Bogers et al. [44] evaluated contrast-enhanced 3D imaging of the prostate vasculature with power Doppler. 3D power Doppler images were obtained before and after intravenous administration of 2.5 g Levovist (Schering, Germany). Subsequently, random and/or directed TRUS-guided biopsies were performed. Prostate vasculature was judged with respect to symmetry and vessel distribution. Eighteen patients with a suspicion of prostate cancer either because of an elevated PSA (greater than 4.0 ng/mL; Tandem-R-assay) or an abnormal DRE were included in the study. Prostate cancer was detected in 13 patients. Vascular anatomy was judged abnormal in unenhanced images in six cases, of which five proved malignant. Enhanced images were considered suspicious for malignancy in 12 cases, including one benign and 11 malignant biopsy results. Sensitivity of enhanced images was 85% (specificity 80%) compared with 38% for unenhanced images (specificity 80%) and 77% for conventional gray-scale TRUS (specificity 60%). Among six patients who showed no gray-scale abnormalities, vascular patterns were judged abnormal in four cases, of which three were malignant. Based on these findings, the authors concluded that contrast-enhanced 3D power Doppler angiography is feasible in patients with potential prostate cancer who are scheduled for prostate biopsies.

A more recent analysis by the same group suggested that 3D contrast-enhanced power Doppler US is a better diagnostic tool than the DRE, PSA level, gray-scale US or power Doppler US alone. The most suitable diagnostic predictor for prostate cancer was a combination of 3D contrast-enhanced power Doppler US and PSA levels [45].

In a further study, we compared contrast-agent enhanced transrectal color Doppler-targeted biopsy with conventional gray-scale US-guided systematic biopsy for the detection of prostate cancer. 90 consecutive screening volunteers with no symptoms, who took part in the PSA screening programme (serum total PSA ≥ 1.25 ng/mL and free to total PSA ratio < 18%) were studied [46]. Six patients were excluded because they did not complete the protocol (due to pain, problems with anesthesia, or imaging). Therefore, 84 patients (mean age: 57 [SD11] years) were included in our study. Two independent investigators assessed each patient. One investigator used contrast agent-enhanced colour Doppler imaging with a Sequoia 512 unit (Siemens Medical Solutions, USA) fitted with an end-fire probe operating at a Doppler frequency of 9 MHz. Biopsy samples were targeted at the hypervascular regions. The number of targeted biopsies was limited to five or fewer per patient. Targeted biopsies were obtained during intravenous infusion of Levovist with a concentration of 300 mg/mL, at an infusion rate of 1 mL/min to a maximum dose of 5 g. The contrast agent-enhanced color Doppler study was done before the systematic biopsy samples were taken, because the reverse could produce hyperemia that would be misleading. Subsequently, a second investigator took ten systematic biopsy samples of the prostate in a standard spatial distribution guided by conventional gray-scale ultrasonography on a Combison 530MT unit (Kretztechnik, Austria). Cancer detection rates for the two techniques were compared. Prostate cancer was present in 24 (29%) of 84 patients, with a mean total PSA of 3.7 ng/mL. Prostate cancer was detected in 23 (27%) of 84 patients with contrast agent-enhanced color Doppler targeted biopsy, and in 17 (20%) of 84 patients with systematic conventional gray-scale US-guided biopsy (Fig. 4). Prostate cancer was detected by contrast agent-enhanced color Doppler in seven (8%) patients with a negative systematic biopsy sample. In one

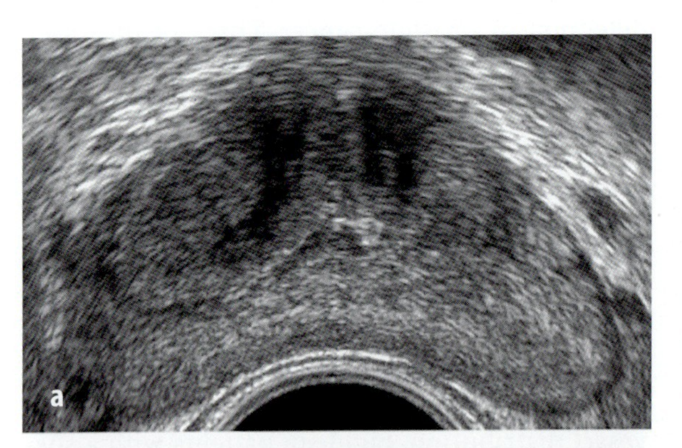

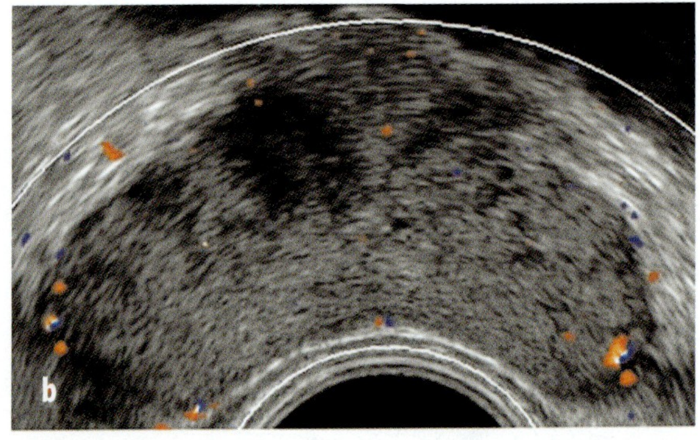

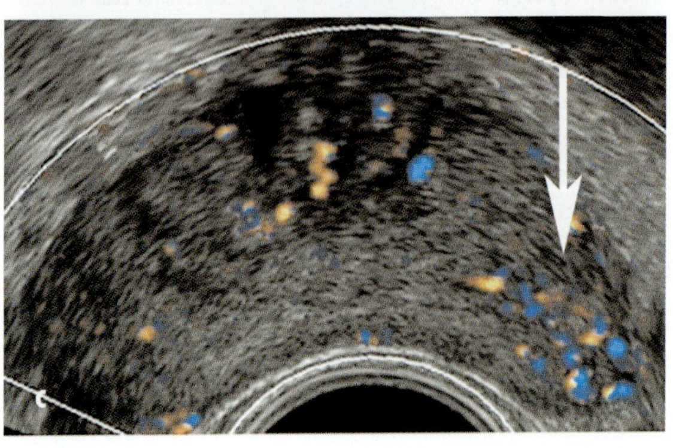

Fig. 4a-c. *Contrast-enhanced color Doppler ultrasound in a patient with an elevated PSA.* **a** Gray-scale ultrasound shows no focal abnormality. **b** Unenhanced color Doppler ultrasound shows no hypervascular lesion. **c** Contrast-enhanced color Doppler ultrasound shows a hypervascular lesion at the left mid-gland. Targeted biopsies out of this lesion were shown to be prostate cancer (Reprinted with permission from [17a])

patient, prostate cancer was detected only on systematic biopsy. The by-patient analysis shows a significant improvement in the detection of prostate cancer with contrast agent-enhanced color Doppler-targeted biopsy compared with systematic conventional gray-scale US-guided biopsy (McNemar's test: $p = 0.034$). On the basis of our analysis of individual biopsy cores, the detection rate of contrast agent-enhanced color Doppler targeted biopsy (13% or 55/409 cores) was better than the detection rate of systematic gray-scale US-guided biopsy (4.9% or 41/840 cores). To compare these detection rates and compensate for the patient-clustered nature of our biopsy data, conditional logistic-regression analysis was done. The odds ratio for detection of cancer by contrast agent-enhanced color Doppler-targeted biopsy versus systematic gray-scale US-guided biopsy was 4.3 ($p < 0.001$ [95% CI 2.6-7.1]). In addition, with respect to cost the targeted biopsy approach in our study resulted in a decrease in core samples and reduction of pathological interpretation costs by more than 50% (US$110 per patient). Furthermore, the reduced number of biopsies generally results in fewer complications (i.e., pain, hematuria, or hematospermia). The Gleason score of all cancers detected by contrast agent-enhanced colour Doppler-targeted biopsy was 6 or higher. The Gleason score provides a histological grade of prostate cancer based upon the degree of glandular differentiation with grades ranging from 2 to 10 (grade 2 = more differentiated, grade 10 = least differentiated). The one cancer that was missed with contrast agent-enhanced imaging showed no hypervascular areas, and a Gleason score of 4. Published studies based upon the Connecticut tumour registry suggest no loss of life expectancy in conservatively treated men with Gleason scores of 2 to 4, and only a modest risk of death at Gleason scores of 5 and 6. Therefore, based on our preliminary data, contrast agent-enhanced color Doppler detected all clinically significant cancers in our series. Therefore, these preliminary suggest that this technique may allow for a limited targeted biopsy approach, which will be cost-effective provided that the cost of the US contrast-agent ($65 per patient) is less than the savings based upon the reduced number of biopsy cores ($110 per patient). However, these results should be confirmed for different populations in other countries to determine whether a limited, targeted biopsy approach is applicable in other clinical settings.

To further evaluate these preliminary data we performed the same approach in an additional 230 male screening volunteers [47]. Cancer was detected in 69 of the 230 patients (30%), including 56 (24.4%) by contrast-enhanced targeted biopsy and in 52 (22.6%) by systematic biopsy (Figs. 5, 6). Cancer was detected by targeted biopsy alone in 17 patients (7.4%) and by systematic biopsy alone in 13 (5.6%). The overall

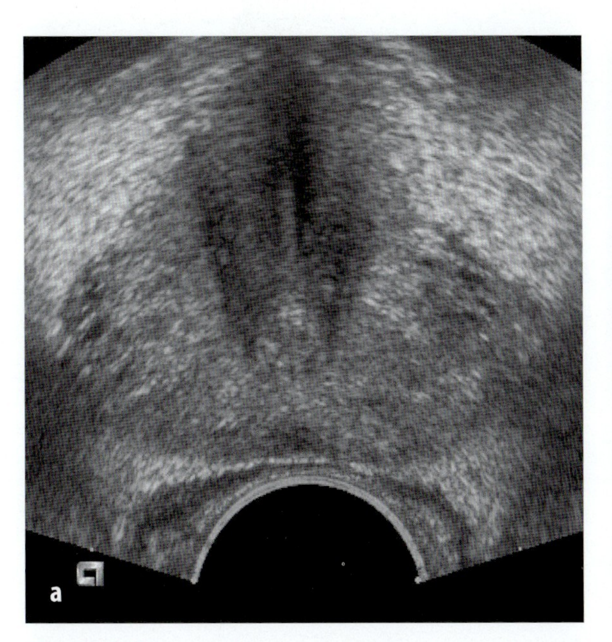
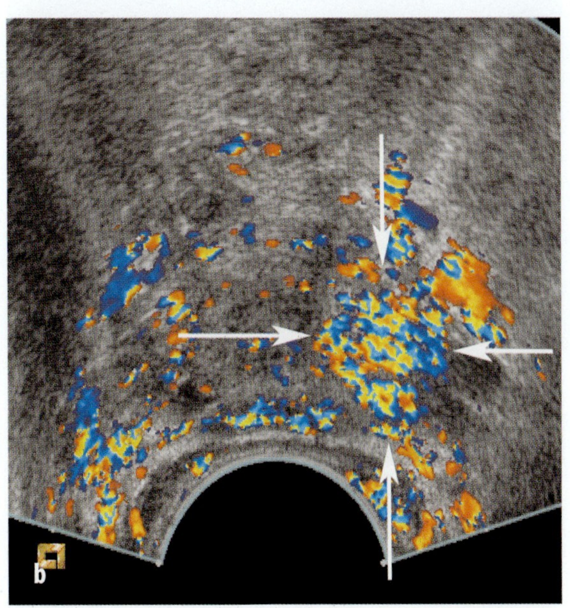

Fig. 5a, b. *Contrast-enhanced color Doppler ultrasound in a patient with an elevated PSA.* **a** Gray-scale ultrasound shows no focal abnormality at the apex. **b** Contrast-enhanced color Doppler ultrasound shows a hypervascular lesion at the left apex, which proved to be prostate cancer (Reprinted with permission from [17a])

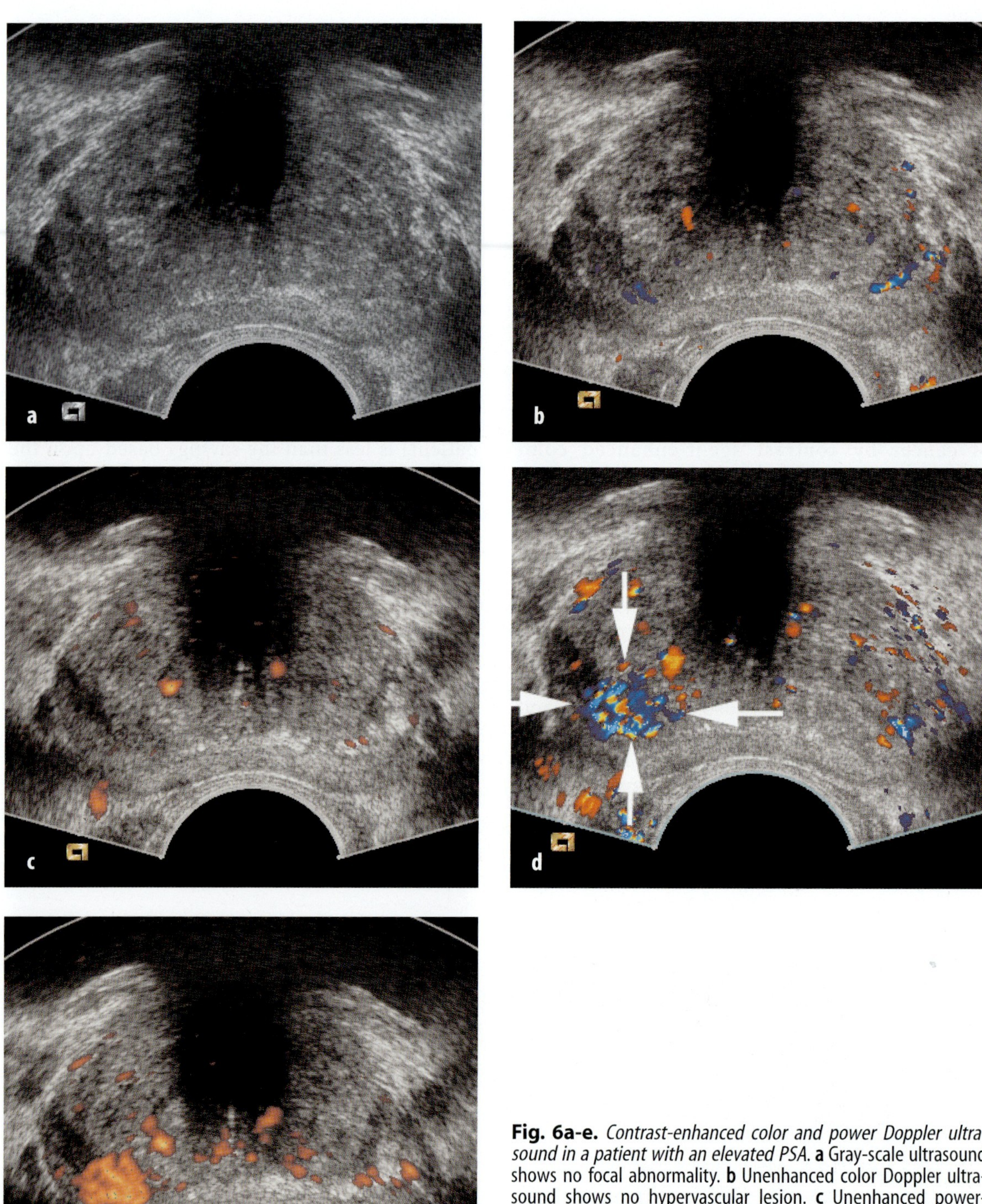

Fig. 6a-e. *Contrast-enhanced color and power Doppler ultrasound in a patient with an elevated PSA.* **a** Gray-scale ultrasound shows no focal abnormality. **b** Unenhanced color Doppler ultrasound shows no hypervascular lesion. **c** Unenhanced power-Doppler ultrasound shows no hypervascular lesion. **d** Contrast-enhanced color Doppler ultrasound shows a hypervascular lesion at the right mid-gland, representing prostate cancer. **e** Contrast-enhanced power Doppler ultrasound shows a hypervascular lesion at the right mid-gland, representing prostate cancer (Reprinted with permission from [47a])

cancer detection rate by patient was not significantly different for targeted and systematic biopsy ($p = 0.58$). However, the detection rate for targeted biopsy cores (10.4% or 118 of 1139 cores) was significantly better than for systematic biopsy cores (5.3% or 123 of 2300 cores, $p < 0.001$). Contrast-enhanced targeted biopsy in a patient with cancer was 2.6-fold more likely to detect prostate cancer than systematic US-guided biopsy, though contrast-enhanced targeted biopsy alone is a reasonable approach for decreasing the number of biopsy cores.

Roy et al. [48] investigated the accuracy of contrast-enhanced color Doppler endorectal US to guide biopsy for the detection of prostate cancer. They studied a total of 85 patients with gray-scale and color Doppler before and during intravenous injection of US contrast agent made of galactose-based air microbubbles. The biopsy protocol was performed during contrast injection. An additional 18 directed cores were obtained based on contrast-enhanced imaging. Diagnostic efficiencies with and without contrast medium injection for detecting prostate cancer were compared based on biopsy results. Cancer was identified in a total of 58 biopsy sites in 54 patients. Gray-scale imaging revealed 96 abnormal hypoechoic nodules or irregular zones inside the outer gland, of which 48 were malignant on pathological evaluation. Contrast-enhanced color Doppler had higher sensitivity (93%) than unenhanced color Doppler (54%), while specificity increased only 79% to 87% for enhanced imaging. Nine of ten isoechoic suspicious zones were depicted with enhancement, while unenhanced Doppler detected seven of them. There was no significant difference between the intensity of enhancement and tumor Gleason scores. Roy et al. concluded that contrast-enhanced color Doppler endorectal US increases the detection of prostate cancer. Improvement in sensitivity was high, while the difference in specificity was not as pertinent. Contrast-enhanced color Doppler endorectal US is an accurate technique, which uses a common US unit. This technique is easy to perform and not time-consuming. Obtaining additional biopsy cores of suspicious enhancing foci significantly improves the detection rate of cancer.

Sedelaar et al. [49] demonstrated the correlation between microvessel density (MVD) and 3D contrast-enhanced power Doppler imaging. In all patients, the enhanced side of the prostate was correlated with a higher MVD count. Concerning the MVD and the color pixel density, we found similar results doing contrast-enhanced color Doppler US using the US contrast agent Levovist (Fig. 7) [50].

Gray-Scale Harmonic Ultrasound

A new approach to contrast-enhanced imaging of the prostate is gray-scale harmonic US using phase- or pulse-inversion, or a single pulse tech-

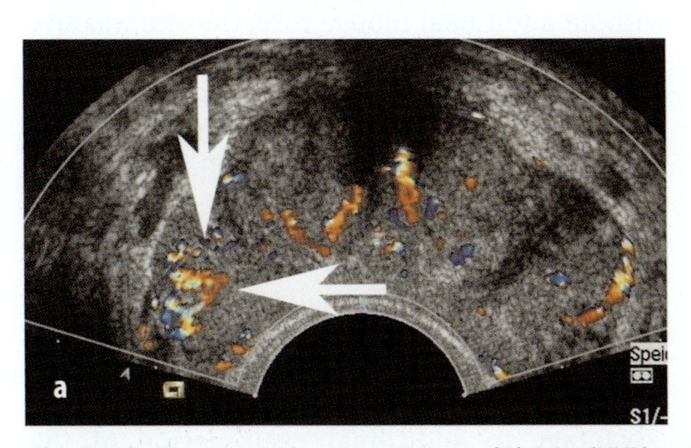

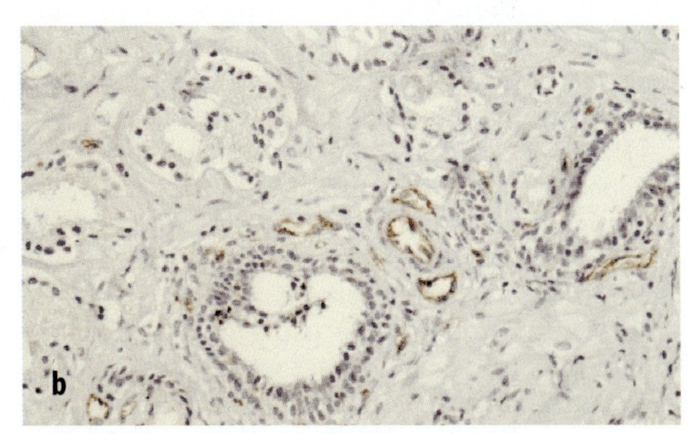

Fig. 7a, b. *Comparison between microvessel density (MVD) and contrast-enhanced color-pixel-density.* **a** Contrast-enhanced color Doppler ultrasound shows a hypervascular lesion representing prostate cancer at the right mid-gland with a high color pixel density. **b** Immunhistochemistry shows a high MVD (vessels outlined in brown) (Reprinted with permission from [17a])

nology to exploit the non-linear behavior of the bubbles in order to differentiate blood flow echoes from background tissue with high contrast, and spatial resolution. Albrecht et al. [51] demonstrated this technique in 39 human subjects. Gray-scale enhancement of vessels and organ parenchyma was seen in all cases. Enhancement occurred from both flowing and stationary microbubbles. Flow-independent enhancement of tissue represents a major advance in contrast-enhanced US with many potential applications, especially in tumor imaging.

In a preliminary study of 26 subjects, Halpern et al. [52] investigated the usefulness of contrast-enhanced US to depict vascularity in the prostate. Continuous gray-scale and intermittent gray-scale imaging were performed at the fundamental frequency. Phase inversion gray-scale imaging was available only for the final few subjects in the study. US findings were correlated with sextant biopsy results. After the administration of the contrast material Imagent (Alliance Pharmaceutical Corp. USA), gray-scale and Doppler images revealed visible enhancement ($p < 0.05$). Using intermittent imaging, the authors found focal enhancement in two isoechoic tumors that were not visible on baseline images. No definite focal area of enhancement was identified in any patient without cancer. Furthermore, contrast-enhanced images revealed obvious enhancement of transient hemorrhage in the biopsy tracts of three patients. They concluded that gray-scale as well as Doppler enhancement of the prostate can be seen on US images after the administration of an intravenous contrast agent, and that contrast-enhanced intermittent US of the prostate may be useful for the selective enhancement of malignant prostatic tissue.

Halpern et al. [53] have recently completed a prospective study of contrast-enhanced TRUS in 60 patients who underwent sextant biopsy of the prostate. All examinations were performed with the Sonoline Elegra (Siemens Medical Systems, Ultrasound Group, USA) using gray-scale harmonic imaging. Each subject was evaluated with conventional gray-scale, harmonic gray-scale and power Doppler US prior to contrast infusion. The evaluation was repeated during intravenous infusion of Definity (DuPont Pharmaceuticals, USA). Gray-scale imaging was performed in continuous mode and with intermittent imaging using interscan delay times of 0.5, 1.0, 2.0 and 5.0 seconds. Each biopsy was scored prospectively as benign or malignant on baseline imaging, and again during contrast-enhanced TRUS. Prostate cancer was present in 37 biopsy sites from 20 subjects. Baseline imaging demonstrated cancer in 14 sites from 11 subjects. Contrast-enhanced TRUS showed cancer in 24 sites from 15 subjects. Each of the five subjects whose prostate cancer was not detected by contrast-enhanced TRUS had only a single positive biopsy core with a Gleason score of 6 or less. The improvement in sensitivity from 38% at baseline to 65% with contrast was significant ($p < 0.004$) (Fig. 7). Specificity was not significantly different at baseline (83%) and during contrast imaging (80%). These results suggest that contrast-enhanced TRUS may improve sensitivity for prostate cancer detection without substantial loss of specificity.

In another study the value of directed biopsy for the detection of prostate cancer during contrast-enhanced endorectal gray-scale harmonic US was assessed. Forty patients were evaluated with harmonic gray-scale US. The evaluation was performed before administration of contrast agent, during continuous intravenous infusion of perflutren lipid microspheres, and again during bolus administration of the microspheres. Sextant biopsy sites were scored prospectively on a six point scale for suggestion of malignancy at baseline during contrast infusion and after bolus administration. An additional directed core was obtained at 20 of the sextant biopsy sites based on contrast-enhanced imaging. Cancer was identified in 30 biopsy sites in 16 of the patients (40%). A suspicious site identified during contrast-enhanced TRUS was 3.5 times more likely to have positive biopsy findings than the adjacent site that was not suggestive of malignancy ($p < 0.025$). When a suspicious site was evaluated with an additional biopsy core, the site was five times more likely to have a biopsy with positive findings than a standard sextant site ($p < 0.01$). No difference in diagnostic accuracy was found between the continuous infusion of contrast material and bolus administration. The authors concluded that contrast-enhanced transrectal gray-scale harmonic US improves the sonographic detection of malignant foci in the prostate. The performance of multiple biopsies of suspicious enhancing foci significantly improves the detection of cancer. However, no advantage to additional examination of the gland after bolus administration of contrast material was found [54].

A more recent analysis by the same group assessed prostate cancer detection and discrimination of benign from malignant prostate tissue with contrast-enhanced US. 301 subjects referred for prostate biopsy were evaluated with contrast-enhanced US using continuous harmonic imaging (CHI) and intermittent harmonic imaging (IHI) with interscan delay times of

0.2, 0.5, 1.0, 2.0 seconds, as well as continuous color and power Doppler. Targeted biopsy cores were obtained from sites of greatest enhancement, followed by spatially distributed cores in a modified sextant distribution. Prostate cancer was detected in 363 biopsy cores from 104 of 301 subjects (35%). Cancer was found in 15.5% (175 of 1133) of targeted cores and 10.4% (188 of 1806) of sextant cores ($p < 0.01$) (Figs. 8, 9). Among subjects with cancer, targeted cores were twice as likely to be positive (odds ratio [OR] = 2.0, $p < 0.001$). Clustered receiver operating characteristic (ROC) analysis of imaging findings at sextant biopsy sites yielded the following Az values: pre-contrast gray scale: 0.58; pre-contrast color Doppler: 0.53; pre-contrast power Doppler: 0.58; CHI: 0.62; IHI (0.2 sec): 0.64; IHI (0.5 sec): 0.63; IHI (1.0 sec): 0.65; IHI (2.0 sec): 0.61; contrast-enhanced color Doppler: 0.60; contrast-enhanced power Doppler: 0.62. A statistically significant benefit was found for IHI over baseline imaging ($p < 0.05$). Prostate cancer detection rate of contrast-enhanced targeted cores is significantly higher when compared with sextant cores. Contrast-enhanced TRUS with IHI provides a statistically significant improvement in discrimination between benign and malignant biopsy sites. However, given the relatively low ROC areas, this technique may not be sufficient to predict which patients have benign versus malignant disease [55].

In a preliminary study we investigated contrast agent dynamics with gray-scale harmonic US. We have investigated 15 patients with biopsy-proven prostate cancer with a Technos MPX unit (Esaote Biomedica, Italy) and gray-scale harmonic imaging (contrast-tuned imaging [CnTI]). We have used the contrast agent SonoVue (Bracco Imaging, Italy) by bolus administration in a dose of 4.8 ml and have evaluated degree, onset, and duration of contrast-enhancement. We found in 14 of 15 prostate cancers (93%) an earlier and higher enhancement with a faster wash-out when compared to normal prostate tissue (unpublished data) (Fig. 10). Therefore these preliminary results demonstrate that assessment of contrast agent dynamics may offer new perspectives in prostate cancer diagnosis.

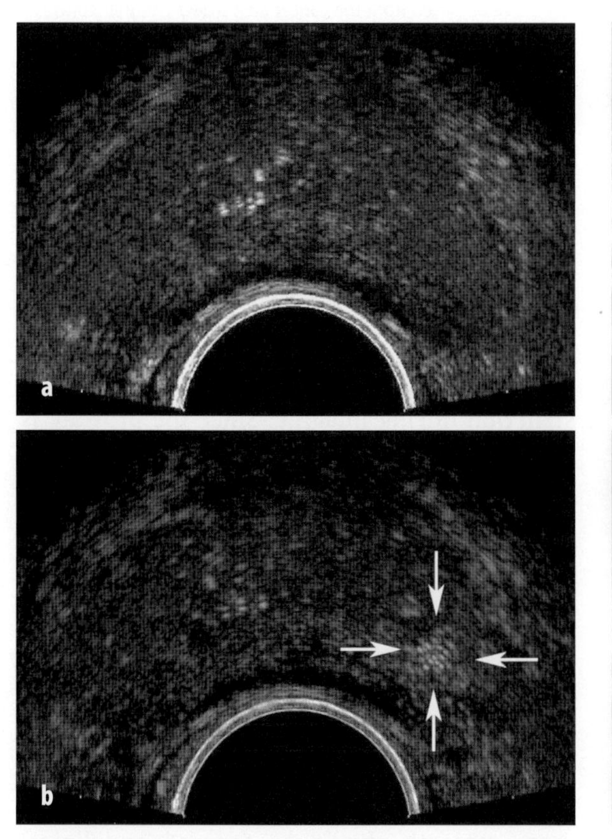

Fig. 8a, b. *Gray-scale harmonic ultrasound in a patient with prostate cancer (CnTI-technique).* **a** Continuous administration of the contrast agent shows no enhancing lesion. **b** Intermittent imaging (interscan delay of 2 s) shows an enhancing area at the left mid-gland, which has been proven to be prostate cancer (Reprinted with permission from [17a])

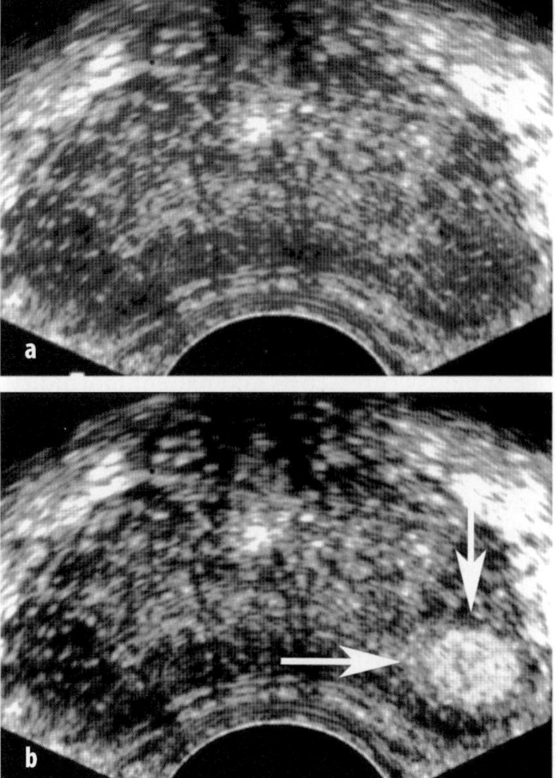

Fig. 9a, b. *Gray-scale harmonic ultrasound in a patient with prostate cancer (ECI-techique).* **a** Intermittent imaging (interscan delay of 0.5 s) shows no enhancing area in the prostate. **b** Intermittent imaging (interscan delay of 2 s) shows an enhancing area at the left mid-gland, which was been proven to be prostate cancer (Reprinted with permission from [17a])

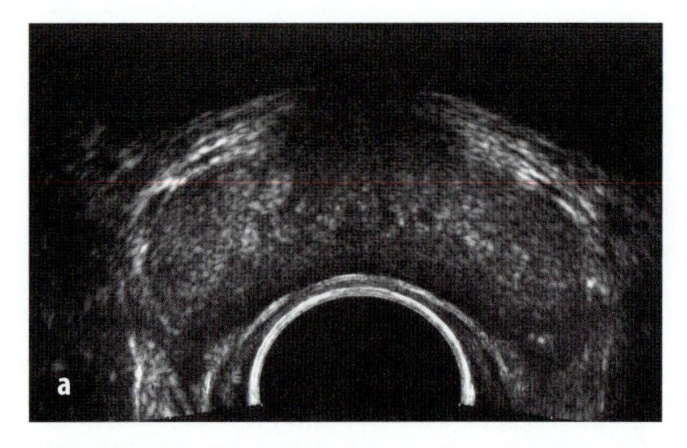

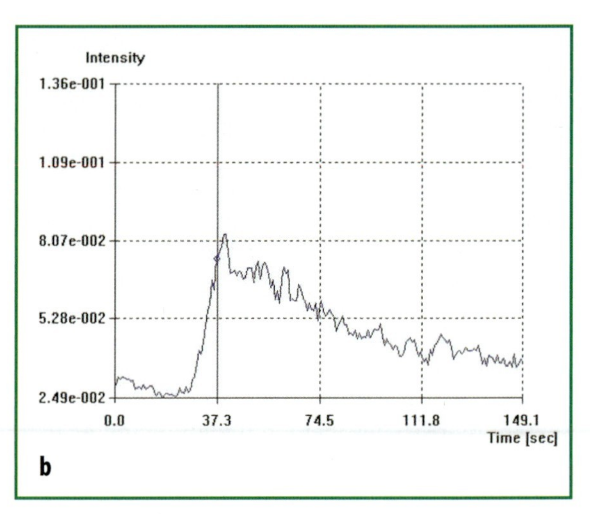

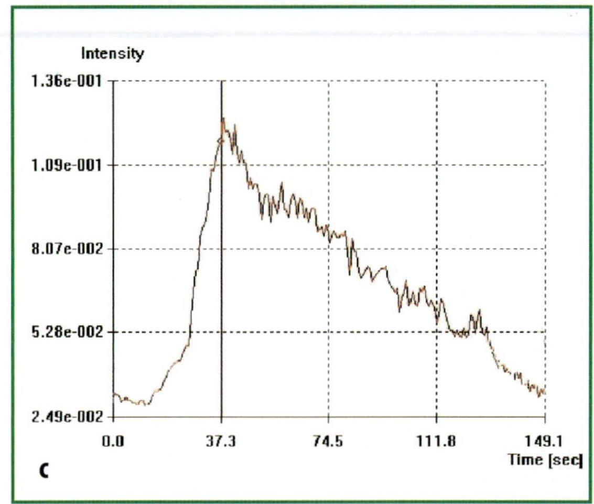

Fig. 10a-c. *Contrast agent dynamics in a patient with prostate cancer.* **a** Gray-scale ultrasound shows no focal abnormality. **b** Time-intensity curve of the right side without cancer **c** Time-intensity curve obtained from the cancer area shows a higher contrast-enhancement and a faster wash-out (Reprinted with permission from [17a])

Conclusion and Perspectives

Overall the detection of prostate cancer is significantly improved by the use of contrast-enhanced US. Contrast-enhanced US allows for targeted biopsies, which significantly reduces the number of biopsy cores, costs and patient morbidity. In addition, contrast-enhanced US has shown an excellent correlation with the Gleason score, which means that contrast-enhanced US improves prostate cancer grading. The good correlation between MVD and color pixel density offers new perspectives for assessment of prostate cancer prognosis. Preliminary data on the assessment of contrast agent dynamics seem to offer new perspectives in discrimination between malignant and benign prostate tissue. However, substantial uncertainty remains in the interpretation of contrast-enhanced TRUS images. In a recent study, 16% (59/360) of contrast-enhanced TRUS images were rated as indeterminate with respect to vascular enhancement. Future studies of contrast-enhanced TRUS should investigate new techniques to optimize the signal from contrast agents in the prostate, and to maximize the difference in signal between benign and malignant tissues. Halpern et al. reported greater enhancement with intermittent imaging and bolus administration of contrast. New imaging techniques may be developed to reduce bubble destruction during imaging. Since the prostate is generally evaluated with a frequency in the range of 5.0-7.5 MHz, newer bubble agents that resonate at higher frequencies may provide better signals. Alternatively, harmonic imaging at lower frequencies or with subharmonics may be useful with current contrast agents [56, 57]. 'Targeted' microbubbles are under development. These microbubbles bind to certain substances or tissues, and could therefore make contrast-enhanced US even more sensitive.

In summary, we have just entered the era of contrast-enhanced US of the prostate. The first clinical evaluations show promising results, and more research should be focused on clinical evaluation of the available techniques. Hopefully, this will result in the accuracy of imaging we urgently need for prostate cancer detection and localization.

Key Points

- The detection of prostate cancer is significantly improved by the use of CEUS.
- CEUS allows for targeted biopsies, which significantly reduces the number of biopsy cores, costs and patient morbidity.
- CEUS has shown an excellent correlation with the Gleason score: CEUS improves prostate cancer grading.
- The good correlation between MVD and color pixel density offers new perspectives for assessment of prostate cancer prognosis.
- Preliminary data on the assessment of contrast agent dynamics seem to offer new perspectives in discrimination between malignant and benign prostate tissue.

References

1. Jemal A, Tiwari RC, Murray T et al (2004) Cancer statistics, CA Cancer J Clin. 54:8-29
2. D'Amico AV, Moul JW, Carroll PR (2003) Surrogate end point for prostate cancer-specific mortality after radical prostatectomy or radiation therapy. J Natl Cancer Inst 95:1376-1383
3. D'Amico AV, Chen MH, Roehl KA, Catalona WJ (2004) Preoperative PSA velocity and the risk of death from prostate cancer after radical prostatectomy. N Engl J Med 351:125-135
4. Carey BM (2005) Imaging for prostate cancer prostate carcinoma. Clin Oncol (R Coll Radiol) 7:553-559
5. Smith DS, Catalona WJ (1994) The nature of prostate cancer detected through prostate specific antigen based screening. J Urol 152:1732
6. Catalona WJ, Smith DS, Ratliff TL et al (1993) Detection of organ-confined prostate cancer is increased through prostate-specific antigen-based screening. JAMA 270:948-954
7. Smith RA, Cokkinides V, Eyre HJ (2003) American Cancer Society guidelines for the early detection of cancer, 2003. CA Cancer J Clin 53:27-43
8. Smith RA, von Eschenbach AC, Wender R et al (2001) American Cancer Society guidelines for the early detection of cancer: update of early detection guidelines for prostate, colorectal, and endometrial cancers. CA Cancer J Clin 51:38-75
9. Carroll PR, Lee KL, Fuks ZY et al (2001) Cancer of the prostate. In: DeVita VT Jr, Hellman S, Rosenberg SA (eds) Cancer: Principles and Practice of Oncology, 6th edn. Lippincott, Williams, & Wilkins, Philadelphia, Chapter 34
10. Partin AW, Hanks GE, Klein EA et al (2002) Prostate-specific antigen as a marker of disease activity in prostate cancer. Oncology (Hunting) 16:1024-1038, 1042, 1047-1048
11. Gretzer MB, Partin AW (2003) PSA markers in prostate cancer detection. Urol Clin North Am 30:677-686
12. Caplan A, Kratz A (2002) Prostate-specific antigen and the early diagnosis of prostate cancer. Am J Clin Pathol 117(suppl):S104-S108
13. DeMarzo AM, DeWeese TL, Platz EA et al (2004) Pathological and molecular mechanisms of prostate carcinogenesis: implications for diagnosis, detection, prevention, and treatment. J Cell Biochem 15:459-477
14. Oh WK, George DJ, Kantoff PW (2002) Rapid rise of serum prostate specific antigen levels after discontinuation of the herbal therapy PC-SPES in patients with advanced prostate carcinoma: report of four cases. Cancer 94:686-689
15. Stamey TA, Kabalin JN, McNeal JE et al (1989) Prostate specific antigen in the diagnosis and treatment of adenocarcinoma of the prostate: II. Radical prostatectomy treated patients. J Urol 141:1076
16. Morgan TO, Jacobsen SJ, McCarthy WF et al (1996) Age-specific reference ranges for prostate-specific antigen in black men. N Engl J Med 335:304-310
17. Carter HB, Coffey DS (1990) The prostate: an increasing medical problem. Prostate 16:39-48

17a. Frauscher F, Pallwein L, Klauser A et al (2005) Ultrasound contrast agents and prostate cancer. Radiologe 45:544-551

18. Hodge KK, McNeal JE, Terris MK, Stamey TA (1989) Random systematic versus directed ultrasound guided transrectal core biopsies of the prostate. J Urol 142:71-74
19. Eskew LA, Bare RL, McCullough DL (1997) Systematic 5 region prostate biopsy is superior to sextant method for diagnosing carcinoma of the prostate. J Urol. 157:199-202
20. Naughton CK, Miller DC, Mager DE (2000) A prospective randomized trial comparing 6 versus 12 prostate biopsy cores: impact on cancer detection. J Urol 164:388-392
21. Rifkin MD, Sudakoff GS, Alexander AA (1993) Prostate: techniques, results, and potential applications of color Doppler US scanning. Radiology 186:509-513
22. Kelly IM, Lees WR, Rickards D (1993) Prostate cancer and the role of color Doppler US. Radiology 189:153-156
23. Newman JS, Bree RL, Rubin JM (1995) Prostate can-

cer: diagnosis with color Doppler sonography with histologic correlation of each biopsy site. Radiology 195:86-90
24. Littrup PJ, Klein RM, Gross ML et al (1995) Color Doppler of the prostate: histologic and racial correlations. Radiology 197:365
25. Ismail M, Petersen R0, Alexander AA et al (1997) Color Doppler imaging in predicting the biologic behavior of prostate cancer: correlation with disease-free survival. Urology 50:906-912
26. Ismail M, Gomella LG, Alexander AA (1997) Color Doppler sonography of the prostate. Tech Urol 3:140-146
27. Alexander AA (1995) To color Doppler image the prostate or not: that is the question. Radiology 195:11-13
28. Rifkin MD, Alexander AA, Helinek TG, Merton DA (1991) Color Doppler as an adjunct to prostate ultrasound. Scand J Urol Nephrol Suppl 137:85-89
29. Sillman F, Boyce J, Fruchter R (1981) The significance of atypical vessels and neovascularization in cervical neoplasia. Am J Obstet Gynecol 139:154-159
30. Srivastava A, Laidler P, Davies RP et al (1988) The prognostic significance of tumor vascularity in intermediate- thickness (0.76-4.0 mm thick) skin melanoma. A quantitative histologic study. Am J Pathol 133:419-423
31. Weidner N, Semple JP, Welch WR, Folkman J (1991) Tumor angiogenesis and metastasis - correlation in invasive breast carcinoma. N Engl J Med 324:1-8
32. Brawer MK, Deering RE, Brown M et al (1994) Predictors of pathologic stage in prostatic carcinoma. The role of neovascularity. Cancer 73:678-687
33. Fleischer AC, Rodgers WH, Rao BK et al (1991) Assessment of ovarian tumor vascularity with transvaginal color Doppler sonography. J Ultrasound Med 10:563-568
34. Cho JY, Kim SH, Lee SE (1998) Diffuse prostatic lesions: role of color and power Doppler ultrasonography. J Ultrasound Med 17:283-287
35. Halpern EJ, Sirup SE (2000) Using Gray-scale and Color and Power Doppler sonography to detect prostatic cancer. Am J Roentgenol AJR 174:623-627
36. Kedar RP, Cosgrove D, McCready VR et al (1996) Microbubble contrast agent for color Doppler US: effect on breast masses. Work in progress. Radiology 198:679-686
37. Forsberg F, Merton DA, Liu JB et al (1998) Clinical applications of ultrasound contrast agents. Ultrasonics 36:695-701
38. Forsberg E, Liu JB, Bums PN et al (1994) Artifacts in ultrasonic contrast agent studies. J Ultrasound Med 13:357-65
39. Goldberg BB, Liu JB, Forsberg F (1994) Ultrasound contrast agents: a review. Ultrasound Med Biol 20:319-333
40. Ragde H, Kenny GM, Murphy GP, Landin K (1997) Transrectal ultrasound microbubble contrast angiography of the prostate. Prostate 32:279-283
41. Watanabe M (1998) Color Doppler enhancement with contrast agents for the detection of prostatic cancer. Nippon Rinsho 56:1040-1044
42. Frauscher E, Helweg G, Gotwald TF et al (1998) The value of contrast-enhanced color Doppler ultrasonography in the diagnosis of prostate cancer. Radiology 209:417 (abstract)
43. Bree RL, DeDreu SE (1998) Contrast-enhanced color Doppler of the prostate as an adjunct to gray-scale identification of cancer prior to biopsy. Radiology 209:418
44. Bogers HA, Sedelaar JP, Beerlage HP et al (1999) Contrast-enhanced three-dimensional power Doppler angiography of the human prostate: correlation with biopsy outcome. Urology 54:97-104
45. Unal D, Sedelaar JP, Aarnink RG et al Three-dimensional contrast-enhanced power Doppler ultrasonography and conventional examination methods: the value of diagnostic predictors of prostate cancer. BJU Int (in press)
46. Frauscher F, Klauser A, Halpern EJ et al (2001) Detection of prostate cancer with a microbubble ultrasound contrast agent. Lancet 357:1849–1850
47. Frauscher F, Klauser A, Volgger H et al (2002) Comparison of contrast-enhanced color Doppler targeted biopsy with conventional systematic biopsy: impact on prostate cancer detection. J Urol 167:1648–1652
47a. Frauscher F, Klauser A, Berger AP (2003) The value of ultrasound (US) in the diagnosis of prostate cancer. Radiologe 43:455-463
48. Sedelaar JP, Van Leenders GJ, Hulsbergen-Van De Kaa CA et al (2001) Microvessel density: correlation between contrast ultrasonography and histology of prostate cancer. Eur Urol 40:285–293
49. Roy C, Buy X, Lang H et al (2003) Contrast-enhanced color Doppler endorectal sonography of prostate: efficiency for detecting peripheral zone tumors and role for biopsy procedure. J Urol 170:69-72
50. Strohmeyer D, Frauscher F, Klauser A et al (2001) Contrast-enhanced transrectal color Doppler ultrasonography (TRCDUS) for assessment of angiogenesis in prostate cancer. Anticancer Res 21:2907–2913
51. Albrecht T, Hoffmann CW, Schettler S et al (2000) B-mode enhancement at phase-inversion US with air-based microbubble contrast agent: initial experience in humans. Radiology 216:273-278
52. Halpern EJ, Verkh L, Forsberg F et al (2000) Initial experience with contrast-enhanced sonography of the prostate. AIR 174:1757-1580
53. Halpern EJ, Rosenberg M, Gomoll LG (2001) Contrast-enhanced sonography of the prostate. Radiology 219:219-225
54. Halpern EJ, Frauscher F, Rosenberg M, Gomella LG (2002) Directed biopsy during contrast-enhanced sonography of the prostate. AJR Am J Roentgenol 178:915-919
55. Halpern EJ, Ramey JR, Strup SE (2005) Directed biopsy during contrast-enhanced sonography of the prostate. Detection of prostate carcinoma with contrast-enhanced sonography using intermittent harmonic imaging. Cancer 104:2373-2383
56. Shi WT, Forsberg F, Hall AL et al (1999) Subharmonic imaging with contrast agents: initial results. Ultrasonics imaging 21:79-94
57. Forsberg F, Shi WT, Goldberg BB (2000) Subharmonic imaging of contrast agents. Ultrasonic 38:93-98

IV.5

Recent Advances in Contrast-Enhanced Ultrasound in Woman Pelvis Lesions

Henri Marret, Stéphane Sauget, Molly Brewer and François Tranquart

Introduction

Ultrasound (US) is the primary imaging modality for the detection and characterization of female pelvis lesions during screening, or for any pelvic symptom. It has been proven that the association of suprapelvic and transvaginal approaches gives a complete view of the female pelvis and provides some specific indicators for a high level confidence diagnosis. As it was demonstrated that Doppler US plays a role in such diagnoses, some research has been conducted to allow better detection of vessels within or surrounding a lesion. The sensitivity of Doppler methods remains limited because of either patient or technical limitations, allowing us to detect vessels larger than 80 μm; not enough for a correct assessment of neoangiogenesis. This has led physicians to propose the use of contrast agents for US in order to enhance contrast between the lesion and parenchyma and thus to improve the quality of information provided by US methods.

The recent introduction of US contrast agents has totally changed the depiction of specific vascular signs for a definite diagnosis by allowing a marked increase in signal from the vessels, especially with modern non-linear imaging techniques. Contrast-enhanced ultrasound (CEUS) allows an adequate depiction of vessels in relation to the pure intravascular characteristics of those agents, reinforced by the real-time assessment of the enhancement after contrast injection. The recent availability of this imaging technique for transvaginal applications has allowed physicians to use CEUS in gynecology, such as in ovarian or uterine lesions, for a better assessment of vascular patterns that could play a role in diagnosis management.

Ovarian Lesions

Ovarian carcinoma represents the second most frequent gynecological cancer observed in women, with a poor long-term outcome largely related to late diagnosis and the frequency, around 15%, of malignant lesions. This is due to the absence of any alarm signal for initiating an US exam to detect any ovarian abnormalities. It has long been proven that US is the most powerful technique for detecting ovarian cancer, with a sensitivity of 80-85%. One of the most common suggestions for an early diagnosis of ovarian cancer is to detect the neovessels that allow the tumor to grow. Vessel changes within the ovary may be visualized before tumor detection itself. Color Doppler has been assessed as one of the US techniques that can be used to describe specific characteristics of ovarian vascularization [1-6]. Power Doppler is useful to map ovarian vessels, including those associated with malignancy (in septa, papillarities and tissular parts of the lesion) while pulsed Doppler is used to measure blood flow velocity [7-9]. Doppler imaging and the subjective evaluation of the gray-scale image improves our ability to make a correct diagnosis prior to surgery [10, 11], which improves patient outcome if a malignancy is present [12-15]. The need for a more powerful US technique is driven by the specific role of US in pelvic lesions and the need for the treatment planning, including chemotherapy and particularly, surgery. Recently, quantification of the vascularization of a tumor using power Doppler has been performed by analysis of images using special software [16-18], allowing us to calculate the number of colored pixels on a digitized image. Until now, subjective evaluation of the gray-scale and Doppler US in experienced hands has been considered the most powerful method for discriminating between benign and malignant adnexal masses [11]. We have demonstrated that power Doppler index (colored pixel number inside the tumor/total pixel of the tumor) is a simple and accurate parameter to discriminate an ovarian malignancy from a benign ovarian mass [19].

Prior Studies

The first-generation US contrast agent used was mainly Levovist (Schering, Germany) [20, 21]. Only a few small studies [22-24] have been published using this contrast agent for gynecological purposes. They validated the feasibility of the technique in ovaries. Orden in 2003 [25] and our team in 2004 [26] first described the kinetics of the agent within the ovary and ovarian tumors in order to define the parameters that can be useful for malignancy discrimination. Our prospective pilot study was conducted, with the following aims: (1) to evaluate the contribution of contrast-enhanced power Doppler and derive objective parameters for the diagnosis of malignancy in ovarian tumors; and (2) to compare these parameters to other variables that have been evaluated to differentiate malignant adnexal masses from benign ones.

The time intensity curves of Levovist can then be derived over 5 minutes for a region of interest (ROI) corresponding to solid tissue from each mass (Fig. 1). The software calculates the total power Doppler intensity, which is determined by the number and intensity of colored pixels inside the ROI for each image. The enhancement quickly achieves a maximum intensity and has a biphasic wash-out phase, with a decrease in intensity down to the baseline level at around 3 minutes. From the time-intensity curve, baseline intensity and peak intensity were noted and the percentage ratio of intensity enhancement (expressed as a fraction of enhancement) was calculated using the following formula: 100*(peak intensity-baseline intensity)/baseline intensity. The time-intensity curves were analyzed for the following indices: uptake time (in seconds), wash-out time, half-intensity wash-out time, and the area under the curve (AUC). Orden [25] and ourselves [26] describe almost the same differences between benign and malignant enhancement curves. After a quick rise to maximum enhancement, the wash-out phase differed between cancers and benign ovarian tumors. The duration of contrast-enhancement or wash-out period and the AUC appeared to have a very important power of discrimination. In our study, AUC and wash-out time were the two discriminate parameters with the highest sensitivity (96%). Only one cancer was missed using these two parameters with the threshold (derived from the received operating characteristic (ROC) curve) fixed at 88 seconds-1 and 175 seconds, respectively. Using the traditional criteria of resistance index (RI) and CA125, the sensitivity was lower, at 86% with four missed cancers (three of the missed cancers were borderline tumors and one was Stage I), but no false positives (specificity = 100%). Orden [25] found that the mean duration of contrast-enhancement was 190 seconds in malignant tumors and 104 seconds in benign tumors, whereas we found 221 seconds versus 114 seconds. These results suggest that kinetic parame-

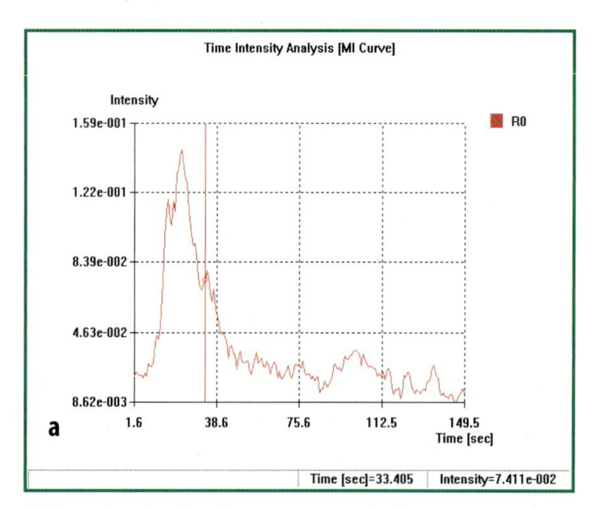

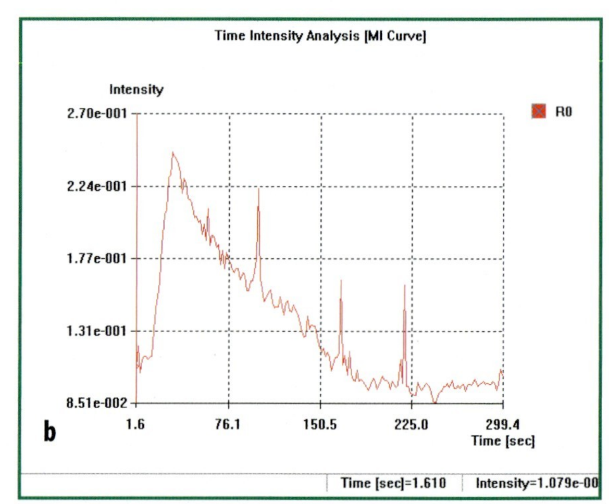

Fig. 1a, b. a Results of Levovist contrast-enhancement in ovarian tumors. Example of a benign tumor showing a short wash-out time. **b** Example of a malignant tumor showing a long wash-out time (peaks are related to movements artifacts)

ters derived from power Doppler enhanced using Levovist provide new valid criteria that appear accurate for the discrimination of benign pelvic masses from malignant primary epithelial ovarian tumors and could improve the pre-operative diagnosis of ovarian cancer.

Second-Generation Agents: SonoVue, Definity

Second generation US contrast agents (SonoVue, Bracco SpA, Italy; Definity, Bristol Myers Squibb, USA) have previously demonstrated their value in the investigation of neovessels in organs other than ovaries with a high degree of safety [27]. In our case, the dose of SonoVue needs to be increased to 4.8 ml, as we use higher US frequencies for the transvaginal approach.

To date no study has been published in human ovaries using SonoVue, except a recent paper from Testa et al. [28], who described some vascular patterns in the female pelvis. We have recently conducted a study to determine whether second-generation contrast agents could characterize changes in ovarian vascularization during the ewe estrus cycle and to select parameters that remained stable with cyclic changes [29]. Following SonoVue injection, wash-out time and AUC were the most stable parameters derived from the time-intensity curve between ovaries and between the follicular and luteal phases. Uptake time and total time of enhancement were also constant. Enhancement ratio and wash-in period changed with corpus luteum formation. Our results reflect menstrual cycle changes and vascular physiology of the normal ovary. One of the limitations of this study is the heterogeneity of the ovarian vascular characteristics. The ovary of the ewe is smaller than that of a woman and the corpus luteum is proportionately larger, which could influence the results of this study; however, the same heterogeneity should be present in women, albeit in a smaller portion of the ovary. Further studies in women should be performed to characterize menstrual changes in enhancement in order to define stable and unstable parameters of enhancement.

We are currently conducting several ovarian studies to validate SonoVue in Europe, and Definity in the United States, for discrimination of human ovarian tumors. In our preliminary experience using both products, we were able to describe the microbubble distribution inside the tumor vessels with high accuracy, resulting in an improvement in the diagnostic confidence for the discrimination of benign from malignant ovarian tumors. For example, the absence of enhancement inside solid tissue or intracystic papillarities can confirm a diagnosis of clots or solid component included within a dermoid cyst. In the first cases, detection of enhancement within septa and/or papillarities is always the sign of malignancy confirmed by histology (Figs. 2, 3). Compared to Levovist, the results appear to be much more precise and accurate without artifacts such as blooming or movement. However, time-intensity curves appear quite similar, with a few differences in the wash-out period, such as a longer return to baseline and a less marked biphasic phase (distribution and elimination phase).

A single injection of SonoVue gives us access to a very precise map of the ovarian and tumor microcirculation in both the ewe and the woman. One of the challenges in detecting small vascular changes is the selection of the ROI. In all published studies, the ROI encompassed the entire ovary and the enhancement curve was based on pixel mapping extracted from this ROI.

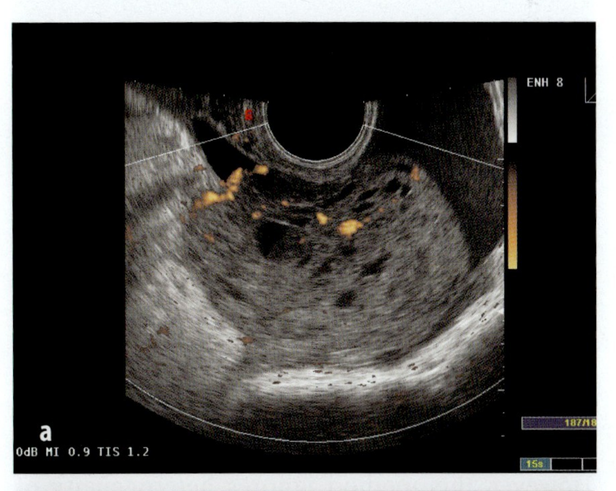

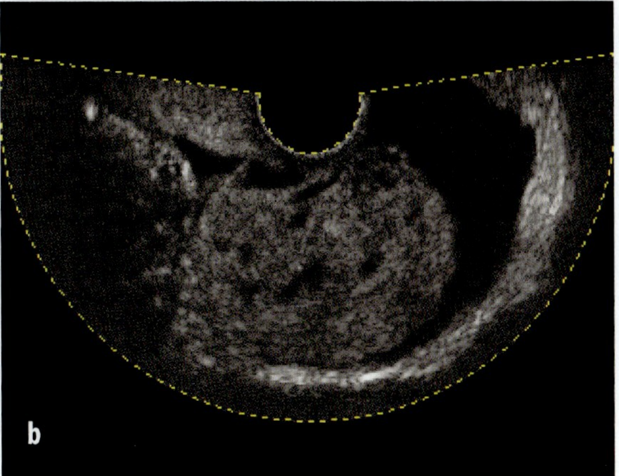

Fig. 2a, b. Arterial enhancement within an ovarian cancer (**a** power Doppler imaging) after SonoVue injection (Esaote system, transvaginal examination), demonstrating a heterogeneous global and intense enhancement from the tissular part (**b**), confirmed by surgery

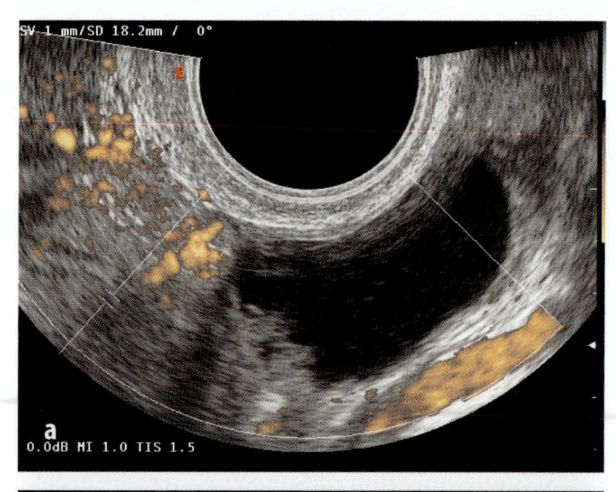

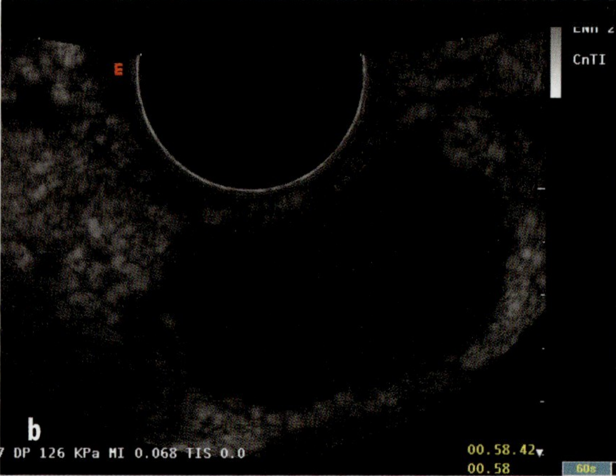

Fig. 3a, b. Absence of arterial enhancement within a wall abnormality in an ovarian cystic lesion (**a**) after SonoVue injection (**b** Esaote system, transvaginal examination) in favor of the diagnosis of a hemorrhagic cyst (confirmed by surgery)

Reproducibility of this procedure is very high and will be higher using CEUS, which allows the ovarian contours to be drawn more accurately. However, this method ignores heterogeneity of tissue components and enhancement. Therefore, selective sampling of regions within the ovary may be required to improve discrimination of lesions. Although visual appreciation of heterogeneity is improved by pixel mapping displays, selection of ROI is operator-dependent. Moreover, it is known that the baseline signal for any given tissue differs with the US machine, the probe used, the movements of the probe and the settings of the US machine, even if identical sequences are used. In addition, the calculation of the ratio of enhancement will differ with different conditions [30]. Consequently, the ratio of enhancement is probably not the best parameter to use, although gray-scale imaging reduces artifacts and improves the reproducibility compared to color Doppler. Wash-out parameters may be more adapted to discriminate regions inside the ovary with high enhancement. Improvement in microvessel detection and increased visibility of nodular areas of enhancement inside the ovary with different enhancement curves could be shown, as has been demonstrated in prostate cancer [31]. Moreover, one case of ovarian cancer with normal-sized ovaries was diagnosed only by CEUS [32], suggesting that contrast agents will improve the ability of US to detect small cancers that are not associated with ovarian enlargement or areas within a mass that have a focus of malignancy.

From an angiogenesis perspective, contrast agents markedly increase the number of visible vessels available for dynamic analysis, and allow us to identify the aberrant vascularity that pathologists visualize in early stage cancers. Any imaging assay of tumor microvascular characteristics must be validated against accepted surrogates of angiogenesis, including histological microvessel density (MVD), vascular endothelial growth factor (VEGF), and VEGF receptors. Correlation of these factors with Doppler US has been previously carried out in other organs, but not in the ovary, and not using CEUS [33]. In addition, CEUS should also be validated against other imaging techniques that measure vascular function, such as magnetic resonance imaging (MRI) [34].

In conclusion, results of all these preliminary studies are in favor of the use of CEUS being applied prospectively in non-invasive studies of ovarian angiogenic function, mainly for the diagnosis of malignancy, but also including response to drug treatment, fertility research, ovarian hyperstimulation syndrome, and early assessment of response to antiangiogenic chemotherapy.

Uterine Lesions

Study of uterine vascularity using power Doppler is nowadays one of the most important tools to describe and discriminate uterine tumors. Macroscopic vascularization of myomas, polyps, endometrial cancer, adenomyosis, or cervical cancer is well known, but some limitations are encountered in therapeutic monitoring of these tumors. Microbubble enhancement affords the direct depiction of tumor neoangiogenesis and may help us to establish a more precise vascular map of the tumor and normal surrounding myometrium. By quantifying time-intensity curves after injection of microbubbles, tumors can be shown to exhibit significantly different enhancement kinetics from normal tissue.

A Myoma Evaluation

Leiomyomas are the most common benign tumors of the uterus in women between 20 and 50 years old. A successful and safe alternative treatment to hysterectomy is uterine artery embolization (UAE) [35-38]. Symptoms are improved or resolved in 90% of women at one year [36, 39]. However, rare potential complications, such as uterine necrosis and premature menopause, have been reported [40, 41]. The polyvinyl alcohol particles, the Embospheres, or other embolic agents injected into each uterine artery tend to reach leiomyomas selectively, but may reduce blood supply to the uterus and induce ischemic uterine necrosis [42]. Moreover, because uterine and ovarian vessels communicate directly via the tubal arteries, once stasis has begun, they may also reach the ovaries, probably by a phenomenon of reflux, reducing ovarian perfusion and even causing infarction [40, 41]. The reported incidence of amenorrhea after UAE is 1-3%. However, these rare cases limited UAE to women with accomplished childbearing. Such complications might be prevented, or at least rapidly detected by comparison of pre- and post-operative assessment of leiomyoma vasculature occlusions.

We successfully used contrast-enhanced sonography with SonoVue during UAE procedures in a patient with multiple large leiomyomas to demonstrate that injected micro-particles were targeted uniquely to leiomyomas [43]. Contrast-enhanced sonography was performed just before UAE, immediately after left UAE, and after bilateral UAE. Pre-UAE images showed a completely perfused uterus with hyperenhanced areas corresponding to the leiomyomas. The next two acquisitions showed hypoperfused areas corresponding to the leiomyomas. The last acquisition, taken after complete bilateral uterine artery occlusion, showed persistent perfusion into normal myometrium but none in the leiomyomas.

Following this first publication, we tested the feasibility of contrast-enhanced US for the diagnosis of fibroids. It is remarkable that this indication could be reached by the use of transvaginal approach for tiny fibroids (with injection of 4.8 ml of SonoVue) but also by the use of the suprapubic approach for large fibroids (with injection of 2.4 ml of SonoVue only). Injection of SonoVue could provide a very precise description of the uterine vascularization more esaily than with angiography and cheaper than MRI. After contrast injection, macro- and microcirculation of the myoma first appeared, followed by the normal myometrial enhancement and finally within the endometrium (Fig. 4). Enhancement patterns vary markedly among the patients, from an absence of enhancement for the whole tumor, to a complete and rapid enhancement after injection. Wash-out was typically complete after 3 minutes, giving a black hole corresponding to the whole lesion. This wash-out helps us to iden-

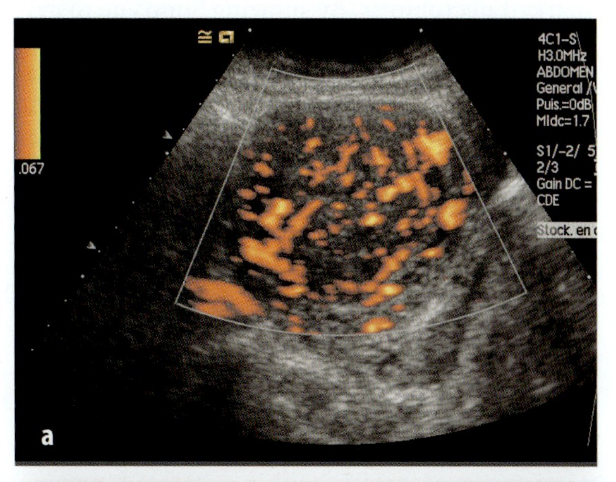

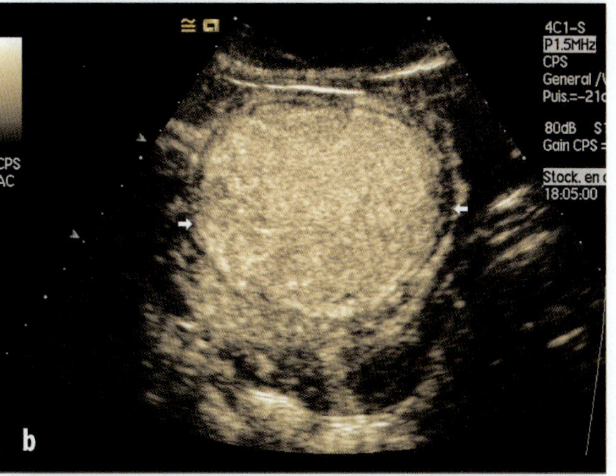

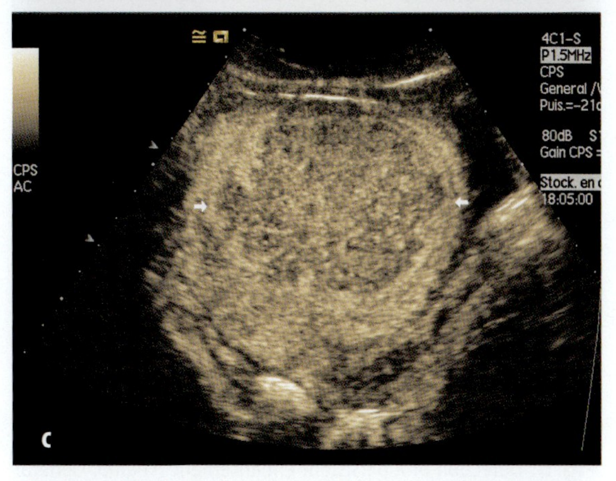

Fig. 4a-c. Arterial enhancement within a uterine fibroid (**a**) after SonoVue injection (Sequoia system, suprapubic examination) demonstrating a quite global and intense enhancement, higher than from normal myometrium (**b**), followed by a marked wash-out (**c**)

tify some tiny fibroids that are not visible on conventional sonography, for a perfect match with MRI detection. Secondly, it is remarkable that most of the endometrium clearly demonstrates an early wash-out after contrast injection, in some cases exceeding the size of endometrium. Third, it clearly shows that microbubbles first arrive in the myoma before the normal myometrium, except in some large myomas with marked necrobiosis. By showing SonoVue distribution within the uterus, we are able to better select fibroids with possible benefit of embolization and we were able to corroborate the approach used by the particles injected for embolization.

Using CEUS, we could quickly assess the efficacy of UAE as well as evaluate local consequences on normal myometrium and ovaries, whereas both uterine arteries were totally occluded. This US method could play a major role in the assessment of early technical failure rate and in the identification of vascular risk factors for clinical failure and late recurrences. Contrast-enhanced US can also be proposed to detect the persistence of vessels within a treated myoma with higher confidence, as it was reported that this precedes the late recurrence confirmed by an increased size of the myomas (Fig. 5). This will be a more sensitive method than color Doppler US for an assessment of induced vascularity changes [44].

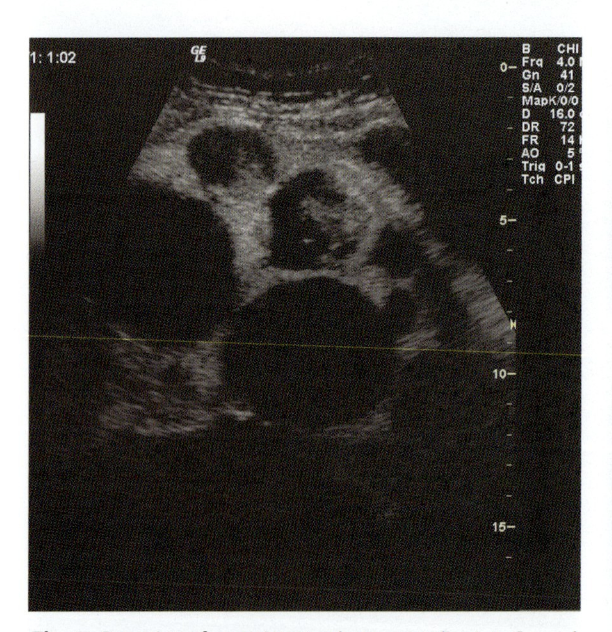

Fig. 5. Detection of a persistent enhancement (Logiq9, General Electric) within two fibroids (arrows) after uterine artery embolization, which corresponds to an incomplete embolization when the other fibroids were totally excluded. This was confirmed six months later by a size increase of these two fibroids, while the other fibroids decreased in size

In conclusion, we can state that contrast-enhanced sonography provides a means to assess tumor response to various therapeutic approaches. Thus, the potential for imaging uterine perfusion with microbubble-enhanced sonography is significant and warrants further investigation.

Cancer of the Cervix

Cancer of the cervix is frequent and is accompanied by local extension or lymph node extension, which guides treatment planning, i.e., the choice between initial treatment by surgery or by radiochemotherapy. An intense enhancement is reported for these lesions before specific treatment, with an improvement in the definition of limits but with some limitations in the positive diagnosis (Fig. 6) as reported by Testa et al. [28]. Local assessment of angiogenesis will be of value to follow local changes under chemotherapy or radiotherapy and to better schedule surgery. This method could be used in place of MRI to assess treatment efficacy and in conjunction with positron emission tomography (PET) for treatment planning.

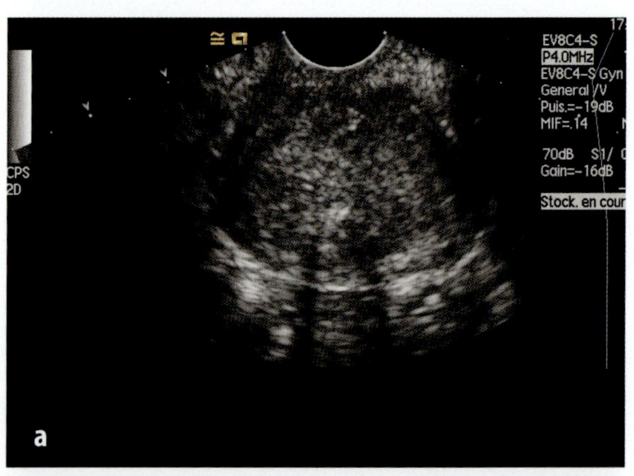

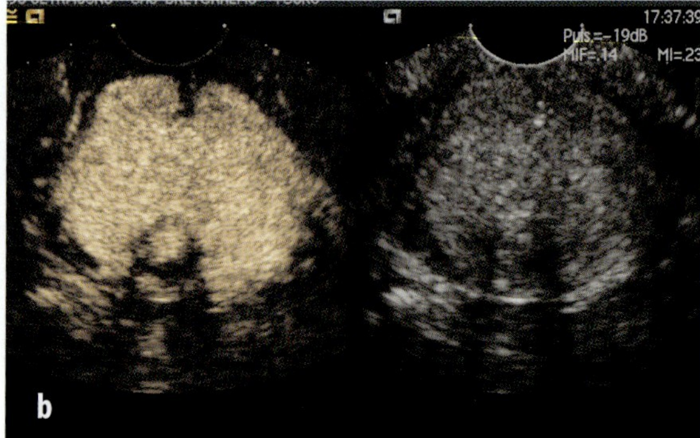

Fig. 6a, b. Typical strong and homogeneous enhancement from a cervical cancer (**a**) after SonoVue injection (**b**) (Sequoia system, transvaginal examination)

Key Points

- Contrast-enhanced ultrasound is useful for the discrimination of malignancy in ovarian disease.
- In cases of myoma, contrast-enhancement is useful for uterine artery embolization monitoring by selecting patients with possible early recurrence.
- In cervical cancer, ultrasound enhancement using contrast agents is useful for monitoring radiochemotherapy, to select patients that present a good or a poor response to treatment.

References

1. Marret H, Tranquart F, Sauget S, Lansac J (2003) Apport du Doppler pour le diagnostic des tumeurs ovariennes. J Radiol 84:1725-1731
2. Zanetta G, Vergani P, Lissoni A (1994) Color Doppler ultrasound in the preoperative assessment of adnexal masses. Acta Obstet Gynecol Scand 73:637-641
3. Timor-Tritsch LE, Lerner JP, Monteagudo A, Santos R (1993) Transvaginal ultrasonographic characterization of ovarian masses by means of color flow-directed Doppler measurements and a morphologic scoring system. Am J Obstet Gynecol 168:909-913
4. Valentin L, Sladkevicius P, Marsal K (1994) Limited contribution of Doppler velocimetry to the differential diagnosis of extrauterine pelvic tumors. Obstet Gynecol 83:425-433
5. Alcazar JL, Ruiz-Perez ML, Errasti T (1996) Transvaginal color Doppler sonography in adnexal masses: which parameter performs best? Ultrasound Obstet Gynecol 8:114-119
6. Valentin L (1999) Prospective cross-validation of Doppler ultrasound examination and gray-scale ultrasound imaging for discrimination of benign and malignant pelvic masses. Ultrasound Obstet Gynecol 14:273-283
7. Timmerman D, Valentin L, Bourne TH et al (2000) Terms, definitions and measurements to describe the sonographic features of adnexal tumors: a consensus opinion from the International Ovarian Tumor Analysis (IOTA) Group. Ultrasound Obstet Gynecol 16:500-505
8. Tailor A, Jurkovic D, Bourne TH et al (1998) Comparison of transvaginal color Doppler imaging and color Doppler energy for assessment of intraovarian blood flow. Obstet Gynecol 91:561-567
9. Merce LT, Caballero RA, Barco MJ et al (1998) B-mode, utero-ovarian and intratumoral transvaginal colour Doppler ultrasonography for differential diagnosis of ovarian tumours. Eur J Obstet Gynecol Reprod Biol 76:97-107
10. Kinkel K, Hricak H, Lu Y et al (2000) US characterization of ovarian masses: a meta-analysis. Radiology 217:803-811
11. Marret H, Ecochard R, Giraudeau B et al (2002) Color Doppler energy prediction of malignancy in adnexal masses using logistic regression models. Ultrasound Obstet Gynecol 20:597-604
12. Junor EJ, Hole DJ, McNulty L et al (1999) Specialist gynaecologists and survival outcome in ovarian cancer: a Scottish national study of 1866 patients. Br J Obstet Gynaecol. 106:1130-1136
13. Eisenkop SM, Spirtos NM, Montag TW et al (1992) The impact of subspecialty training on the management of advanced ovarian cancer. Gynecol Oncol 47:203-209
14. Kehoe S, Powell J, Wilson S, Woodman C (1994) The influence of the operating surgeon's specialisation on patient survival in ovarian carcinoma. Br J Cancer 70:1014-1017
15. Carney ME, Lancaster JM, Ford C et al (2002) A population-based study of patterns of care for ovarian cancer: who is seen by a gynecologic oncologist and who is not? Gynecol Oncol 84:36-42
16. Epstein E, Skoog L, Isberg PE et al (2002) An algorithm including results of grey-scale and power Doppler ultrasound examination to predict endometrial malignancy in women with postmenopausal bleeding. Ultrasound Obstet Gynecol 20:370-376
17. Fleischer AC, Wojcicki WE, Donnelly EF et al (1999) Quantified color Doppler sonography of tumor vascularity in an animal model. J Ultrasound Med 18:547-551
18. Amso NN, Watermayer SR, Pugh N et al (2001) Quantification of power Doppler energy and its future potential. Fertil Steril 76:583-587
19. Marret H, Sauget S, Giraudeau B et al (2005) Power Doppler vascularity index for predicting malignancy of adnexal masses. Ultrasound Obstet Gynecol 25:508-513
20. Correas JM, Bridal L, Lesavre A et al (2001) Ultrasound contrast agents: properties, principles of action, tolerance, and artifacts. Eur Radiol 11:1316-1328
21. Suren A, Osmers R, Kulenkampff D, Kuhn W (1994) Visualization of blood flow in small ovarian tumor vessels by transvaginal colour Doppler sonography after echo enhancement with injection of Levovist. Gynecol Obstet Invest 38:210-212
22. Orden MR, Gudmundsson S, Kirkinen P (2000)

Contrast-enhanced sonography in the examination of benign and malignant adnexal masses. J Ultrasound Med 19:783-788
23. Szymanski M, Szymanski W, Grabiec M, Korenkiewicz J (1999) Evaluation of using Levovist in the differential diagnosis of ovarian tumors. Ginekol Pol 70:444-449
24. Kupesic S, Kurjak A (2000) Contrast-enhanced, three-dimensional power Doppler sonography for differentiation of adnexal masses. Obstet Gynecol 96:452-458
25. Orden MR, Jurvelin JS, Kirkinen PP (2003) Kinetics of a US contrast agent in benign and malignant adnexal tumors. Radiology 226:405-410
26. Marret H, Sauget S, Giraudeau B et al (2004) Contrast-enhanced sonography helps in discrimination of benign from malignant adnexal masses. J Ultrasound Med 23:1629-1639
27. Morel DR., Schwieger I, Hohn L (2000) Human pharmacokinetics and safety evaluation of SonoVue, a new contrast agent for ultrasound imaging. Invest Radiol 35:80-85
28. Testa A, Ferrandina G, Fruscella E et al (2005) The use of contrasted transvaginal sonography in the diagnosis of gynecologic diseases. J Ultrasound Med 24:1261-1266
29. Marret H, Brewer M, Giraudeau B et al (2005) Ovine model to evaluate ovarian vascularization using contrast-enhanced sonography. Comparative Medicine 55:150-155
30. Seidel G, Vidal-Langwasser M, Algermissen C et al (1999) The influence of Doppler system settings on the clearance kinetics of different ultrasound contrast agents. Eur J Ultrasound 9:167-175
31. Halpern EJ, Rosenberg M, Gomella LG (2001) Prostate cancer: contrast-enhanced US for detection. Radiology 219:219-25
32. Emoto M, Fujimitsu R, Hiwasaki H, Kawarabayashi T (2003) Normal sized ovarian cancer detected by colour Doppler Ultrasound using a microbubble contrast agent. J Clin Oncol 21:3703-3705
33. Cheng WF, Lee CN, Chen CA et al (1999) Vascularity index as a novel parameter for the in vivo assessment of angiogenesis in patients with cervical carcinoma. Cancer 85:651-657
34. Padhani AR (2002) Dynamic contrast-enhanced MRI in clinical oncology: current status and future directions. J Magn Reson Imaging 16:407-422
35. Watson GM, Walker WJ (2002) Uterine artery embolisation for treatment of symptomatic fibroids in 114 women: reduction in size of the fibroids and women's views of success treatment. BJOG 109:129-135
36. Brunereau L, Herbreteau D, Gallas S et al (2000) Uterine artery embolization in the primary treatment of uterine leiomyomas: technical features and prospective follow-up with clinical and sonographic examinations in 58 patients. AJR Am J Roentgenol 175:1267-1272
37. Spies JB, Scialli AR, Jha RC et al (1999) Initial results from uterine fibroid embolization for symptomatic leiomyomata. J Vasc Interv Radiol 10:1149-1157
38. Pelage JP, Le Dref O, Soyer P et al (2000) Fibroid related menorrhagia: treatment with superselective embolization of the uterine arteries and midterm follow-up. Radiology 215:428-431
39. Tranquart F, Brunereau L, Cottier JP et al (2002) Prospective sonographic assessment of uterine artery embolization for the treatment of fibroids. Ultrasound Obstet Gynecol 19:81-87
40. Amato P, Roberts AC (2001) Transient ovarian failure: a complication of uterine artery embolization. Fertil Steril 75:438-439
41. Stringer NH, Grant T, Park J, Oldham L (2000) Ovarian failure after uterine artery embolization for treatment of myomas. J Am Assoc Gynecol Laparosc 7:395-400
42. Spies JB (2003) Uterine artery embolization for fibroids: understanding the technical causes of failures. J Vasc Interv Radiol 14:11-14
43. Marret H, Tranquart F, Sauget S et al (2004) Contrast-enhanced sonography during Myomas embolization Ultrasound Obstet Gynecol 23:77-79
44. Muniz CJ, Fleischer AC, Donnelly EF, Mazer MJ (2002) Three-dimensional color Doppler sonography and uterine artery arteriography of fibroids: assessment of changes in vascularity before and after embolization. J Ultrasound Med 21:129-133

IV.6

Role of Contrast Ultrasound in Breast Lesions and Sentinel Lymph Nodes

Giorgio Rizzatto and Roberta Chersevani

Introduction

The use of perfusion imaging has resulted in new interest in both research and clinical applications of contrast agents in breast ultrasound (US). The basics of contrast-enhanced US of breast cancers are similar to those for all tumors, and are based on the detection of tumor-associated neoangiogenesis. In the breast, neoangiogenesis is characteristic of both invasive disease and *in situ* cancer, including high-grade ductal carcinoma *in situ* (DCIS).

Most breast tumors have increased vascular density, irregular and often chaotic branching and penetrating vessels, with irregular calibers and velocities.

All these patterns reflect the abnormalities that are specific to rapidly growing tumors: irregular and variable vessel caliber, elongated and coiled vessels, arterio-venous shunts, disturbed dichotomous branching and decreasing caliber, and incomplete vascular wall [1]. The correlation between the vascular disorganization and the grade of tumoral anaplasia is very close.

Baseline Ultrasound

The relative risk for malignancy is higher as detected by conventional breast US when the vessels exhibit irregular morphology and irregular velocities: these two characteristics contribute to define a typical 'mosaic' pattern.

In contrast, fibroadenomas, the most common benign tumor in the breast, generally have poor vascularity; vessels are peripheral, regular and small, with a nest arrangement.

There is some overlap, however, in the vascular properties of breast lesions, but this gray area represents less than 10% of all pathologies. Inflammatory lesions, proliferating and juvenile fibroadenomas and phylloid tumors may have rich vascularity; only inflammations and malignant phyllodes usually exhibit 'mosaic' patterns. Small tubular or ductal lesions with intense fibrosis may have very poor blood supplies. Intraductal carcinoma is covered by the original basement membrane and is supplied by perfusion only from capillary vessels out of the ducts; the only exception is a papillary form with fibrovascular cores [2]. In invasive carcinoma, tumoral cells are accompanied by surrounding angiogenesis, and are supplied from capillary vessels in the circumference.

With conventional US, these patterns are better imaged when Doppler frequency is higher than 5 MHz, pulse repetition frequency (PRF) is between 600 and 800 Hz, and the area of interest is scanned with minimal compression.

Vascular assessment has progressed enough to depict vessels in almost all the tumors and in most fibroadenomas [3]. With optimal technique, blood flow may be detected through small blood vessels of 1 mm or less in diameter and with blood flow in the order of 1 cm/s. This allows visualization of arterioles and venules, but it is not enough to reveal flow through smaller blood vessels at the capillary level.

In most cases, vascularity acts as major alert for inflammation and malignancy. Ozdemir et al. [4] prospectively examined 112 lesions originally identified by mammography and US with Doppler. Doppler studies increased the specificity of mammography and gray-scale sonography for lesions 10 mm and smaller (from 88.9% to 100%) and for those larger than 10 mm (from 70% to 96.6%). Abnormal vascularity has also been demonstrated using color Doppler in areas of DCIS in which mammography showed only microcalcifications [5].

Flow visualization indicates a higher possibility of malignancy but must not be considered the main US parameter for malignancy [3, 6]. Doppler software may also assess quantitative parameters such as flow velocity, pulsatility and resistivity indexes. Quantitative analysis offers adjunctive information to differentiate malignant from benign tumors [6] and to monitor the chemotherapeutic response of locally advanced breast cancers [7].

In the beginning, contrast-enhanced US was used in breast imaging to increase the sensitivity and specificity of color Doppler scanning [8]. The use of contrast agents markedly improved visualization of the intratumoral vascular architecture. Now similar images are obtained with medium level technology and accurate scanning techniques.

Using the presence of vascularity as criterion for malignancy, Moon et al. [9] found an increase in sensitivity (36% to 95%) and positive and negative predictive values, but a reduction in specificity (86% to 79%), due to the hypervascularity of some benign lesions. Weind et al. [10] had already demonstrated an overlap in the microvessel distribution between carcinomas and fibroadenomas. Ellis [11], re-evaluating their results, pointed out that the higher the grade of tumor in their series, the higher the distribution ratio, and that fibroadenomas and grade I tumors had no substantial difference in vascular distribution. These results confirm that frequently there is little functional difference between low-grade invasive tumors and benign tumors.

Schroeder et al. [12] compared the different published studies with unenhanced and enhanced color Doppler and found that diagnostic accuracy improves with contrast-enhancement. This was mainly caused by better assessment of the vascular architecture and better depiction of the hypervascularity of malignancies.

Stuhrmann et al. [13] tested the possibility of improving the evaluation of benign breast lesions at Doppler sonography in patients scheduled for surgical resection. They measured the degree of enhancement provided by Levovist (scored on an ad hoc 5-point scale), the number of tumour vessels, the time to maximal enhancement, and vascular morphology and course (classified as avascular lesions; lesions with monomorphic or peripheral vessels; and lesions with irregular penetrating vessels). They observed more vessels and faster, stronger enhancement in malignant tumors compared to benign lesions, but the best distinction was afforded by vascular morphology and course, with a 90% sensitivity. However, the 81% specificity limited the clinical utility of this approach. Later reports confirmed that irregularities in the morphology and course of tumoral vessels may be highly suggestive of malignancies leading to a sensitivity of 95% and specificity of 83% or higher [14, 15]. As reported by Zdemir et al. [16], only in the category BI-RADS 4 could the combination of mammography-gray-scale US and contrast-enhanced Doppler achieve a higher specificity (71%) and positive predictive value (70%) than mammography-gray-scale US (39% and 53%, respectively).

Contrast-enhanced Doppler was also assessed in the difficult differentiation between post-operative scar and tumor recurrence. Many studies have confirmed that contrast-enhanced hypervascularity may suggest recurrence [12]. Contrast-enhanced US was found to substantially reduce biopsy rates [17] and was suggested as an alternative to magnetic resonance imaging (MRI), particularly in the first 18 post-operative months, when nodular scars or granulomas may also be vascularized with decreasing tendency parallel to the increasing age of the scar [18].

Unfortunately, most of the results originating from all the published series on breast masses did not correlate well with the microvessel density determined histopathologically, and so far this imaging modality has not translated into increased diagnostic accuracy. Since the breast is a relatively superficial organ, diagnostic biopsy is considered safe and is performed as a gold standard. Thus, there is less demand for an imaging technique to differentiate between malignant and benign lesions.

The relatively poor correlation between Doppler flow parameters and histopathological analysis of microvessel density confirms that Doppler US mainly visualizes tumoral macrovasculature.

The specificity and sensitivity of evaluating breast lesions with MRI is improved by performing quantitative imaging with the aid of contrast agents: malignant tumors show early enhancement followed by wash-out or plateau, whereas benign lesions exhibit a gradual increase in enhancement from early to late phases. To determine if this phenomenon is also observed during dynamic contrast-enhanced ultrasonography, Huber et al. [19] studied 47 patients with breast lesions and measured color pixel density on Doppler US for 3 minutes after injection of Levovist. They reported a shorter time to peak enhancement for carcinoma than for benign tumors. More recently, the same group [20] confirmed a shorter time to peak for malignancies ($p < 0.01$) and a higher peak color-pixel-density ($p < 0.03$). Different time-intensity curves have been found for carcinomas, fibroadenomas and scars [21]. Focal inflammations, due to their markedly increased vascularity, showed the same curves as malignancies. But with first generation agents the wash-out behaviour, although different, was adversely influenced by the continuous bubble destruction induced by the high US mechanical pressure induced by conventional Doppler imaging.

Contrast Ultrasound Features

New contrast agents are less fragile and allow use of specific softwares that reveal the perfusion flow even in the smallest vessels [22].

Current experience is based on the use of a blood-pool echo-contrast agent. SonoVue (Bracco, Italy) consists of microbubbles containing sulphur-hexafluoride (SF6) encapsulated by a flexible phospholipid-shell. These microbubbles have a mean diameter of 2.5 µm, with 99% of the bubbles smaller than 11 µm, allowing a free passage in the capillaries but keeping the agent within the vascular lumen.

Tumor angiogenesis is a sequential process. During the organization of tumor-associated capillary networks, neovessels progressively acquire their distinctive structural and functional characteristics [23]. Their lining is formed by fenestrated endothelial cells limited by a discontinuous basement membrane; as a result the neoangiogenetic vessels are more permeable than the normal ones.

Vascular endothelial growth factor directly stimulates endothelial cell division and migration; it strongly increases permeability, allowing the extravasation of plasma proteins and resulting in the formation of an extravascular gel conducive to neovascular growth [24].

In contrast-enhanced MRI, the actual tracers cross the tumor microvessels and extravasate in the extravascular tumoral space. On the contrary, the diameter of SonoVue microbubbles keeps the agent within the vascular lumen (intravascular tracer). Therefore, the area of the perfusion and the correlated time-intensity curves strictly correspond to the neoangiogenetic vascular bed, and not to the extravascular tumor space.

The microbubble suspension contains 8 µl/ml SF6 gas. The best results in the breast are obtained with bolus injections of 4.8 ml administered intravenously through a three-way connector, followed by an injection of 5 ml saline solution for flushing.

Due to the flexibility of the microbubbles' phospholipid-shell, the reflectivity of SonoVue is very high. This results in a strong echo-enhancement. Due to the poor solubility and diffusivity of SF6, this agent is also highly resistant to pressure.

Depending on the frequency and amplitude (the mechanical index [MI]) of the ultrasound wave, SonoVue microbubbles may reflect the incident wave repeatedly without being altered (low MI continuous imaging). The reflected wave contains harmonic frequency components caused by the non-linear bubble oscillations. The microbubbles are very flexible, so significant harmonic response is obtained even at very low MI.

Although harmonics are also generated during propagation of ultrasound waves in tissues, SonoVue microbubbles generate echoes that are considerably larger than tissue echoes at harmonic frequencies. Contrast-specific imaging modes have been developed in order to accurately discriminate between the harmonic response from microbubbles and the response from tissue.

This results in perfusional images of the tumoral microcirculation based only on the microbubbles response. Microvascular blood velocities in the order of 0.1-10 mm/s, that cannot be detected with conventional Doppler methods, can be demonstrated with this technique.

Actual experience is based on the use of Contrast-Tuned Imaging (CNTI) that is a low MI technique proposed by Esaote (Italy), in which the fundamental echo is filtered out and only the second harmonic echo is detected by the US probe.

The best perfusion imaging in the breast is obtained with MI values between 0.1 and 0.08, without reducing the field of view too much to avoid superficial artifacts and with the focal zone positioned just behind the deeper lesion's margin. Compression must be minimized.

Perfusion is seen as an area of enhancement on the background of a nearly absent tissue signal and with minimal microbubble destruction (Fig. 1). Unfortunately, the resolution is rather poor in harmonic mode, and may be problematic for detecting small lesions. However, linear hyperechoic structures, like ligaments, often act as reference structures to keep the right scanning position.

CNTI has the capability to render the time-intensity curves. The signal perfusion intensity is monitored over time in selected tumor regions of interest (ROIs) and plotted on a final graph. Curves can be filtered and normalized according to the baseline signal intensity in the selected ROIs (Fig. 1).

Role of Contrast Ultrasound in Clinical Practice

A number of European physicians are participating in the multicenter project Perfusion Ultrasound Multicenter European Breast study (PUMEB 04-06) to determine the appropriate uses of low MI contrast tuned imaging in the evaluation of breast cancers. Participants include G. Rizzatto, R. Chersevani, E. Cassano, A. Gambaro (Italy), J. Camps Herrero (Spain), S. Paebke (Germany) and G. Ralleigh (United Kingdom). Initially the group decided to focus on five clinically relevant topics: lesion characterization, lesions first identified on

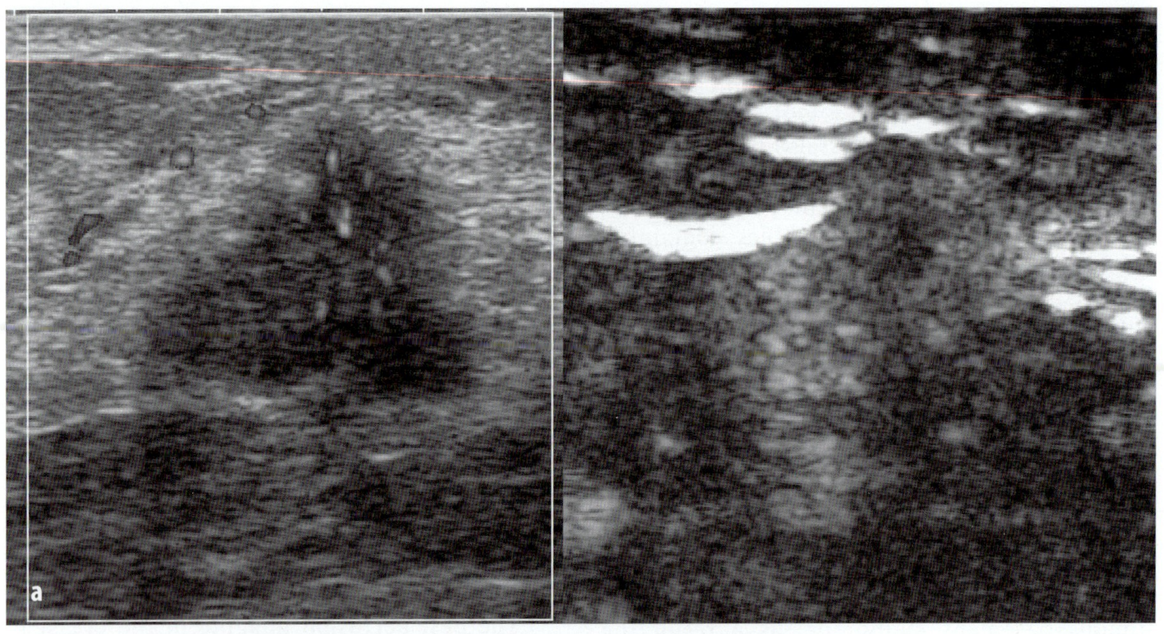

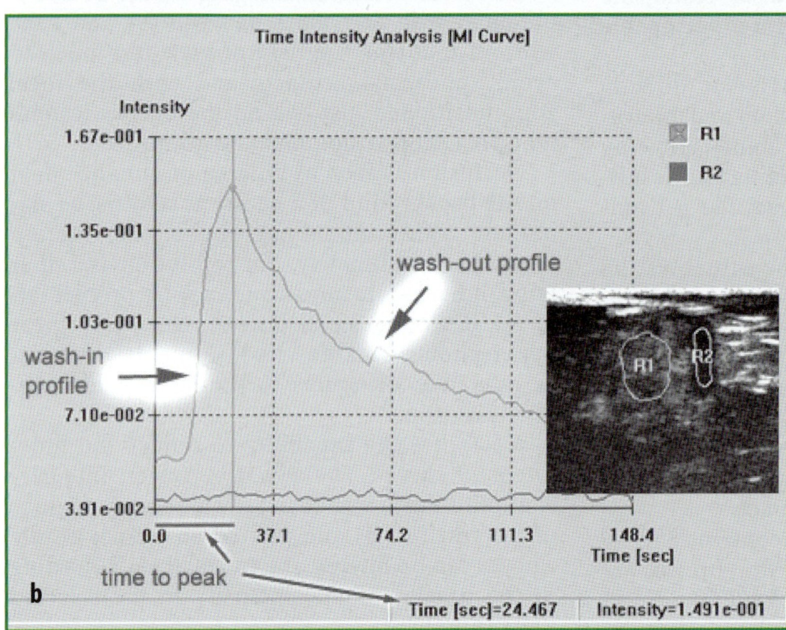

Fig. 1a, b. **a** Infiltrating ductal carcinoma. Baseline Doppler imaging shows few intratumoral vessels; adjoining tissues are hyperechoic and Cooper's ligaments are thickened and retracted. Perfusion imaging (at 24 seconds from microbubble injection) demonstrates intense enhancement. Due to poor spatial resolution, perfusion US completely misses all the morphological alterations of the surrounding tissues and ligaments. **b** Time-intensity analysis shows a high peak intensity value and a very short time-to-peak (24.4 seconds); both patterns indicate a very high possibility of malignancy. Wash-out profile is very steep due to the arterio-venous shunts

MRI, microcalcifications in DCIS, lymph node metastases and lesion response to neoadjuvant therapy in locally advanced breast cancers (LABC). The preliminary results of this multicenter study were published [25] and presented at the 90th Scientific Assembly and Annual Meeting of the Radiological Society of North America (Chicago, November 2004).

Experience reveals that contrast agents cannot be used to increase the sensitivity of US in the detection of small cancers occult on mammography. The motion artifacts and the intrinsic limitation of the US field of view do not allow a comprehensive assessment of the whole breast volume. Moreover, morphologic imaging becomes less efficient than in conventional US; small calcifications and tiny lesions often escape detection, therefore preventing perfusion assessment.

Future developments are needed both for technology and contrast agents.

Large matrix transducers will probably help to acquire larger three-dimensional volumes and computer aided detection (CAD) will increase the recognition of small enhancing lesions, therefore assisting screening procedures. The properties of tracers must change, however, providing both longer recirculating times and higher resolution without movement artifacts.

Breast Lesions

Actually, perfusion imaging is not yet mature enough to become a substitute for conventional US plus US-guided biopsy. This limitation is similar as for other contrast-enhanced imaging, such as MRI or nuclear medicine. The information that can be obtained through simple pathologic sampling is accurate enough for it to continue being the gold standard.

However, actual perfusion imaging gives some interesting results; its future developments will certainly give rise to new applications both in diagnosis and therapy.

Some new characteristics that have issue from the clinical use of CNTI are:

- avascular lesions (adenosis, fibrotic changes, scars) do not exhibit internal perfusion (Fig. 2);
- fibroadenomas usually have only a peripheral rim of perfusion (Fig. 3);
- some fibroadenomas have a diffuse perfusion and a peripheral rim during the latest phases (75 seconds and more);
- the perfused area in malignancies is always larger that the vascular area seen with contrast-enhanced Doppler (Fig. 4). Conspicuity differs mainly in infiltrating tumors with acoustic shadowing and in lobular carcinomas growing without mass;
- tumoral perfusion may be nonhomogeneous, mainly in larger or treated tumors;
- tumoral perfusion slightly differs in the same patient with different injections; this might be related to the differences induced by the manual injection and/or the correlation with the cardiac cycle;
- tumoral perfusion is lower in older patients (60 years and above);
- time-to-peak is usually shorter for malignancies (20-25 seconds) than for benign lesions (30 seconds and more) (Fig. 5);
- time-to-peak is slightly increased for *in situ* and low-grade invasive carcinomas;
- time-intensity curves in invasive tumors, probably due to the presence of important arteriovenous shunts, exhibit a very rapid wash-out (Figs. 1, 5);
- time-intensity curves in benign lesions or *in situ* carcinomas have a longer plateau and/or a less steep gradient during the early wash-out phase (70-150 seconds).

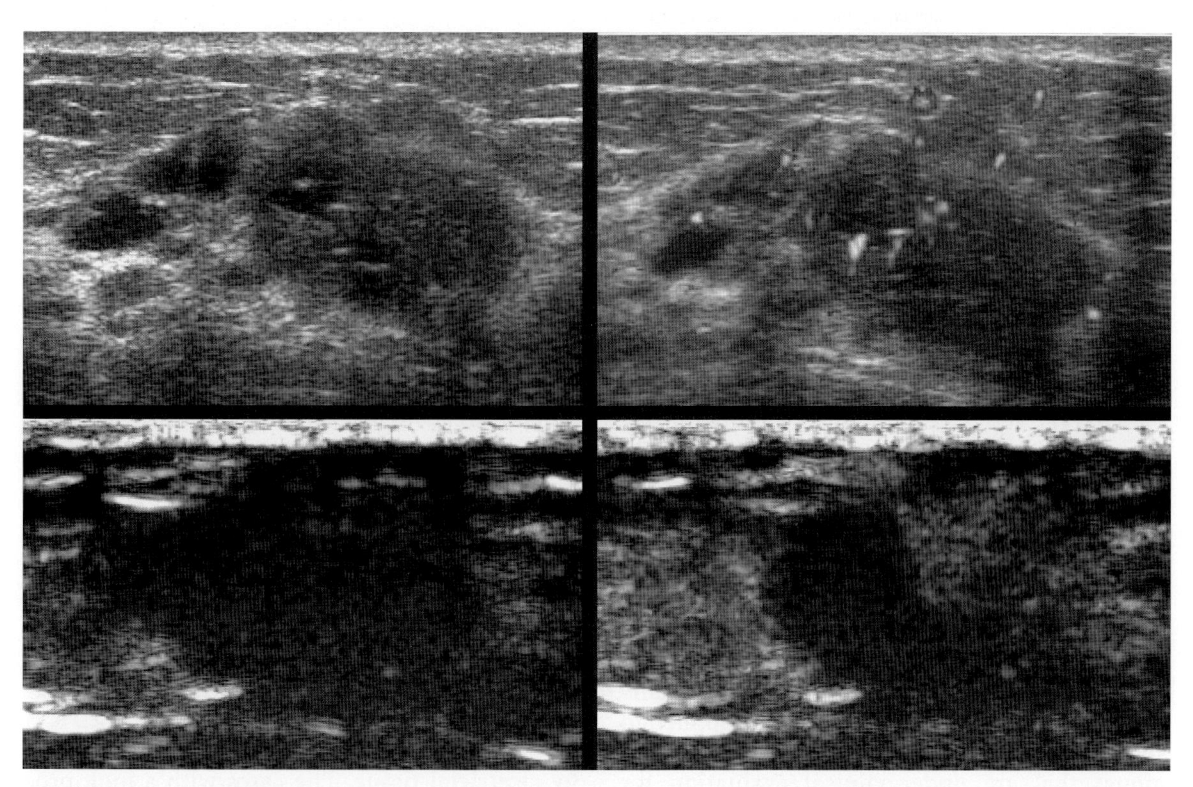

Fig. 2. Focal area of benign adenosis presenting as a palpable lump. Conventional imaging and Doppler (top) show a hypoechoic area with multiple small cysts, tiny calcifications and irregular vessels. Perfusion imaging (baseline and 50 seconds after the injection-bottom right) shows only minimal peripheral enhancement

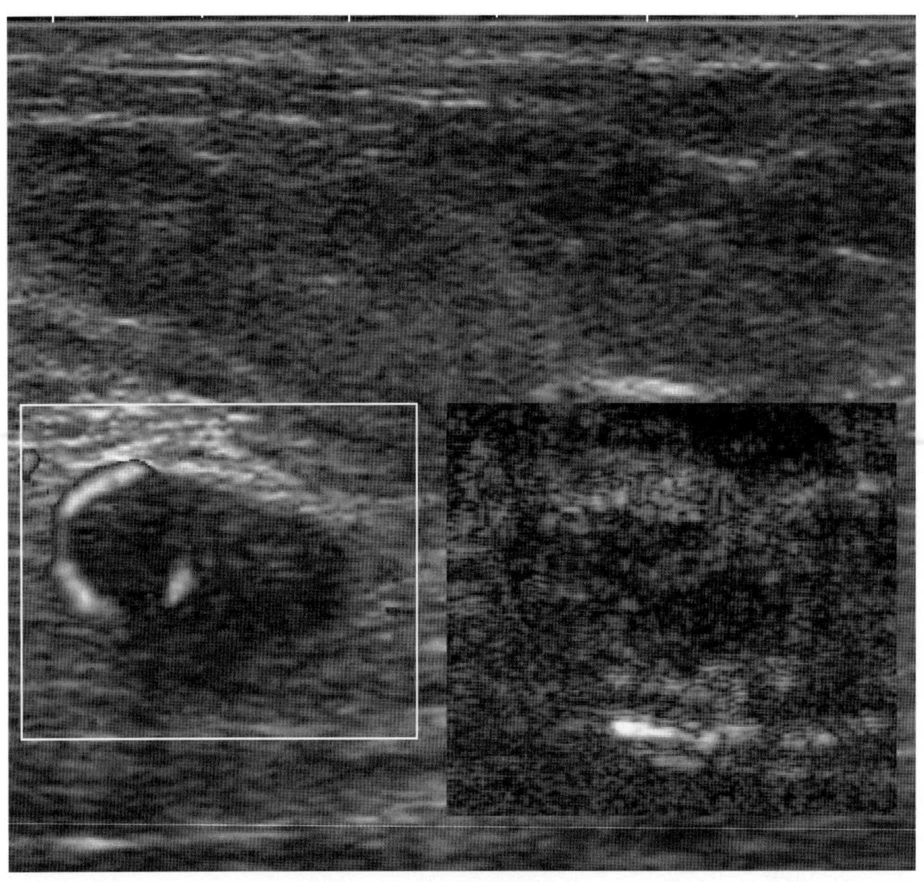

Fig. 3. Deeply located fibroadenoma with multilobulated margins. Most fibroadenomas show only a peripheral rim of perfusion; this pattern is more evident in the late wash-out phase (90-180 seconds)

Using Optison as a contrast agent, Jung et al. [26] observed a diffuse contrast medium accumulation in the late phase (8-18 min, mean 12 min) in 90% of all malignant tumors (30/33), but only in one benign lesion.

Many of these characteristics correlate well with the different vascular arrangements of breast pathologies.

A larger series is now under evaluation for quantitative analysis, using new off-line software in order to define standards ranges. This will probably lead to a better understanding of tumoral kinetics and support the use of perfusion US to monitor the results of therapies on tumoral vascularity.

One niche example of therapy monitoring is the use of perfusion software in the early evaluation of radio-frequency in breast cancer recurrence [27]; the same protocol might be applied to all the other minimally invasive ablation techniques that are under clinical evaluation for small breast cancers.

Currently, the monitoring field is mostly restricted to advanced breast cancers (ABC), including local recurrence, disseminated disease or LABC. This type of presentation is quite common in developing countries or areas without structured screening programs. In this last stage, the tumor in the breast is usually more than 5 cm across, it has destroyed the superficial fascia and invaded the subcutaneous lymphatic network, or it has spread to the axillary nodes or to other nodes or tissues near the breast.

Neoadjuvant therapy includes standard cytotoxic and/or hormonal manipulation. About 75% of LABC regress with cytotoxic treatment, allowing surgery with disease-free margins. In more than 50% of these patients there is no tumor, or only a microscopic tumor, remaining [28]. In the responsive area, cancer tissue is transformed to a xanthogranulomatous lesion with the infiltrations of macrophages and lymphocytes [2]. It is replaced by myxomatous fibrous tissue and then by cicatricial tissue. The cases with a high proportion of intraductal components have lower response [2]; the larger number of residual can-

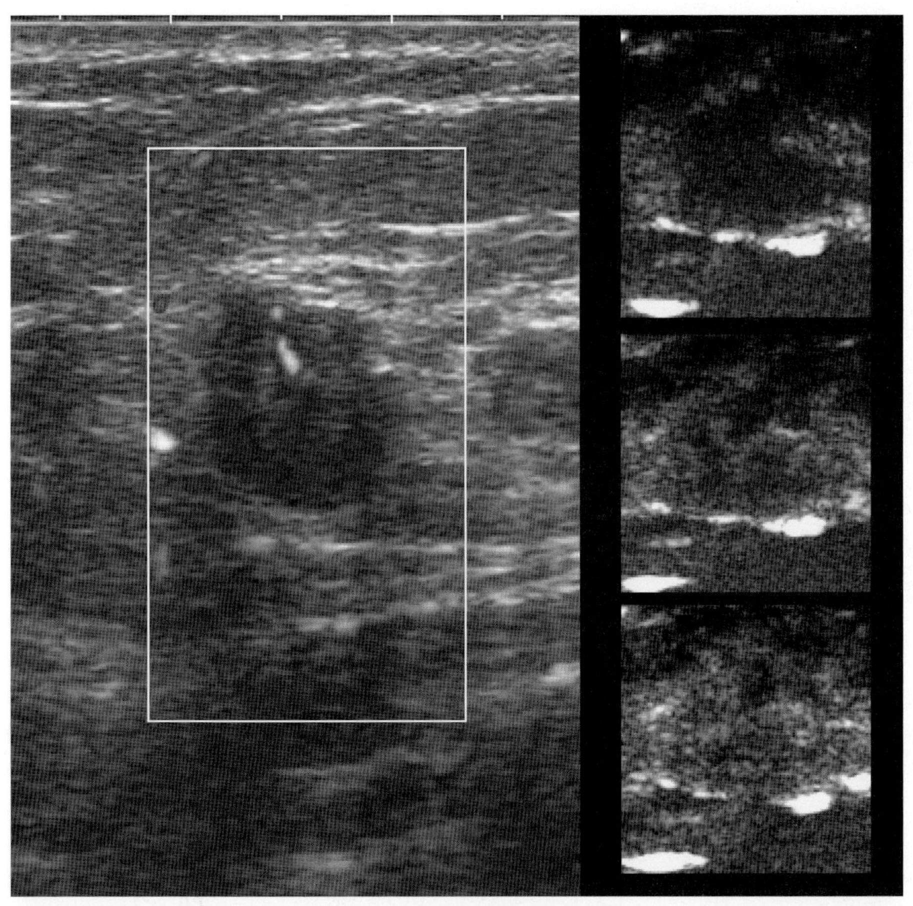

Fig. 4. Small infiltrating ductal carcinoma, 8 mm in size, with only one internal vessel at the baseline. Perfusion is not very homogeneous, but is very intense (baseline, 17 and 24 seconds after the injection)

cer cells are found within the ducts and preserve their proliferative activity. In all the tumors there is a consistent reduction in mitotic activity and in global microvessel density. Complete response to neoadjuvant chemotherapy is documented also for axillary nodal metastases. Kuerer et al. [29] reported complete axillary conversion in 23% of patients. Arimappamagan et al. [30] found a complete response in 22% of patients, while in 10% conversion was complete for both axilla and primary tumor.

The management of ABC is an expanding field. Many trials are now going on to evaluate also the potential of novel combinations of new cytotoxins like anthracyclines and taxanes, or the effects of monoclonal antibodies like excerptin. Future developments will include host response modifiers, such as agents that suppress angiogenesis.

The challenges for breast imaging lie in the ability to incorporate technologies to ensure both accurate staging and effective monitoring of tumor response.

Mammography and conventional US have limited efficiency; they usually measure the tumor response, evaluating the changes in its diameter, morphology and echopattern. MRI seems to be the most accurate imaging modality [31]. The correlation between tumor diameter measured by histopathology and MRI is very high; a clear reduction in size is usually seen only after the third cycle. Size reduction is usually associated with a decrease of the contrast-enhancement parameters.

MRI is not universally available. Optimization of a US protocol to monitor treatment outcomes would be advantageous both clinically and economically.

Huber et al. [32] have already documented an increased US efficiency when color Doppler flow imaging is added to conventional US. A good efficiency has also proved for very short interval monitoring of the neoangiogenetic vascularity of inflammatory lesions undergoing antibiotic therapy [8].

More recently, Pollard et al. [33] have documented the potentials of a destruction-replen-

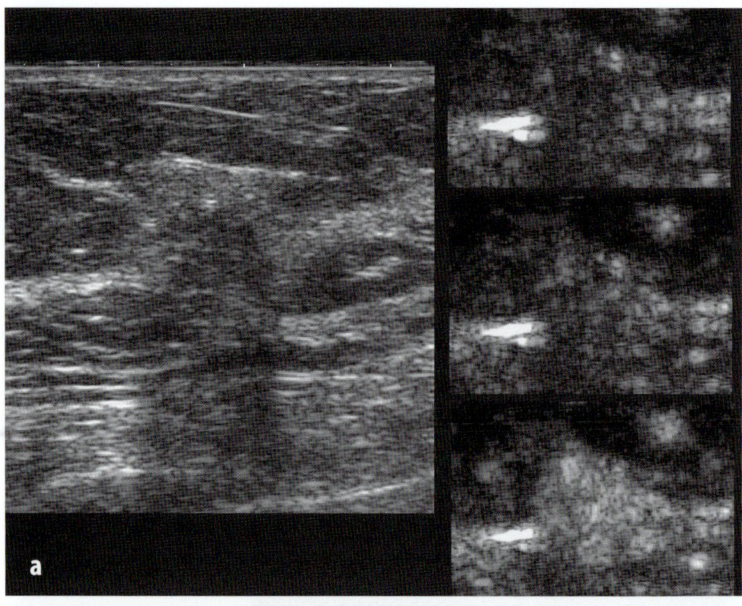

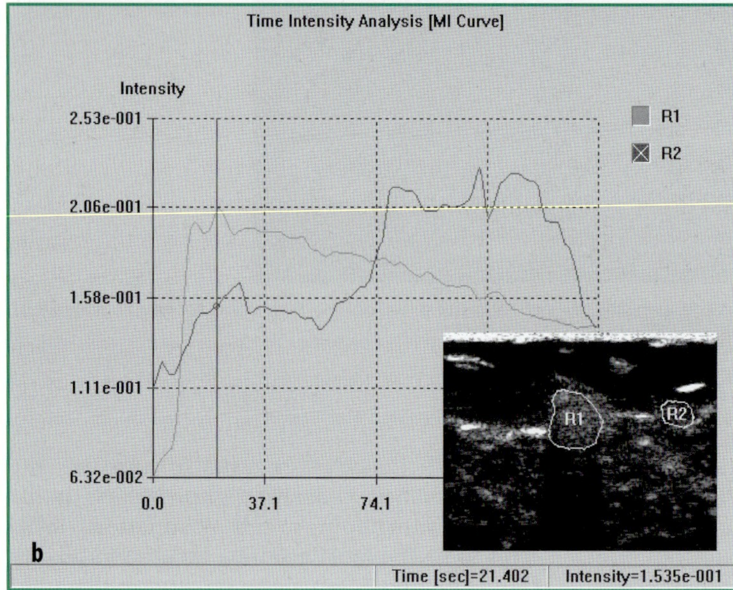

Fig. 5a, b. a Small infiltrating lobular carcinoma, 6 mm in size, seen as a round low echogenic area with acoustic shadowing. Perfusion imaging (baseline, 16 and 21 seconds after microbubble injection) shows an intense enhancement. **b** Time-intensity analysis shows a wash-in profile characteristic for malignancy (R1), but with a long wash-out phase. The tumor is very small and has fewer arterio-venous shunts than larger carcinomas

ishment US technique in monitoring the anti-neoangiogenetic effects of therapy in rat models.

The experience with CNTI demonstrates that contrast-enhanced Doppler may give false negative vascular patterns, while perfusion imaging still registers important residual intratumoral vascularity [25]. In almost all cases, the degree and the distribution of the US perfusion correlates well with the pathologic changes (Fig. 6).

Currently, perfusion US must be considered as the only alternative to MRI; it also offers the possibility of guiding further biopsies on the residual areas. In the future, with the clinical introduction of new therapies, it will be very important to understand if monitoring should be restricted to the tumoral vessels or also include the extravascular bed. This decision will determine the choice in favor of perfusion US or MRI.

Broumas et al. [34] have developed a new US perfusion method that yields information about the vascular volume and flow rate in each voxel, as well as the spatial distribution of blood flow within an imaging plane. This system offers good capabilities for therapy monitoring; as contrast bubbles are confined to the blood pool, US probably provides the most accurate assessment of microvessel location and fractional vascular volume.

Two major interests are linked to the near future of US perfusion imaging.

The first of these is the capability to vehiculate drugs or other components within the microbubble. The bubbles will be targeted and linked to specific tissues, they will be monitored up to the peak perfusion within the tumor, or

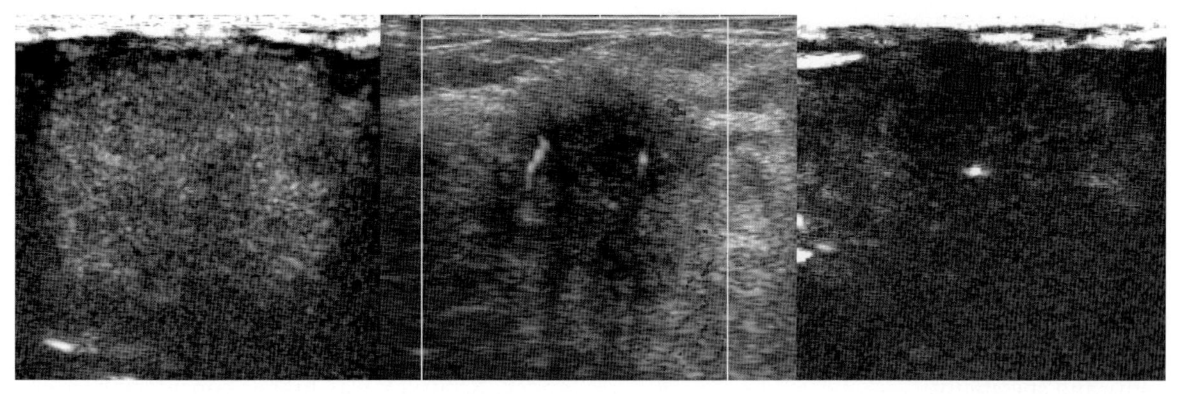

Fig. 6. Lobular carcinoma presenting as locally advanced breast cancer. Perfusion is very intense before neoadjuvant therapy (left). After 4 cycles of cytotoxic treatment the tumoral volume has significantly reduced; at conventional Doppler there are only marginal vessels. Perfusion imaging (right) confirms the good therapeutic result, showing an almost complete absence of enhancement. The patient was immediately scheduled for surgery

within benign pathologies like inflammations. Fusion with molecular imaging and optical probes might be part of this future. The same transducer will use higher energies to destroy the microbubbles or to partially fragment their shells and to release the drug in the proper time. The same perfusion US imaging will monitor the effects of therapy.

Sentinel Lymph Nodes

A second improvement will be the capability of new contrast agents to enter the lymphatic stream and to fully replace radiotracers in the sentinel lymph node (SLN) procedure.

Some of these future applications are already being used in ongoing projects on animal models [35-41].

Today, most patients with breast cancer undergo local resection or mastectomy, as well as axillary lymph node dissection if a SLN procedure has provided evidence of malignancy. This procedure involves biopsy and histopathological analysis of the first draining (sentinel) lymph node, identified by following the clearance through the lymphatic system of a radioactive or colored dye injected into the breast near the tumor.

Actually, the use of the SLN procedure is a standard for breast surgery and oncology [42]. This behaviour is justified by the knowledge that when the sentinel node is negative for malignancy, there is very low likelihood that the tumor has metastasized to the axillary nodes; in this case many surgical groups now avoid axillary dissection.

In general, SLN is an accurate procedure, but pitfalls do exist. Studies correlating the results of SLN biopsy with axillary dissection in more than 3000 patients have shown that SLN biopsy has a technical success rate of 88%, sensitivity of 93%, and accuracy of 97% [43]. Veronesi et al. [44] have found 32% of positive SLNs in 516 patients with primary breast cancer in whom the tumor was less than, or equal to, 2 cm in diameter; in 34% the SLNs were seeded only by micrometastases (foci ≤ 2 mm in diameter).

Sonography can usually identify enlarged reactive or metastatic nodes. *In vitro* studies demonstrate that metastatic disease is often indicated by an enlarged and round-shaped node, the absence of an echogenic hilum, a marginal bulging or a small hypoechoic area within the echogenic cortex [45, 46]. Doppler studies show a reduced vascularity inside the metastatic deposits; in case of massive metastatic infiltration the remaining vessels are displaced at the periphery of the node [47]. Similarly Esen et al. [48] found that in nodes smaller than 1 cm, only asymmetrical cortical thickening and peripheral flow were significant.

The prevalence of peripheral flow is explained by the pathologic behaviour of breast metastases. Cancer cell emboli occur in the lymphatic capillaries of primary sites, flow in the collecting lymphatics, enter the lymph node via afferent or efferent lymphatics, are deposited in the sinus, proliferate, and spread over all parts of the node. Angiogenic factors produced by the neoplastic cells induce peripheral neovascularity, with atypical anastomoses and various grades of distortion and infiltration during the centripetal course of the vessels [49]. The mechanism is completely different for lymphoma that colonizes the central part of the node where lymphatic follicles are located and spares both the hilum and peripheral structures. Development of new vessels from the main artery and its branches produces vessel enlargement and an increase in blood flow; there are no signs of peripheral neovascularity.

Conventional US has a great potential; both specificity and positive predictive value are high [3, 48, 50]. US-guided biopsy can confirm a positive diagnosis [51] and these patients can be immediately scheduled for nodal dissection.

Actual accuracy is mainly linked to morphologic and structural alterations and abnormal vascularity. US resolution is within the range of macrometastases (4 mm or more); this situation is expected in around 20 to 25% of all the breast cancer patients.

Perfusion US certainly increases both sensitivity and specificity.

Some new characteristics issuing from the clinical use of CNTI are:

- a normal or reactive cortex always has an intense, homogeneous perfusion;
- marginal bulgings without lack of perfusion may reflect normal morphologic variability;
- in the early phase of metastatic seeding the node is highly reactive, with diffuse and homogeneous enhancement;
- CNTI does not have enough resolution to depict micrometastases (≤ 2 mm in diameter) but small deposits larger than 3 mm are clearly seen as non-perfused 'black' areas not always predictable on the basis of conventional imaging and Doppler;
- in case of massive infiltration, there is no enhancement (Fig. 7) and/or the perfused uninvolved area is always larger than shown with conventional imaging and Doppler;
- in the case of enlarged nodes with Doppler massive vascularity, the behaviour of the perfusion progression may suggest different pathologies.

In a recent group of 65 breast cancer patients that underwent both SLN and perfusion US procedures, pathology assessed the presence of metastases in 42.1% of all nodes; preliminary perfusion US correctly identified 62.5% of these metastatic nodes. Accuracy was higher considering nodes with macrometastases (88.2%) but no node with only micrometastases was correctly assessed. Preliminary perfusion US gave true positive metastatic assessment in 26.3% of these patients.

Many imaging groups dealing with a large number of breast cancers have already appreciated the accuracy and the advantages offered by sonography [3, 48, 50]. Nodes can be assessed in a very early phase and US can very precisely guide a needle to the suspicious areas.

Perfusion imaging offers a unique capability in picking up the metastatic areas in all the different nodal locations that may be involved by breast carcinoma. Small deposits, 3 mm and more, located in the normal cortex are easily discovered and

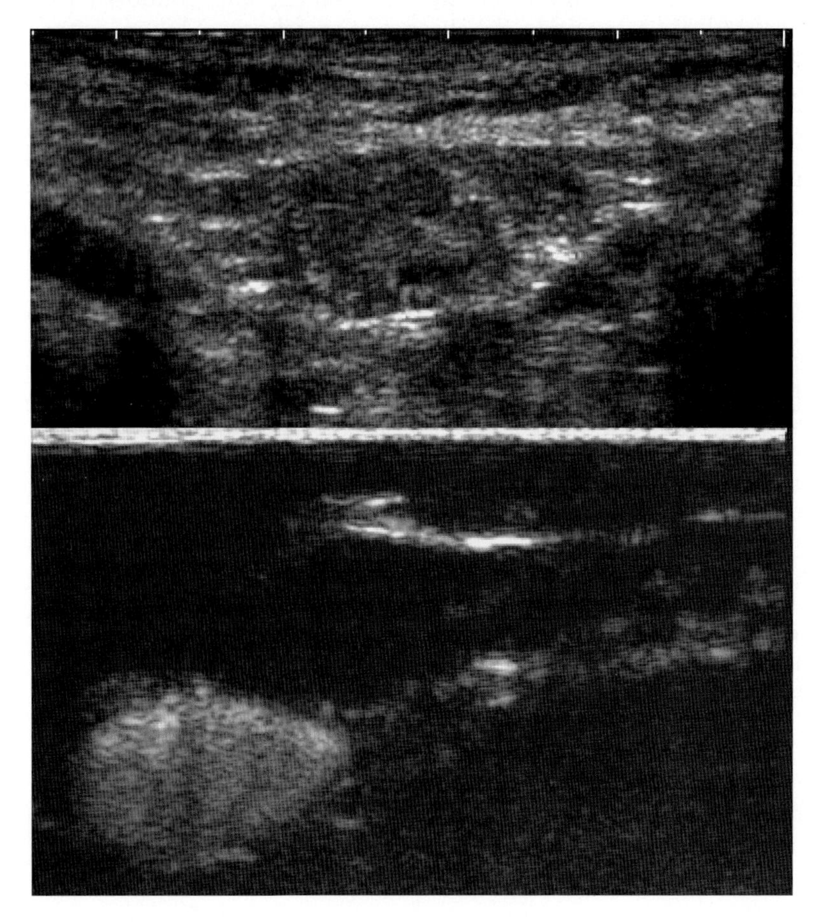

Fig. 7. Two adjacent axillary nodes in a patient with a 12 mm lobular carcinoma of the lower outer quadrant of the right breast. Nodes are only slightly enlarged and keep their regular oval shape; but the hilum is no longer visible and the cortex is not homogeneous. Perfusion imaging (*bottom*) shows an intense enhancement of the axillary artery but no perfusion was assessed inside the nodes. Pathology revealed that both the nodes were completely filled by metastatic deposits

are precisely assessed with biopsy. False positives may be related to small fibrotic changes or granulomas. In cases of enlarged nodes that exhibit poor vascularity on conventional Doppler, the needle is guided in the metastatic areas that are usually smaller than when viewed with conventional imaging. In other cases the intense but inhomogeneous speckled enhancement in the early arterial phase, that seems to be mostly related to non Hodgkin lymphomas [52], is accurate enough to readdress the patient.

Perfusion imaging actually increases the already high positive predictive value of US in nodal assessment. When a node is positive on US and biopsy the patient is scheduled for axillary dissection and a SLN procedure is avoided. Depending upon the staging distribution and the US technique used in the different series, a SLN procedure might be avoided in 10-25% of patients with breast cancer. Imaging impact is very high because of the reduced cost of the diagnostic procedure and the better scheduling of the operation room.

In the future, new contrast agents will be injected with the same technique used in radiotracer procedure. Goldberg et al. [53] tested an agent consisting of lipid-stabilized perfluorobutane microbubbles on animal models with reticuloendothelial system-specific uptake capability. Subcutaneous, submucosal and parenchymal injections were used. Massaging the injection site caused both an increased rate of movement of the contrast within the lymphatic channels and an increased reflectivity of the SLN. The mean time required to visualize the nodes was 15 minutes. They established the regional drainage pathways, showing continuity of the channels between the injection site and the enhanced node; lymphatic channels were traced for distances of up to 38 cm. In all cases, contrast-enhancement was confined to the SLN; nodes as small as 3 mm were detected. Goldberg et al. [41] had already demonstrated that the metastatic deposits are represented as non-perfused areas. If this technique will give the same results in clinical practice it will certainly simplify SLN assessment.

Key Points

- Conventional US without contrast agents is limited in its ability to detect metastases and The best perfusion imaging in the breast is obtained with MI values between 0.1 and 0.08, without reducing the field of view too much, thus avoiding superficial artifacts, and with the focal zone positioned just behind the deeper lesion's margin. Compression must be minimized.
- Perfusion imaging is not yet developed enough to become a substitute for conventional US plus biopsy.
- Fibroadenomas usually have only a peripheral rim of perfusion, while the perfused area in malignancies is always larger than that of the vascular area seen with contrast-enhanced Doppler.
- Time-to-peak is usually shorter for malignancies (20-25 sec) than for benign lesions (30 secand longer).
- Perfusion ultrasound must be considered as the only alternative to MRI for evaluating the efficacy of the neoadjuvant therapy in advanced cancers; it also offers the possibility of guiding further biopsies on the residual areas.
- Perfusion imaging actually increases the already high positive predictive value of US in sentinel node (SLN) assessment. Small deposits, 3 mm and larger, located in the normal cortex are easily discovered and are precisely assessed with biopsy.
- When a node is positive on US and biopsy, the patient is scheduled for axillary dissection and a SLN procedure is avoided.
- In the future, new contrast agents will be injected with the same technique as used in radiotracer procedures.

References

1. Less JR, Skalak TC, Sevick EM et al (1991) Microvascular architecture in a mammary carcinoma: branching patterns and vessel dimensions. Cancer Res 51:265-273
2. Wu W, Kamma H, Ueno E et al (2002) The intraductal component of breast cancer is poorly responsive to neo-adjuvant chemotherapy. Oncol Rep 9:1027-1031
3. Rizzatto G (2001) Towards a more sophisticated use of breast ultrasound. Eur Radiol 11:2425-2435
4. Ozdemir A, Ozdemir H, Maral I et al (2001) Differential diagnosis of solid breast lesions. Contribution of Doppler studies to mammography and gray scale imaging. J Ultrasound Med 20:1091-1101
5. Teh WL, Wilson AR, Evans AJ et al (2000) Ultrasound guided core biopsy of suspicious mammographic calcifications using high frequency and power Doppler ultrasound. Clin Radiol 55:390-394
6. del Cura JL, Eligararay E, Zabala R et al (2005) The use of unenhanced Doppler sonography in the evaluation of solid breast lesions. AJR Am J Roentgenol 184:1788-1794
7. Singh S, Pradhan S, Shukla RC et al (2005) Color Doppler ultrasound as an objective assessment tool for chemotherapeutic response in advanced breast cancer. Breast Cancer 12:45-51
8. Rizzatto G, Chersevani R (1998) Breast ultrasound and new technologies. Eur J Radiol 27:S242-S249
9. Moon WK, Im JG, Noh DY et al (2000) Nonpalpable breast lesions: evaluation with power Doppler US and a microbubble contrast agent-initial experience. Radiology 217:240-246
10. Weind KL, Maier CF, Rutt BK et al (1998) Invasive carcinomas and fibroadenomas of the breast: comparison of microvessel distributions. Implications for imaging modalities. Radiology 208:477-483
11. Ellis RL (1999) Differentiation of benign versus malignant breast disease. Radiology 210:878-880
12. Schroeder RJ, Bostanjoglo M, Rademaker J et al (2003) Role of power Doppler techniques and ultrasound contrast-enhancement in the differential diagnosis of focal breast lesions. Eur Radiol 13:68-79
13. Stuhrmann M, Aronius R, Roefke C et al (1998) Vascularization of breast tumors: use of ultrasound contrast medium in evaluating tumor entity. Preliminary results. Rofo Fortschr Geb Rontgenstr Neuen Bildgeb Verfahr 169:360-364
14. Schroeder RJ, Maeurer J, Vogl TJ et al (1999) D-galactose based signal-enhanced color Doppler sonography of breast tumors and tumorlike lesions. Invest Radiol 34:109-115
15. Sehgal CM, Arger PH, Rowling SE et al (2000) Quantitative vascularity of breast masses by Doppler imaging: regional variations and diagnostic implications. J Ultrasound Med 19:427-440
16. Zdemir A, Kilic K, Ozdemir H et al (2004) Contrast-enhanced power Doppler sonography in breast lesions: effect on differential diagnosis after mammography and gray scale sonography. J Ultrasound Med 23:183-195
17. Winehouse J, Douek M, Holz K et al (1999) Contrast-enhanced color Doppler ultrasonography in suspected breast cancer recurrence. Br J Surg 86:1198-1201
18. Stuhrmann M, Aronius R, Schietzel M (2000) Tumor vascularity of breast lesions: potentials and limits of contrast-enhanced Doppler sonography. AJR Am J Roentgenol 175:1585-1589
19. Huber S, Helbich T, Kettenbach J et al (1998) Effects of a microbubble contrast agent on breast tumors: computer-assisted quantitative assessment with color Doppler US-early experience. Radiology 208:485-489
20. Kettembach J, Helbich TH, Huber S et al (2005) Computer-assisted quantitative assessment of power Doppler US: effects of microbubble contrast agent in the differentiation of breast tumors. Eur J Radiol 53:238-244
21. Rizzatto G, Chersevani R, Ralleigh G (2005) Breast. In : Quaia A (ed) Contrast media in ultrasonography : basic principles and clinical applications. Springer, Berlin Heidelberg New York, pp 301-314
22. Rizzatto G (2003) Contrast-enhanced ultrasound examination of breast lesions. Eur Radiol 13:D63-D65
23. Scoazec J (2000) Tumor angiogenesis. Ann Pathol 20:25-37
24. Rosen LS (2002) Clinical experience with angiogenesis signaling inhibitors: focus on vascular endothelial growth factor (VEGF) blockers. Cancer Control 9:36-44
25. Rizzatto G, Martegani A, Chersevani R et al. (2001) Importance of staging of breast cancer and role of contrast ultrasound. Eur Radiol 11 (Suppl 3):E47-E52
26. Jung EM, Jungius KP, Rupp N et al (2005) Contrast-enhanced harmonic ultrasound for differentiating breast tumors - first results. Clin Hemorheol Microcirc 33:109-120
27. Lamuraglia M, Lassau N, Garbay JR et al (2005) Doppler US with perfusion software and contrast medium injection in the early evaluation of radiofrequency in breast cancer recurrences : a prospective phase II study. Eur J Radiol 56:376-381
28. Honkoop AH, Pinedo HM, De Jong JS et al (1997) Effects of chemotherapy on pathologic and biologic characteristics of locally advanced breast cancer. Am J Clin Pathol 107:211-218
29. Kuerer HM, Sahin AA, Hunt KK et al (1999) Incidence and impact of documented eradication of breast cancer axillary lymph node metastases before surgery in patients treated with neoadjuvant chemotherapy. Ann Surg 230:72-78
30. Arimappamagan A, Kadambari D, Srinivasan K et al (2004) Complete axillary conversion after neoadjuvant chemotherapy in locally advanced breast cancer: a step towards conserving axilla? Indian J Cancer 41:13-17
31. Wasser K, Klein SK, Fink C et al (2003) Evaluation of neoadjuvant chemotherapeutic response of breast cancer using dynamic MRI with high temporal resolution. Eur Radiol 13:80-87
32. Huber S, Medl M, Helbich T et al (2000) Locally advanced breast carcinoma: computer assisted semiquantitative analysis of color Doppler ultrasonography in the evaluation of tumor response to neoadjuvant chemotherapy (work in progress). J Ultrasound Med 19:601-607
33. Pollard RE, Sadlowski AR, Bloch SH et al (2003) Contrast-assisted destruction-replenishment ultrasound for the assessment of tumor microvasculature in a rat model. Technol Cancer Res Treat 1:459-470
34. Broumas AR, Pollard RE, Bloch SH et al (2005) Con-

trast-enhanced computed tomography and ultrasound for the evaluation of tumor blood flow. Invest radiol 40:134-147
35. Allen JS, May DJ, Ferrara KW (2002) Dynamics of therapeutic ultrasound contrast agents. Ultrasound Med Biol 28:805-816
36. Dayton PA, Ferrara KW (2002) Targeted imaging using ultrasound. J Magn Reson Imaging 16:362-377
37. May DJ, Allen JS, Ferrara KW (2002) Dynamics and fragmentation of thick-shelled microbubbles. IEEE Trans Ultrason Ferroelectr Freq Control 49:1400-1410
38. Mattrey RF, Kono Y, Baker K et al (2002) Sentinel lymph node imaging with microbubble ultrasound contrast material. Acad Radiol 9 (Suppl 1):S231-S235
39. Wisner ER, Ferrara KW, Short RE et al (2003) Sentinel node detection using contrast-enhanced power Doppler ultrasound lymphography. Invest Radiol 38: 358-365
40. Choi SH, Kono Y, Corbeil J et al (2004) Model to quantify lymph node enhancement on indirect sonographic lymphography. AJR Am J Roentgenol 183:513-517
41. Goldberg BB, Merton DA, Liu JB et al (2004) Sentinel lymph nodes in a swine model with melanoma: contrast-enhanced lymphatic US. Radiology 230:727-734
42. Lyman GH, Giuliano AE, Somerfield MR et al (2005) American Society of Clinical Oncology guideline recommendations for sentinel lymph node biopsy in early-stage breast cancer. J Clin Oncol 23:7703-7720
43. Liberman L (2003) Lymphoscintigraphy for lymphatic mapping in breast carcinoma. Radiology 228:313-315
44. Veronesi U, Paganelli G, Viale G et al (2003) A randomized comparison of sentinel-node biopsy with routine axillary dissection in breast cancer. N Engl J Med 349:546-553
45. Feu J, Tresserra F, Fabregas R et al (1997) Metastatic breast carcinoma in axillary lymph nodes: in vitro US detection. Radiology 205:831-835
46. Tateishi T, Machi J, Feleppa EJ et al (1999) In vitro B-mode ultrasonographic criteria for diagnosing axillary lymph node metastasis of breast cancer. J Ultrasound Med 18:349-356
47. Yang WT, Chang J, Metreweli C (2000) Patients with breast cancer: differences in color Doppler flow and gray-scale US features of benign and malignant axillary lymph nodes. Radiology 215:568-573
48. Esen G, Gurses B, Yilmaz MH et al (2005) Gray scale and power Doppler US in the preoperative evaluation of axillary metastases in breast cancer patients with no palpable lymph nodes. Eur Radiol 15:1215-1223
49. Giovagnorio F, Galluzzo M, Andreoli C et al (2002) Color Doppler sonography in the evaluation of superficial lymphomatous lymph nodes. J Ultrasound Med 21:403-408
50. Mobbs LM, Jannicky ES, Weaver DL et al (2005) The accuracy of sonography in detecting abnormal axillary lymph nodes when breast cancer is present. JDMS 21:297-303
51. de Kanter AY, van Eijck CH, van Geel AN et al (1999) Multicentre study of ultrasonographically guided axillary node biopsy in patients with breast cancer. Br J Surg. 86: 1459-146251.
52. Rubaltelli L, Khadivi Y, Tregnaghi A et al (2004) Evaluation of lymph node perfusion using continuous mode harmonic ultrasonography with a second-generation contrast agent. J Ultrasound Med 23: 829-83652.
53. Goldberg BB, Merton DA, Liu JB et al (2005) Contrast-enhanced sonographic imaging of lymphatic channels and sentinel lymph nodes. J Ultrasound Med 24:953-965

IV.7

Value of Contrast-Enhanced Ultrasound in Rheumatoid Arthritis

Andrea S. Klauser

Introduction

Rheumatoid arthritis (RA) is a chronic systemic disease of unknown origin, characterized by articular inflammation and destruction, and leading to substantial disability and morbidity. The prevalence of RA is between 0.5 and 1% of the population. Women are affected two to three times more often than men, and the peak age of affliction is 45 to 65 years [1, 2].

RA predominantly involves the synovial tissue of synovial joints and tendon sheaths. In the subsequent course of the disease, adjacent structures such as bone, tendons, capsules, and ligaments may be affected. The long-term consequences of RA and related disorders have been underestimated in the past. Most patients need long-term chronic treatment to slow down the progression of the disease and control acute exacerbations, while many patients also require expensive surgery. Apart from these direct costs, RA causes indirect expenses secondary to disability, loss of productivity and early retirement. Patients with RA have a mean reduction in life expectancy of about five to ten years. Prior to the introduction of new treatment strategies, Sokka et al. [3] reported a disability rate of 44% after a ten year follow-up period.

Irreversible joint destruction and late sequelae of the disease can be reduced by early diagnosis and proper treatment. Clinical and laboratory tests are the first step in the diagnostic evaluation of patients with inflammatory disease and imaging methods are also used, as they play a key role in the early diagnosis. Furthermore, imaging is particularly helpful in view of the fluctuating course of the disease, to detect patients with mild clinical and laboratory inflammatory signs and minor pain and impairment, which then progress to a high degree of damage and destruction of joints and tendons. In addition, if treatment is ineffective the disease may prove to be disabling and mutilating, leading to ankylosis, deformity, and severe secondary osteoarthritis. Therefore, apart from early detection, careful monitoring of disease activity is important.

Currently Available Imaging Techniques

Radiography is routinely used to diagnose RA, assess the degree of articular destruction, and follow the disease. Together with laboratory data and clinical findings, radiography is one of the American College of Rheumatology (ACR) criteria as established in 1987 [4]. It relies on indirect and non-specific signs for RA such as joint-space widening, soft tissue swelling, dislocation and effacement of fat pads, and specific signs such as juxta-articular osteoporosis and bone erosions. However, its sensitivity and specificity in the assessment of soft tissue inflammation and early erosive disease are low [5, 6]. Indeed, the assessment of structural damage by radiography in early RA relates poorly to function. Changes become evident after a minimum period of 6-12 months. Moreover, this technique has a number of limitations such as projectional superimposition, which may obscure erosions and mimic cartilage loss, and the use of ionizing radiation.

Magnetic resonance imaging (MRI) allows excellent viewing of all joint components simultaneously. MRI depicts soft tissue changes and damage to cartilage and bone earlier and better than conventional radiography. It is an excellent tool to assess synovial swelling and volume. Non-enhanced MRI is significantly superior to radiography in detecting bone damage, while contrast-enhanced MRI is used to identify vascularized synovial proliferation and erosions [7, 8]. Synovial membrane enhancement by gadolinium-DPTA is strongly correlated to numerical density of synovial blood vessel. Synovial hyperemia and synovial enhancement detected by MRI depends on tissue perfusion and tissue permeability [7, 9]. The degree of enhancement can be assessed qualitatively and quantitatively and is successfully used for early detection and characterization of inflammatory disease [10-13]. However, its routine use to establish early diagnosis and for multiple follow-up examination at different joints, is limited by its cost and relatively long examination time, non-availability at some centers, and by patients experiencing claustrophobia, which affects nearly 10% of patients.

Baseline Ultrasound

Ultrasound is a readily available imaging modality, available at relatively low cost and acceptable to all patients. US is able to depict minimal bone erosions in early target areas and delineate synovial thickening in peripheral joints affected in the course of RA [6, 14].

Color and power Doppler US (CDUS, PDUS) demonstrate vascularity in synovial proliferations, which is correlated with inflammatory activity, and add additional information to the clinical examination [15-21]. Doppler techniques permit the assessment of synovial vascularization via signals generated by flowing blood cells, but blood flow in microvessels is slow and not easily detected. Several studies found weak correlation between imaging findings and clinical indices of disease activity or pathohistological number of vessels, because the performance of Doppler techniques in the detection of slow flow and flow in small vessels, such as those that are formed in angiogenesis, is still poor [22-24].

Angiogenesis is a basic principle of inflammatory disease and refers to the growth of new capillary blood vessels. Microscopic examination of synovial biopsies shows angiogenesis from the very beginning of disease [25, 26]. Proliferation of hypervascularized pannus can be seen before joint destruction, correlates with disease activity and appears to be crucial to RA's invasive and destructive behavior [27, 28]. Serum vascular endothelial growth factor (VEGF) concentrations are elevated in RA and are known to correlate with disease activity. Furthermore, a correlation between VEGF concentration and radiographic progression between first presentation of RA patients and the subsequent year has been described. Synovial tissues expressing VEGF show a significantly higher microvascular density [29]. Therefore, vascular imaging and serologic markers may be a more sensitive test of disease activity than clinical assessment only. Functional imaging of intra-articular vascularization is thought to improve grading of disease activity. Blood flow at the microvascular level, which is of interest in inflammatory disease, is at a lower velocity and is therefore less readily detectable by conventional CDUS/PDUS.

Contrast-Enhanced Ultrasound

Contrast-enhanced CDUS increases the intensity of Doppler signals from blood through the administration of microbubble contrast agents. It enhances the signal-to-noise ratio and may improve a non-diagnostic Doppler examination by raising the intensity of weak signals to a detectable level [30]. CDUS and PDUS allow better visualization of small vessels with low volume blood flow and have been proven to improve detection of synovial vascularity. In a prospective study, contrast-enhanced CDUS was used to evaluate intra-articular vascularization in 198 finger joints of 46 patients with active RA and 80 finger joints of 10 healthy volunteers. In patients, intra-articular vascularization was detected in 35.3% of joints by non-enhanced CDUS, versus 78.3% of joints by enhanced CDUS. Neither technique detected any intra-articular vascularization in healthy controls. Treatments were modified in 24% of patients on the basis of enhanced CDUS findings [31]. Several contrast-enhanced CDUS studies with first-generation contrast agents have shown to improve the detection of synovial intra-articular vascularity. Contrast-enhanced CDUS has shown promising results in the hands, feet and knee joints and, recently, in sacroiliitis as well [32-37]. In a further small study, contrast-enhanced CDUS was superior to CDUS for the assessment of inflammatory edema, effusion and synovitis [38]. However, its performance is still not ideal because near field application is needed to visualize small joints, where inflammatory changes of RA are mainly located.

Contrast-enhanced gray-scale US (CEUS) is used to maximize contrast and spatial resolution, resorting to particular techniques based on a very low mechanical index (MI) and the higher harmonic emission capabilities of 'second-generation' contrast agents, such as SonoVue (Bracco, Italy). The main advantage of these techniques is that they use lower, non-destructive US power with a very low MI range and a low acoustic output. This results in better detection of microvessel perfusion. The capacity of CEUS to detect vascularity in joints was compared to that of gray-scale US and PDUS by the International Arthritis Contrast Ultrasound (IACUS) study group in a multicenter trial of five European centers comprising 113 consecutive adult patients of both genders with clinically diagnosed RA. A total of 113 joints were examined. The endpoints were the number of joints with active and inactive synovitis, and the measurement of synovial thickness. CEUS achieved substantially better differentiation between active and inactive synovitis (97.3% of joints), compared to US and PDUS (60.1% of joints). The measurement of overall thickness related to active synovia was significantly improved after the administration of contrast medium [39] (Fig. 1).

Quantitative and semi-quantitative MRI analysis of synovial volume have been reported to be able to assess disease activity. Quantitative assessment of synovial enhancement was found to correlate well with histological findings and clinical markers of disease activity [7, 11, 40, 41]. However, all these procedures to quantify contrast-enhancement of MRI as well as US examination, are time-consuming and were not used in clinical routine in the past. Currently, objective quantification by CEUS is a quick modality, well-suited for clinical routine use [42] (Fig. 2). CEUS also provides better spatial resolution, therefore this technique also allows better characterization of the pannus in terms of differentiating between hypervascularity, hypovascularity and avascularity.

However, special designed microbubbles for high frequencies will open up new horizons.

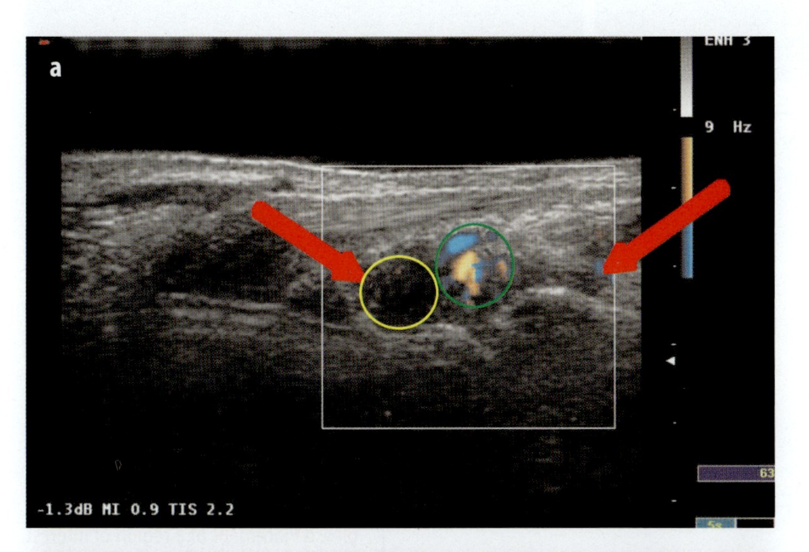

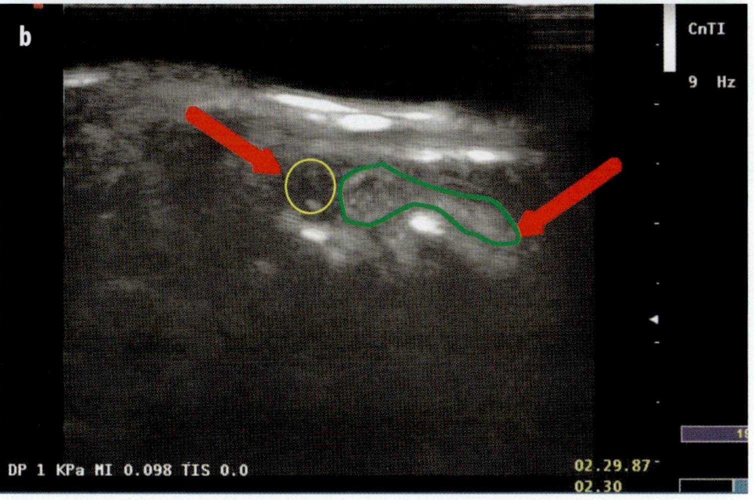

Fig. 1a, b. *Longitudinal US scan over the dorsal radiocarpal joint, showing improved thickness measurement of active synovitis (green) after US contrast administration as demonstrated by the multicenter study of the IACUS group.* **a** PDUS shows hypervascularity only in a small area of the synovial proliferation. **b** CEUS shows diffuse enhancement of the main part of the synovial proliferation

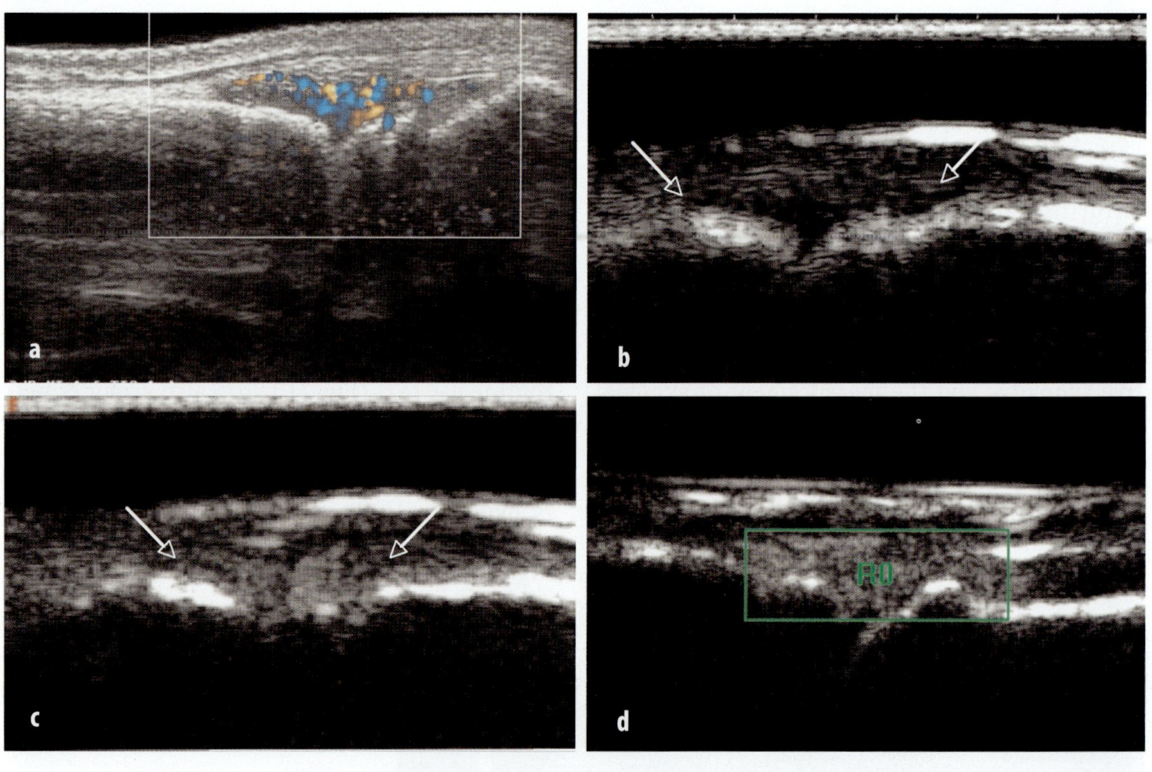

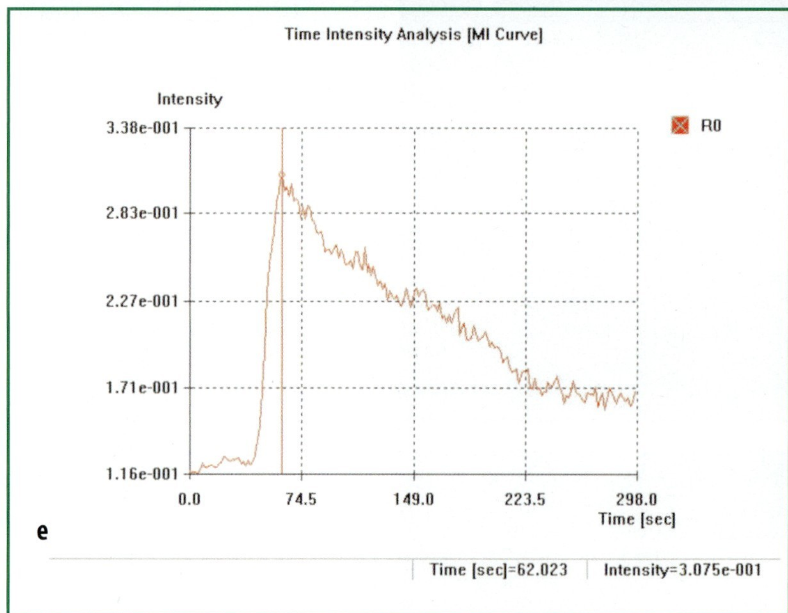

Fig. 2a-e. *Longitudinal dorsal scan of he MCP joint in a patient with very early RA and no palpable synovitis at clinical examination.* **a** PDUS shows hypervascularity in a small synovial proliferation of 9 mm, consistent with high activity. **b** Low MI Imaging before contrast administration. **c** CEUS shows enhancement with complete filling of contrast bubbles. **d** Placement of a region of interest (ROI) for objective quantification of the contrast-enhancement. **e** Time-intensity curve shows a rapid high peak of enhancement, demonstrating objective measurement of the high maximal intensity, consistent with high disease activity

Role of Contrast US in Clinical Practice

Synovitis

Synovial proliferation and the development of pannus, a tumor-like focal proliferation of inflammatory tissue, are crucial in the pathogenesis of RA.

Synovial proliferation is accompanied by the growth of new blood vessels. Hyperemia, the first step in the inflammatory cascade, can be identified by imaging procedures. Microscopic examination of synovial biopsies has shown that the first sign of disease is angiogenesis in the synovial membrane, which correlates with inflammatory activity and occurs before any bone erosion. Recent studies have shown that no bone damage occurs in the absence of synovitis, and that the presence of synovitis is a prognostic indicator of bone damage, thus stressing the importance of early synovitis assessment [43, 44]. Early detection of vascularized synovia should be one of the primary goals in the assessment of RA, as early therapy is important to control disease progression [45]. It may be difficult to distinguish between synovitis and joint fluid because both can demonstrate hypoechoic to echoic characteristics on gray-scale US. US contrast administration allows not only for significantly better differentiation of active articular synovitis, but also allows a better characterization of the synovitis around tendons (Fig. 3). In tendinopathy of early RA patients, MRI has been used to quantify synovitis at the wrist. High scores were predictive of tendon rupture in a small group of patients. Therefore, sensitive assessment of peritendinous synovitis might be of clinical relevance to predict the course of tendon involvement and the risk of tendon rupture in later disease [46]. US allows for excellent assessment of tendon and tendon gliding during active and passive motion. Detection of persistent peri-tendinous vascularized synovitis with vessels entering the tendon might be consistent with aggressive disease, resulting in the development of tendon rupture (Fig. 4). US contrast can improve detection of pathologic intra- and peritendinous vascularity associated with aggressive tenosynovitis.

Even in bursitis or the suprapatellar recess, the administration of contrast may show peripheral enhancement and thus help to distinguish between fluid, fibrous and hypervascular synovial thickening (Fig. 5).

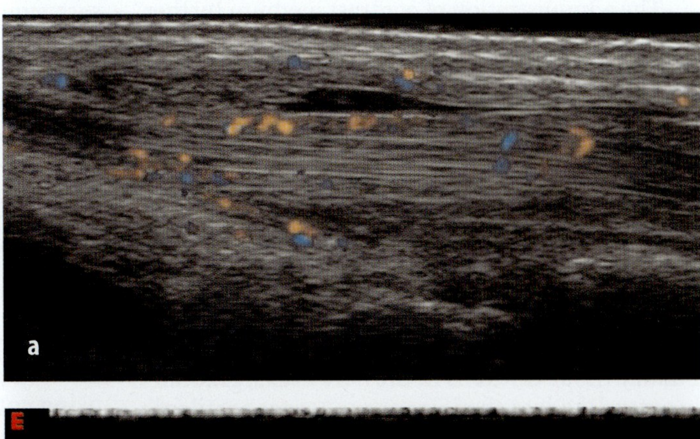

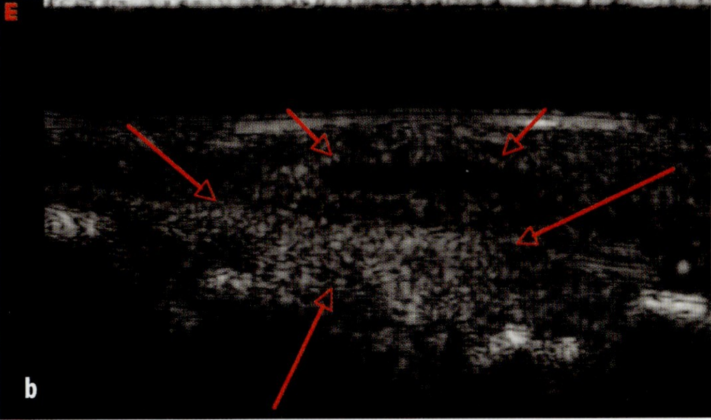

Fig. 3a, b. a Tenosynovitis of extensor tendons of the hand with synovial thickening, fluid in tendon sheath and increased vascularity at PDUS. **b** CEUS shows enhancement in the area where PDUS vessels were detected, but also extending into the tendon and radiocarpal joint (*long arrows*). Only the area suggestive of fluid shows no enhancement (*short arrows*)

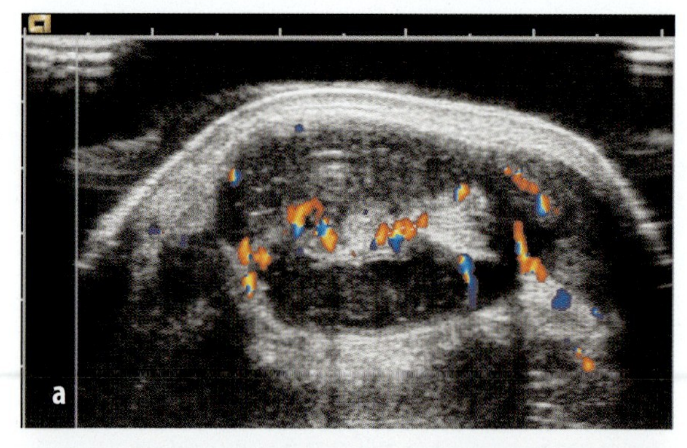

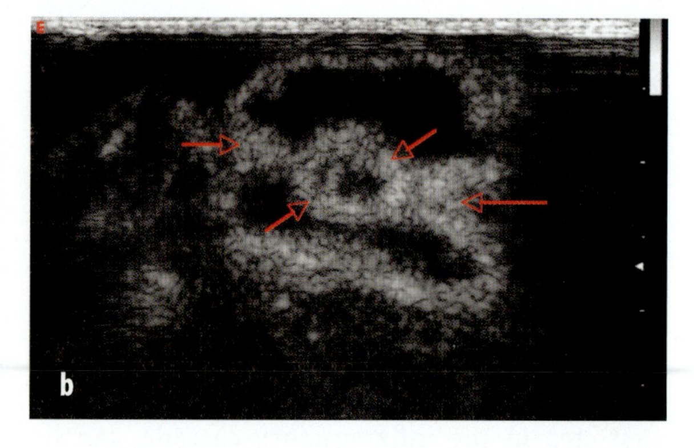

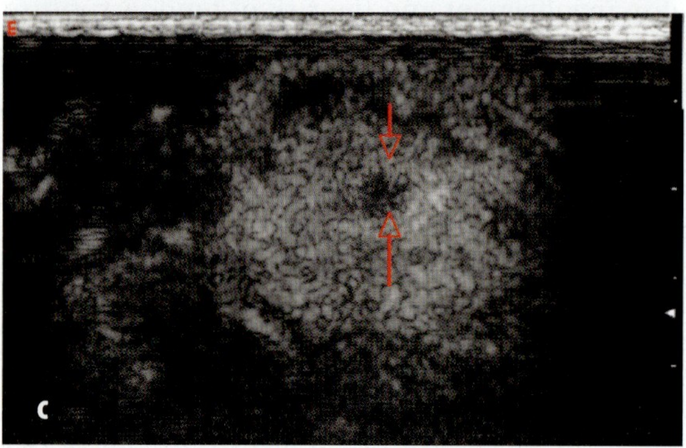

Fig. 4a-c. *Patient with RA (5 yrs), recently with a finger flexor tendon rupture, shows synovial proliferation of the extensor tendons.* **a** Extensive tenosynovitis of extensor tendons, suggestive of aggressive infiltrating synovitis, but only minor vascularity at CDUS. **b** Early post-contrast shows peripheral enhancement (*arrows*). **c** Later post-contrast imaging shows complete filling of the synovitis and the tendons, excluding only one preserved intact extensor tendon (*arrows*)

Synovitis is a hallmark of acute inflammation and is also seen in exacerbated chronic disease. The degree of vascularization is indicative of synovial proliferation and disease activity and therefore could be helpful for prognosis of the disease.

The administration of contrast medium further helps to detect hypervascularization in patients with only mild synovial proliferation (Fig. 6). In the wake of complete disease remission, hyperemia may resolve completely and this can be proven by contrast administration on a very sensitive level (Fig. 7).

Pannus and Erosions

At the beginning of the course of RA, the inflammatory tissue thickens in the bare areas, gradually extending into the joint space across cartilaginous surfaces. Bare areas are small areas easily accessible to US, where bones are covered only by synovium and not by cartilage, and hence are exposed to synovitis-induced bone destruction.

Exact assessment of the severity of active synovitis is an important issue, as MRI studies have shown that the amount of pannus correlates with the aggressiveness of the disease. In these cases, time is of major importance, as erosive destruction usually occurs within the first months of disease if the patient is left untreated. Furthermore, within the first year after RA onset, up to 47% of patients develop erosive disease. Four months after the onset of symptoms, McQueen et al. [47, 48] reported carpal erosions in 45% of patients on MRI, while only 15% of patients had erosions on plain radiographs. Other studies confirm the superiority of MRI and US over conventional radiography to assess synovial activity as a predictor for erosions and joint destruction [5, 6, 44]. The use of contrast agents may be of value in the presence of erosive disease; vascularized erosions are a sign of progressive active disease, thus contrast administration may help to exclude active vascularized erosions.

Therapeutic Follow-up and Advanced Stage

Prevention of structural damage is one of the most important issues in RA. Long-term studies using conventional US and MRI have shown that successful therapy results in fibrotic and/or necrotic pannus and reduction of vascularity. Thus, monitoring disease activity requires imaging techniques that allow a distinction between fibrotic pannus with no residual vascularity, and fibrotic pannus with residual vascularity.

In advanced stages, the inflammatory process may lead to massive erosions and bone mutilation, subluxation or luxation and, eventually, fibrous and bony ankylosis. In this stage, synovial thickening may be especially difficult to stage clinically regarding volume and disease activity. Furthermore, volume does not reflect the aggressiveness

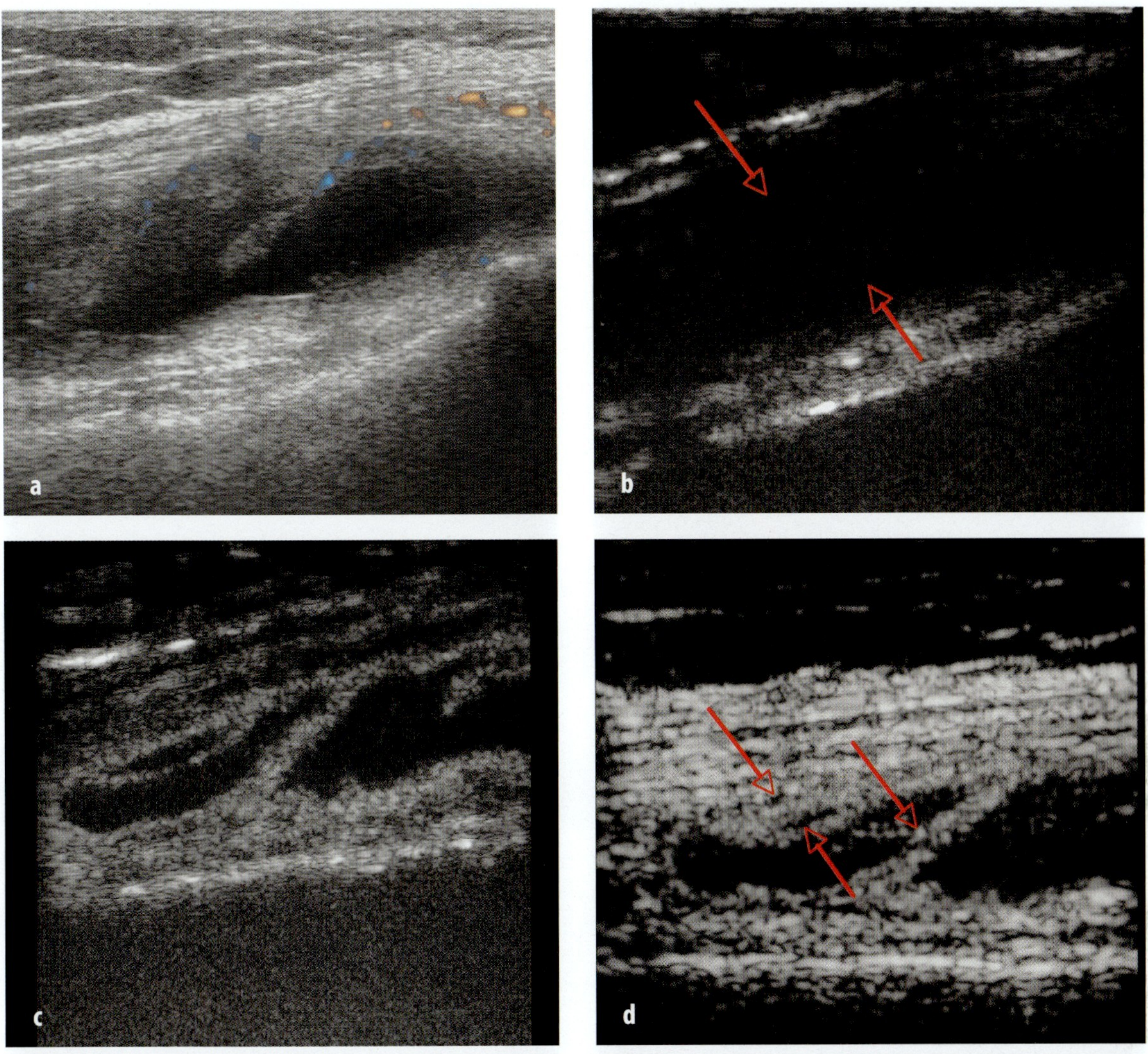

Fig. 5a-d. *Longitudinal US scan at the suprapatellar recess of the left knee in a 37 year-old patient with RA.* **a** Synovial proliferation at the suprapatellar recess, showing only few vascularized spots by PDUS. **b** Baseline pre-contrast low MI image. **c** After contrast administration, improved detection of diffuse enhancement in the synovial proliferation can be observed, with delineation of multiple vascularized septa using a high-end machine to assess the suprapatellar synovitis. **d** Handheld US system now enables contrast application. After contrast administration, improved detection of synovial activity and detection of synovial vascularized septation can be documented at the suprapatellar recess. Using PDUS in a high-end US machine only minor vascularity in the synovial proliferation, mainly effusion, suitable for fluid aspiration could be detected. Contrast administration shows multiple vasularized septation, suggesting that aspiration should not be performed at this site

of the disease, because it can be related not only to active synovitis, but also to effusion or fibrous inactive synovitis. Rather, highly active synovitis leads to even greater mutilation or tendon involvement and tendon rupture. The same applies here as for early disease activity: sensitive detection of decreased vascularity is necessary in order to establish remission of the disease. In treated RA patients with long-standing disease, serum VEGF concentrations have been described to be lower than in patients with early RA. Furthermore, changes in serum VEGF concentration and changes in synovial vascularity assessed by PDUS in patients receiving tumor necrosis factor (TNF) inhibitors have been described [48, 49]. Terslev et al. [50] found a reduction of color pixel per region of interest (ROI) to be a sign of decreased vascular permeability and vasodilatation in the synovial proliferation and further, Ribbens and colleagues used PDUS as an outcome measure of response to anti-TNF alpha treament in synovitis [51]. Also, in the study by Hau et al., a reduction of PDUS flow signals were reported after therapy [52]. Therefore, PDUS seems to be capable of evaluating synovial vascularity to determine prognosis and assess treatment response, but up to now few imaging studies have been available for the therapeutic follow-up of inflammatory disease.

If the patient presents with full remission in terms of resolved vascularity and improved clin-

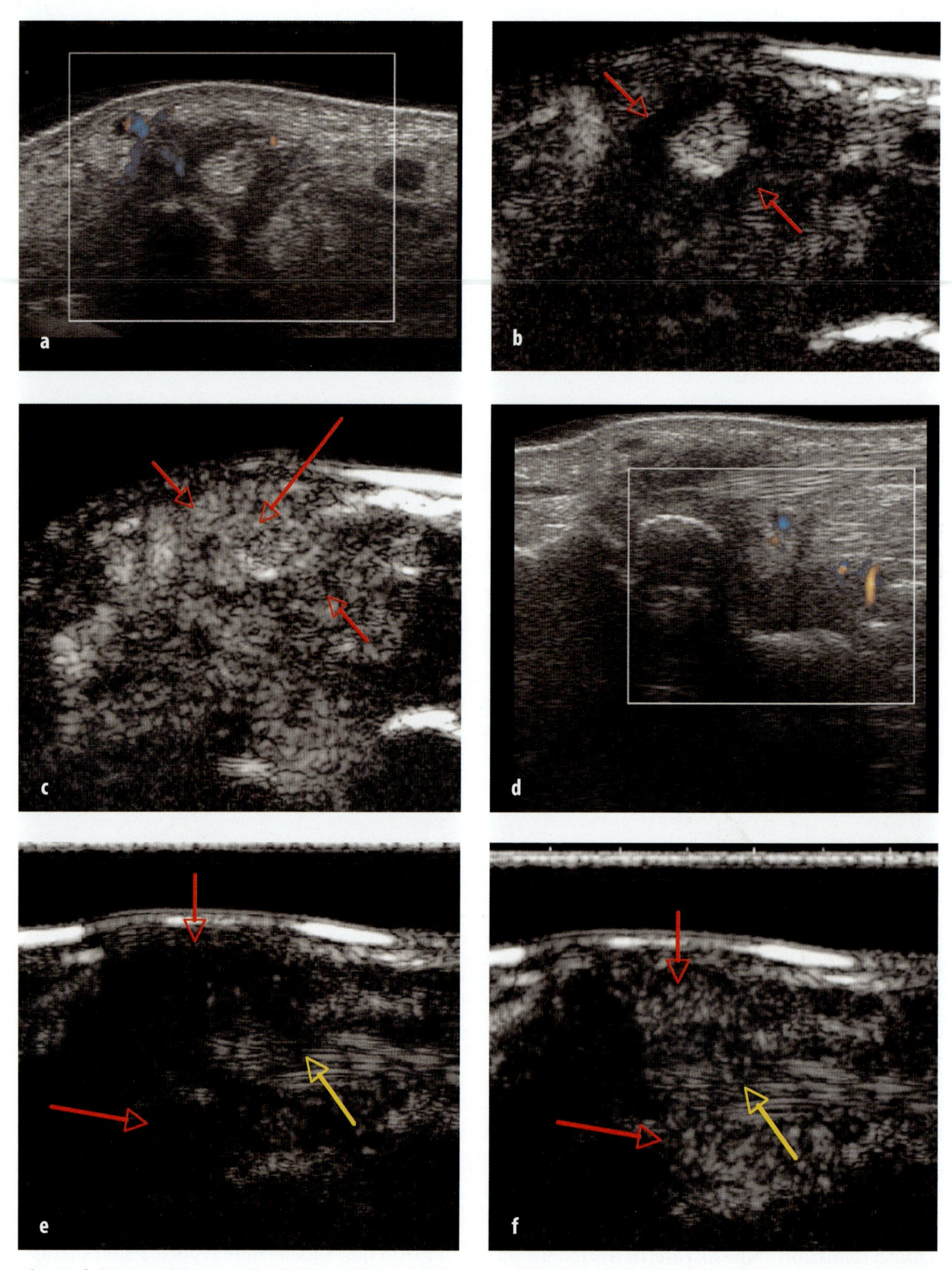

Fig. 6a-f. *Patient with long standing RA (15 yrs), shows clinically minor swelling over the flexor carpi radialis (FCR) tendon.* **a** Axial PDUS shows hypoechoic thickening of FCR tendon sheath with only minor vascularity. **b** Pre-contrast axial scan shows hypoechoic thickening of the synovia around the FCR tendon. **c** Postcontrast axial scan shows increased vascularity around tendon and a few bubbles entering the tendon itself. **d** Longitudinal PDUS shows synovial thickening of FCR tendon sheath and the radiocarpal joint with only minor vascularity. **e** Pre-contrast longitudinal scan. **f** Post-contrast longitudinal scan showing clear articular and peri-tendinous enhancement close to the tendon and a few bubbles entering the tendon, corresponding to high intra-articular and peri-tendinous vascularity at the microvessel level and therefore a high degree of inflammatory activity, which could only be demonstrated by contrast administration. This inflammatory activity may affect also the tendon itself, and therefore cause tendon rupture

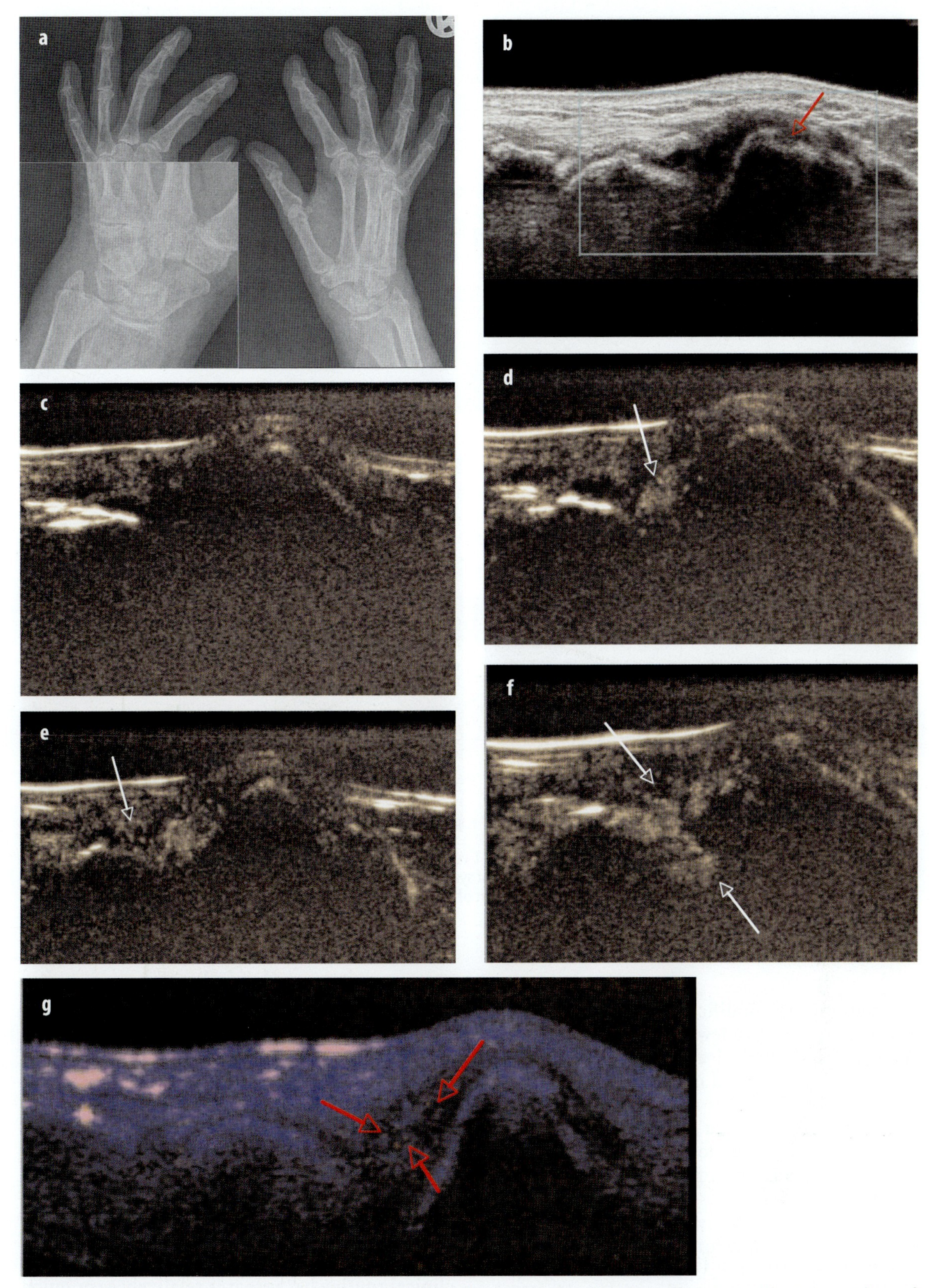

Fig. 7a-g. *Patient with late onset RA under therapy, clinically in disease remission.* **a** Hand X-ray of a patient, without clear evidence of erosions only small cystic alteration. **b** CDUS shows an open-mouthed cortical defect at the processus styloideus ulnae, consistent with the finding of extensive erosive disease and a high amount of synovial proliferation with no vascularity. **c** CEUS: baseline pre-contrast image. **d** CEUS: the first detectable synovial enhancement is located near the processus styloideus ulnae. **e** and **f** CEUS: progressive synovial enhancement with some bubbles in the distal part of synovial thickening. **g** CEUS: late phase, with color-coding for bubbles in orange, showing only very few bubbles remaining

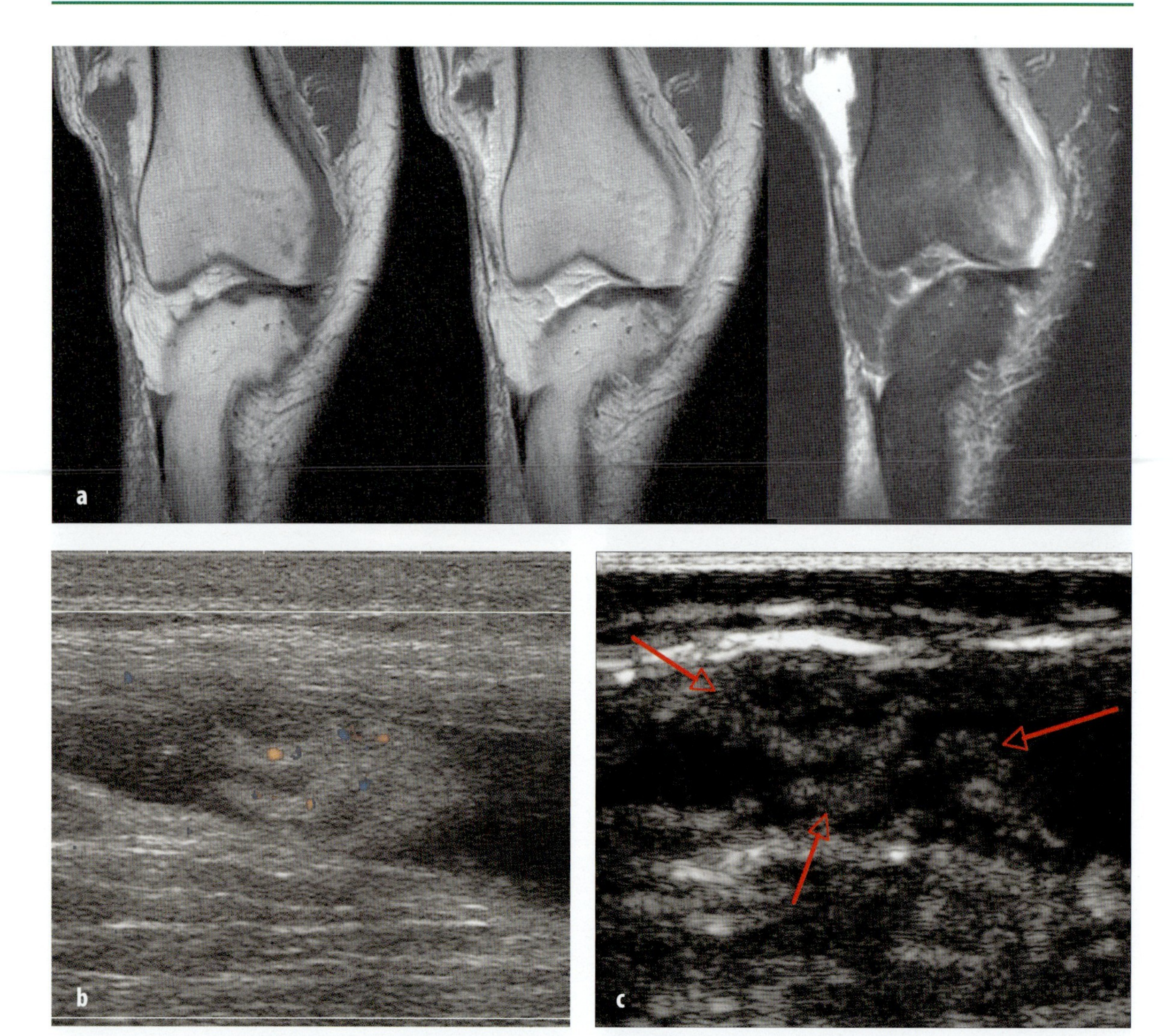

Fig. 8a-c. *US scan of the suprapatellar recess at the knee in a 61 year-old patient with RA.* **a** Coronal gadolinium-enhanced MRI (T1-weighted 722|20; T2-weighted 5035|30) delineates the extension of synovial proliferation in the suprapatellar recess after contrast administration. **b** CDUS shows minor vascularity in the delineated amount of synovial proliferation. **c** CEUS shows improved detection of diffuse vascularity

ical parameters, modification of therapy can be considered. If only a few joints are involved and no significant clinical activity is present, local injections may be used instead of increased systemic medication. This requires close monitoring and therefore good availability of imaging, because the disease does not follow a linear course, especially when potent therapy is initiated early.

In terms of feasibility and costs, US is an ideal imaging technique for long-term monitoring, which is essential in RA patients. Monitoring of multiple joints, which is well performed by US, is also essential for adequate management of RA. The value of using US contrast in monitoring decreased vascularity under effective treatment needs to be evaluated in controlled clinical trials.

Limitations and Advantages

Quantification of contrast-enhancement is important for longitudinal assessments. Some authors have employed subjective grading of vascularity on pre- and post-therapy images. Good correlation was established between subjective grading based on US, using non-enhanced CDUS, and histology [21, 31]. In our experience, subjective grading before and after the application of contrast is an excellent tool in clinical routine because it is relatively easy, quick to perform, and reliable [39]. Quantitative computer-based quantification was not found to be superior. Other investigators used software with digital image analysis to count the number of pixels in a chosen ROI, resulting in a quantitative score [15, 19]. These studies were performed without the use of a US contrast agent. However, the image acquisition procedure has to be standardized and the quality of the examination is highly dependent upon the skill of the operator and the use of optimal equipment. Furthermore, there are potential problems with reproducibility based on intra- and inter-observer variability and the use of different machines. Therefore standardization of measurements and particularly, interpretation of time-intensity curve characteristics, need further investigation.

Disadvantages and Advantages

Bone marrow edema, which is identified by MRI alone, is described as possessing a high predictive value for the development of erosions. It has been suggested that bone marrow is an additional aspect of the disease process in RA [48, 53]. However, bone marrow edema is not specific for RA; it is seen in other conditions as well.

Para-articular osteoporosis diagnosed by radiography is an early sign of joint involvement in RA. It presents as a secondary indirect sign of synovitis and this can be demonstrated directly using MRI or US, as both methods provide sensitive delineation of synovial pathology.

Advantages of US over MRI can be found in terms of costs and examination time; contrast-enhanced US is more economical than contrast-enhanced MRI. The total cost of contrast-enhanced US is still 30-50% less than that of contrast-enhanced MRI. The cost of US contrast can be reduced by slow infusion, which enables imaging of multiple joints. Recently, handheld systems have been developed that allow US contrast examination, which may be a further promising aspect in the rheumatological bedside assessment of RA patients (Figs. 5, 5d).

Further advantages consists of the fact that US contrast agents are less likely to leak into the synovial fluid and diffuse into the tissue than MRI contrast agents and they therefore reflect changes in the intravascular compartment with greater accuracy (Fig. 8). Delayed MRI sequences may present as an enhancement of synovial effusion secondary to the diffusion of gadolinium into the intracellular space.

The variability of joint involvement and disease activity in the examined areas, the occasionally low correlation of clinical symptoms with radiological results, and the fact that different sites may respond differently to RA therapy, call for imaging modalities that allow examination of several joints within a relatively short period of time or during one patient visit. The disease starts in a single joint only in 20% of cases. The most common sites of involvement are the hands, marked by symmetrical arthritis in the fingers, but also the feet, knees, shoulders and elbows. The hips and the sacroiliac joints are usually not affected in the initial stage. The bursa may be involved and there may be changes in tendons as well. All of these regions can be investigated effectively by US within a single examination session. A larger time window to perform contrast-enhanced US would be helpful for the examination of multiple sites.

Perspectives: Grading, Full Remission and Prognosis

Grading of RA

Soft tissue changes have not been adequately classified, as they are not depicted on conventional radiographs based on routinely used grading scores.

A more refined classification encompassing inflammatory changes in soft tissue rather than grading based on conventional radiography is required. The identification of prognostic factors such as persistent synovial hyperemia, is important for adequate management of the disease.

Furthermore, in view of the fact that especially in early RA the use of appropriate therapeutic regimens is important, an acceptable and usable grading system for clinical routine and scientific approach, as established for the use of MRI by Outcome Measures in Rheumatoid Arthritis Clinical Trials (OMERACT), is essential to score synovitis when performing US in RA patients [45, 47, 54].

Achieving full remission is a definite aim when treating RA. However, true remission remains rare in RA and minimal disease activity is advocated as a satisfactory state [55, 56]. Sensitive imaging using contrast-enhanced US might be of important value to predict those patients most at risk of accelerated joint destruction or tendon rupture, when in follow-up no decrease of activity in terms of minimal disease activity or even full remission is present.

Conclusions

Disease activity in RA is reported to be visualized better through the use of US contrast media than by unenhanced US. However, the routine use of contrast for US examinations is not established as for MRI in the assessment of synovitis. The main obstacles to using US contrast media are high costs, technical limitations (for instance in near fields), a relatively short time window of examination, and the need for optimally designed bubbles for near field investigation at higher frequencies. New therapies targeting the microvascular level are demanding an improved diagnostic potential to provide sensitive detection of vascularity. Such methods are required for scientific research as well as in daily clinical examinations. Reliable imaging techniques for the early detection of pannus, as well as for monitoring synovial vascularization and early bone erosions, are necessary for the appropriate management of patients with RA. In addition, there is a need for a grading system that includes synovial activity, which can be obtained by sensitive US assessment of synovial vascularity. This should encompass an assessment of soft tissues in the initial assessment of the disease, as well as subsequent monitoring.

Key Points

- US contrast in RA improves sensitive detection of intra-articular and peritendinous synovial vascularity at the microvascular level.
- US contrast media might be helpful for determining full disease remission by a sensitive assessment of vascularity decrease under adequate therapy.

References

1. Gabriel SE (2001) The epidemiology of rheumatoid arthritis Rheum Dis Clin North Am 27:269-282
2. MMWR (1999) Impact of Arthritis and other rheumatic conditions on the Healty-Care System-United States. JAMA 281:2177
3. Sokka T, Kautiainen H, Mottonen T (1999) Work disability in rheumatoid arthritis 10 years after the diagnosis. J Rheumatol 26:1681-1685
4. Arnett FC, Edworthy SM, Bloch DA et al (1988) The American Rheumatism Association 1987 revised criteria for the classification of rheumatoid arthritis. Arthritis Rheum 31:315-324
5. Backhaus M, Kamradt T, Sandrock D et al (1999) Arthritis of the finger joints: a comprehensive approach comparing conventional radiography, scintigraphy, ultrasound, and contrast-enhanced magnetic resonance imaging. Arthritis Rheum 42:1232-1245
6. Wakefield RJ, Gibbon WW, Conaghan PG et al (2000) The value of sonography in the detection of bone erosions in patients with rheumatoid arthritis. Arthritis Rheum 43:2762-2770
7. Hermann KG, Backhaus M, Schneider U et al (2003) Rheumatoid arthritis of the shoulder joint: comparison of conventional radiography, ultrasound, and dynamic contrast-enhanced magnetic resonance imaging. Arthritis Rheum 48:3338-3349
8. McQueen F, Stewart N, Crabbe J et al (1998) Magnetic resonance imaging of the wrist in early rheumatoid arthritis reveals a high prevalence of erosions at 4 months after symptom onset. Ann Rheum Dis 57:350-356
9. Gaffney K, Cookson J, Blades S et al (1998) Quantitative assessment of the rheumatoid synovial microvascular bed by gadolinium-DTPA enhanced magnetic resonance imaging. Ann Rheum Dis 57:152-157
10. Jorgensen C, Cyteval C, Anaya JM et al (1993) Sensitivity of magnetic resonance imaging of the wrist in very early rheumatoid arthritis. Clin Exp Rheumatol 11:163-168
11. Huang J, Stewart N, Crabbe J et al (2000) A 1-year follow- up study of dynamic magnetic resonance imaging in early rheumatoid arthritis reveals synovitis to be increased in shared epitope-positive patients and predictive of erosions at 1 year. Rheumatology 39:407-416
12. Sugimoto H, Takeda A, Kyodoh K (2000) Early-stage rheumatoid arthritis: prospective study of the effectiveness of MR imaging for diagnosis. Radiology 216:569-575
13. Cimmino MA, Innocenti S, Livrone F et al (2003) Dynamic gadolinium-enhanced magnetic resonance imaging of the wrist in patients with rheumatoid arthritis can discriminate active from inactive disease. Arthritis Rheum 48:1207-1213
14. Grassi W, Filippucci E, Farina A et al (2001) Ultrasonography in the evaluation of bone erosions. Ann Rheum Dis 60:98-103
15. Hau M, Schultz H, Tony HP et al (1999) Evaluation of pannus and vascularization of the metacarpophalangeal and proximal interphalangeal joints in rheumatoid arthritis by high-resolution ultrasound (multidimensional linear array). Arthritis Rheum 42:2303-2308
16. Naredo E, Bonilla G, Gamero F et al (2005) Assessment of inflammatory activity in rheumatoid arthritis: a comparative study of clinical evaluation with grey scale and power Doppler ultrasonography. Ann Rheum Dis 64:375-381

17. Szkudlarek M, Narvestad E, Klarlund M et al (2004) Ultrasonography of the metatarsophalangeal joints in rheumatoid arthritis: comparison with magnetic resonance imaging, conventional radiography, and clinical examination. Arthritis Rheum 50:2103-2112
18. Szkudlarek M, Court-Payen M, Strandberg C et al (2001) Power Doppler ultrasonography for assessment of synovitis in the metacarpophalangeal joints of patients with rheumatoid arthritis: a comparison with dynamic magnetic resonance imaging. Arthritis Rheum 44:2018-2023
19. Qvistgaard E, Rogind H, Torp-Pedersen S et al (2001) Quantitative ultrasonography in rheumatoid arthritis: evaluation of inflammation by Doppler technique. Ann Rheum Dis 60:690-693
20. Weidekamm C, Koller M, Weber M et al (2003) Diagnostic value of high-resolution B-mode and doppler sonography for imaging of hand and finger joints in rheumatoid arthritis. Arthritis Rheum 48:325-333
21. Walther M, Harms H, Krenn V et al (2001) Correlation of power Doppler sonography with vascularity of the synovial tissue of the knee joint in patients with osteoarthritis and rheumatoid arthritis. Arthritis Rheum 44:331-338
22. Forsberg F, Ro RJ, Potoczek M et al (2004) Assessment of angiogenesis: implications for ultrasound imaging. Ultrasonics 42:325-30.
23. Schmidt WA, Volker L, Zacher J et al (2000) Colour Doppler ultrasonography to detect pannus in knee joint synovitis. Clin Exp Rheumatol 18:439-444
24. Taylor PC (2003) The value of sensitive imaging modalities in rheumatoid arthritis. Arthritis Res Ther 5:210-213
25. Koch AE (1998) Angiogenesis: implications for rheumatoid arthritis. Arthritis Rheum 41:951-962
26. Bodolay E, Koch AE, Kim J et al (2002) Angiogenesis and chemokines in rheumatoid arthritis and other systemic inflammatory rheumatic diseases. J Cell Mol Med 6:357-376
27. FitzGerald O, Bresnihan B (1995) Synovial membrane cellularity and vascularity. Ann Rheum Dis 54:511-515
28. Zvaifler NJ, Firestein GS (1994) Pannus and pannocytes: alternative models of joint destruction in rheumatoid arthritis. Arthritis Rheum 37:783-789
29. Taylor PC (2005) Serum vascular markers and vascular imaging in assessment of rheumatoid arthritis disease activity and response to therapy. Rheumatology (Oxford) 44:721-728
30. Blomley MJK, Cooke JC, Unger EC et al (2001) Microbubble contrast agents: a new era in ultrasound. BMJ 322:1222-1225
31. Klauser A, Frauscher F, Schirmer M et al (2002) The value of contrast-enhanced color Doppler ultrasound in the detection of vascularization of finger joints in patients with rheumatoid arthritis. Arthritis Rheum 46:647-6453
32. Carotti M, Salaffi F, Manganelli P et al (2002) Power Doppler sonography in the assessment of synovial tissue of the knee joint in rheumatoid arthritis: a preliminary experience. Ann Rheum Dis 61:877-882
33. Doria AS, Kiss MH, Lotito AP et al (2001) Juvenile rheumatoid arthritis of the knee: evaluation with contrast-enhanced color Doppler ultrasound. Pediatr Radiol 31:524-531
34. Fiocco U, Cozzi L, Rubaltelli L et al (1996) Long term sonographic follow-up of rheumatoid and psoriatic proliferative knee joint synovitis. Br J Rheumatol 35:155-163
35. Magarelli N, Guglielmi G, Di Matteo L et al (2001) Diagnostic utility of an echo-contrast agent in patients with synovitis using power Doppler ultrasound: a preliminary study with comparison to contrast-enhanced MRI. Eur Radiol 11:1039-1046
36. Wamser G, Bohndorf K, Vollert K et al (2003) Power Doppler sonography with and without echo-enhancing contrast agent and contrast-enhanced MRI for the evaluation of rheumatoid arthritis of the shoulder joint: differentiation between synovitis and joint effusion. Skeletal Radiol 32:351-359
37. Klauser A, Halpern EJ, Frauscher F et al (2005) Inflammatory low back pain: high negative predictive value of contrast-enhanced color Doppler ultrasound in the detection of inflamed sacroiliac joints. Arthritis Rheum 53:440-444
38. Klauser A, Frauscher F, Halpern EJ et al (2005) Remitting seronegative symmetrical synovitis with pitting edema of the hands: ultrasound, color doppler ultrasound, and magnetic resonance imaging findings. Arthritis Rheum 53:226-33.
39. Klauser A, Demharter J, De Marchi A et al (2005) Contrast-enhanced gray-scale sonography in assessment of joint vascularity in rheumatoid arthritis: results from the IACUS study group. Eur Radiol 16 [Epub ahead of print]
40. Klarlund M, Ostergaard M, Lorenzen I (1999) Finger joint synovitis in rheumatoid arthritis: quantitative assessment by magnetic resonance imaging. Rheumatology 38:66-72
41. Tamai K, Yamato M, Yamaguchi T, Ohno W (1994) Dynamic magnetic resonance imaging for the evaluation of synovitis in patients with rheumatoid arthritis. Arthritis Rheum 37:1151-1157
42. Klauser A (2005) Contrast-enhanced Ultrasound in rheumatic joint disease. In: Baert AL, Sartor K (ed) Contrast Media in Ultrasonography. Springer, Berlin, Heidelberg, New York, pp 365-379
43. Ostergaard M, Stoltenberg M, Lovgreen-Neilsen P et al (1997) Magnetic resonance imaging-determined synovial membrane and joint effusion volumes in rheumatoid arthritis and osteoarthritis: comparison with the macroscopic and microscopic appearance of the synovium. Arthritis Rheum 40:1856-1867
44. Ostergaard M, Hansen M, Stoltenberg M et al (1999) Magnetic resonance imaging-determined synovial membrane volume as a marker of disease activity and a predictor of progressive joint destruction in the wrists of patients with rheumatoid arthritis. Arthritis Rheum 42:918-929
45. Nell VP, Machold KP, Eberl G (2004) Benefit of very early referral and very early therapy with disease-modifying anti-rheumatic drugs in patients with early rheumatoid arthritis. Rheumatology 43:906-914
46. McQueen F, Beckley V, Crabbe J et al (2005) Magnetic resonance imaging evidence of tendinopathy in early rheumatoid arthritis predicts tendon rupture at six years. Arthritis Rheum 52:744-751

47. McQueen FM, Benton N, Crabbe J et al (2001) What is the fate of erosions in early rheumatoid arthritis? Tracking individual lesions using x-rays and magnetic resonance imaging over the first 2 years of disease. Ann Rheum Dis 60:859–868
48. McQueen F, Stewart N, Crabbe J et al (1999) Magnetic resonance imaging of the wrist in early rheumatoid arthritis reveals progression of erosions despite clinical improvement. Ann Rheum Dis 58:156-163
49. McQueen F, Lassere M, Edmonds J et al (2003) Related OMERACT Rheumatoid Arthritis Magnetic Resonance Imaging Studies. Summary of OMERACT 6 MR Imaging Module. J Rheumatol 30:1387-1392
50. Terslev L, Torp-Pedersen S, Qvisgaard E et al (2003) Effects of treatment with etanercept (Enbrel, TNFR:Fc) on rheumatoid arthritis evaluated by Doppler ultrasonography. Ann Rheum Dis 62:178-181
51. Ribbens C, Andre B, Marcelis S et al (2003) Rheumatoid hand joint synovitis: gray-scale and power Doppler US quantifications following anti-tumor necrosis factor-alpha treatment: pilot study. Radiology 229:562-569
52. Hau M, Kneitz C, Tony H-P et al (2002) High resolution ultrasound detects a decrease in pannus vascularisation of small finger joints in patients with rheumatoid arthritis receiving treatment with soluble tumour necrosis factor alpha receptor (etanercept). Ann Rheum Dis 61:55-58
53. Jimenez-Boj E, Redlich K, Turk B et al (2005) Interaction between Synovial Inflammatory Tissue and Bone Marrow in Rheumatoid Arthritis. J Immunol 175:2579-2588
54. Scheel AK, Hermann KG, Kahler E et al (2005) A novel ultrasonographic synovitis scoring system suitable for analyzing finger joint inflammation in rheumatoid arthritis. Arthritis Rheum 52:733-743
55. Aletaha D, Ward MM, Machold KP et al (2005). Remission and active disease in rheumatoid arthritis: defining criteria for disease activity states. Arthritis Rheum 52:2625-2636
56. Wells GA, Boers M, Shea B et al (2005) Minimal disease activity for rheumatoid arthritis: a preliminary definition. J Rheumatol 32:2016-2024